Call the Midwife

Above: A nursing and midwife recruitment poster from the Second World War (1939–45).

Call the Midwife

A True Story of the East End in the 1950s

JENNIFER WORTH

Clinical Editor
Terri Coates MSc, RN, RM, ADM, Dip Ed

WEIDENFELD & NICOLSON
LONDON

This book is dedicated to Philip, my dear husband

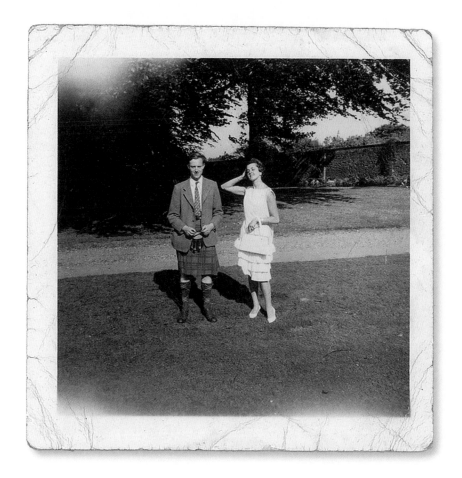

The history of "Mary" is also dedicated to the memory of
Father Joseph Williamson and Daphne Jones

Above: Jennifer Worth with her husband, Philip, at Mill Hill Preparatory School (summer, 1963).

CONTENTS

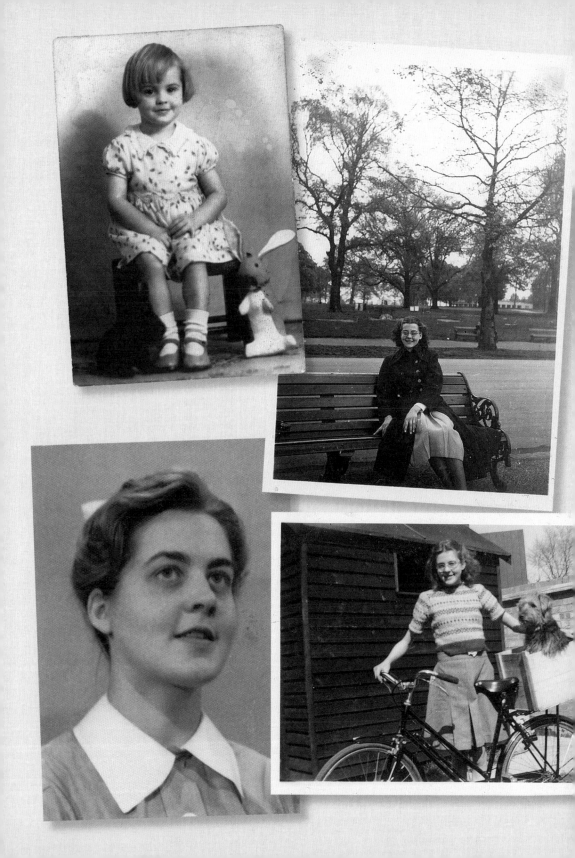

Opposite page: A young Jennifer in the early 1940s (*top far left*); in the late 1940s (*top right*); with her dog, Bryn, in the late 1940s (*bottom right*); in her nurse's uniform in 1957 (*bottom left*).

This page: Jennifer and Philip Worth on their wedding day, 4 April 1963 (*below*); with Philip and baby Suzannah, spring 1965 (*bottom right*); with her daughters in the late 1960s (Suzannah on her knee and Juliette standing next to her; *right*).

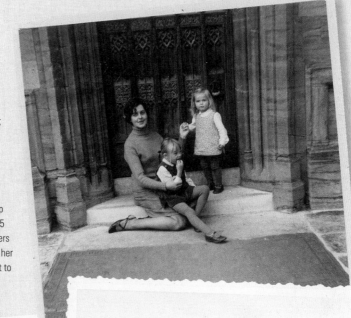

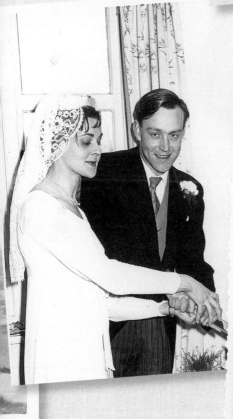

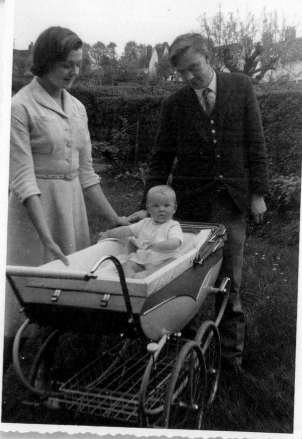

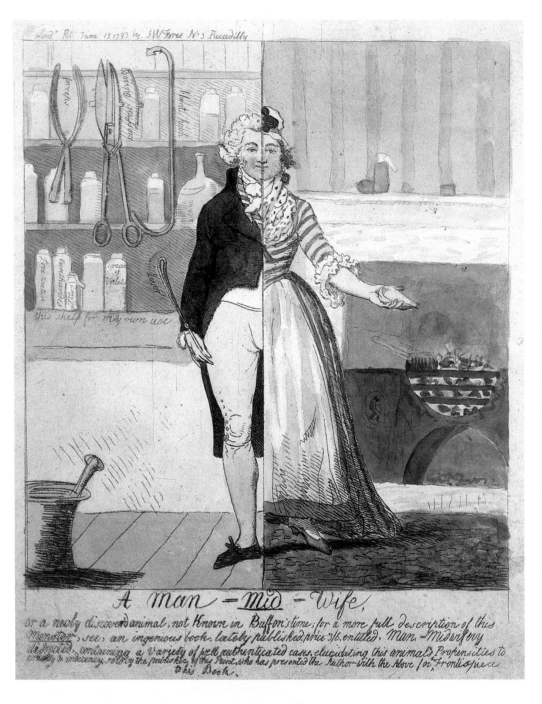

Above: Midwives were often caricatured as this cartoon from 1793 shows. It depicts a midwife bisected into male and female halves.

INTRODUCTION

In the Victorian era, social reform had swept through the country. For the first time authors wrote about iniquities that had never before been exposed, and the public conscience was stirred. Among these reforms, the need for good nursing care in hospitals gained the attention of many farsighted and educated women. Nursing and midwifery were in a deplorable state. It was not considered a respectable occupation for any educated woman, and so the illiterate filled the gap. The caricature figures of Sairey Gamp and Betsy Prig – ignorant, filthy, gin-swilling women – created by Charles Dickens, may seem hilarious as we read about them, but would not have been funny if you had been obliged, through poverty, to place your life in their hands.

Florence Nightingale is our most famous nurse, and her dynamic organisational skills changed the face of nursing for ever. But she was not alone, and the history of nursing records many groups of dedicated women who devoted their lives to raising the standards of nursing. One such group was the Midwives of St Raymund Nonnatus*. They were a religious order of Anglican nuns, devoted to bringing safer childbirth to the poor. They opened houses in the East End of London, and in many of the slum areas of the great industrial cities of Great Britain.

---

* The Midwives of St Raymund Nonnatus is a pseudonym. I have taken the name from St Raymund Nonnatus, the patron saint of midwives, obstetricians, pregnant women, childbirth and newborn babies. He was delivered by Caesarean section ("*non natus*" is the Latin for "not born") in Catalonia, Spain, in 1204. His mother, not surprisingly, died at his birth. He became a priest and died in 1240.

In the nineteenth century (and earlier, of course) no poor woman could afford to pay the fee required by a doctor for the delivery of her baby. So she was forced to rely on the services of an untrained, self-taught midwife, or "handywoman" as they were often called. Some may have been quite effective practitioners, but others boasted a frightening mortality rate. In the mid-nineteenth century, maternal mortality amongst the poorest classes stood at around 35–40 per cent, and infant mortality was around 60 per cent. Anything like eclampsia, haemorrhage, or malpresentation, would mean the inevitable death of the mother. Sometimes these handywomen would abandon a patient to agony and death if any abnormality developed during labour. There is no doubt that their working practices were insanitary, to say the least, and thereby spread infection, disease and often death.

Not only was there no training, but there was also no control over the numbers and practice of these handywomen. The Midwives of St Raymund saw that the answer to this social evil lay in the proper training of midwives and control of their work by legislation.

It was in the struggle for legislation that these feisty nuns and their supporters encountered the fiercest opposition. From about 1870 the battle raged; they were called "an absurdity", "time wasters", "a curiosity", and "an objectionable body of busy-bodies". They were accused of everything from perversion to greed for unlimited financial gain. But the Nonnatus Nuns would not be put down.

For thirty years the battle continued, but in 1902 the first Midwives Act was passed and the Royal College of Midwives was born.

The work of the Midwives of St Raymund Nonnatus was based upon a foundation of religious discipline. I have no doubt that this was necessary at the time, because the working conditions were so disgusting, and the work so relentless, that only those with a calling from God would wish to undertake it. Florence Nightingale records that when she was in her early twenties she saw a vision of Christ, telling her that her life was required for this work.

The St Raymund midwives worked in the slums of the London Docklands[†] amongst the poorest of the poor and for about half of the nineteenth century they were the only reliable midwives working there. They laboured tirelessly through epidemics of cholera, typhoid, polio,

---

† Nonnatus House was situated in the heart of the London Docklands. The practice covered Stepney, Limehouse, Millwall, the Isle of Doggs, Cubitt Town, Poplar, Bow, Mile End and Whitechapel.

and tuberculosis. In the early twentieth century, they worked through two world wars. In the 1940s, they remained in London and endured the Blitz with its intensive bombing of the docks. They delivered babies in air-raid shelters, dugouts, church crypts and underground stations. This was the tireless, selfless work to which they had pledged their lives, and they were known, respected and admired throughout the Docklands by the people who lived there. Everyone spoke of them with sincere love.

Such were the Midwives of St Raymund Nonnatus when I first knew them: an order of nuns, fully professed and bound by the vows of poverty, chastity, and obedience, but also qualified nurses and midwives, which is how I came to be among them. I did not expect it, but it turned out to be the most important experience of my life.

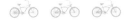

Call the Midwife Chapter I

'Why did I ever start this? I must have been mad!' There were dozens of other things I could have done - modelling, air hostess, ships stewardess, The ideas ran through my head, all glamorous highly paid jobs. Only an idiot would choose to be a nurse. And now a midwife!

2.30 in the morning! I struggled, half asleep, into my uniform. Only 3 hours sleep after a 17 hour working day. Who would do such a job? It was bitterly cold and raining outside. The Mission House was cold enough, and the bicycle shed even colder. In the dark I wrenched at a bicycle and cracked my shin. With blind force of habit I fitted my delivery bag on to the bicycle, and pushed it out into deserted little street.

Round the corner, across the East India Dock Road and onto the Isle of Dogs. The rain had woken me up, and the steady pedalling calmed my temper. Why had I ever started nursing? My thoughts flitted back

CALL THE MIDWIFE

W hy did I ever start this? I must have been mad! There were dozens of other things I could have been – a model, air hostess, or a ship's stewardess. The ideas run through my head, all glamorous, highly paid jobs. Only an idiot would choose to be a nurse. And now a midwife …

Two-thirty in the morning! I struggle, half asleep, into my uniform. Only three hours sleep after a seventeen-hour working day. Who would do such a job? It is bitterly cold and raining outside. Nonnatus House itself is cold enough, and the bicycle shed even colder. In the dark I wrench at a bicycle and crack my shin. Through blind force of habit, I fit my delivery bag on to the bicycle, and push it out into the deserted street.

Round the corner, Leyland Street, across the East India Dock Road and then on to the Isle of Dogs. The rain has woken me up and the steady pedalling calms my temper. Why did I ever go into nursing? My thoughts flit back five or six years. Certainly there had been no feeling of vocation, none of the burning desire to heal the sick that nurses are supposed to feel. What was it then? A broken heart certainly, the need to get away, a challenge, the sexy uniform with the cuffs and ruffs, the pinched-in waists and pert little caps. Were they reasons though? I can't tell. As for the sexy uniform, that's

Opposite: The first page of Chapter 1 from the original manuscript of *Call the Midwife*. The author said that she would think about her books "for months and months and then write 5–7,000 words a day for 3 or 4 hours by hand and then my dear husband types it up for me. I use a fountain pen because I love the feel of a gold nib on paper."

a laugh, I think as I pedal through the rain in my navy gabardine, with the cap pulled down well over my head. Sexy, indeed.

Over the first swing bridge that closes off the dry docks. All day they teem with noise and life, as the great vessels are loaded and unloaded. Thousands of men: dockers, stevedores, drivers, pilots, sailors, fitters, crane drivers, all toiling ceaselessly. Now the docks are silent, the only sound is the movement of water. The darkness is intense.

Past the tenements where countless thousands sleep, probably four or five to a bed, in their little two-room flats. Two rooms for a family of ten or twelve children. How do they manage it?

I cycle on, intent on getting to my patient. A couple of policemen wave and call out their greetings; the human contact raises my spirits no end. Nurses and policemen always have a rapport, especially in the East End. It's interesting, I reflect, that they always go around in pairs for mutual protection. You never see a policeman alone. Yet we nurses and midwives are always alone, on foot or bicycle. We would never be touched. So deep is the respect, even reverence, of the roughest, toughest docker for the district midwives that we can go anywhere alone, day or night, without fear.

The dark unlit road lies before me. The road around the Isle is continuous, but narrow streets lead off it, criss-crossing each other, each containing thousands of terraced houses. The road has a romantic appeal because the sound of the moving river is always present.

Soon I turn off the West Ferry Road into the side streets. I can see my patient's house at once – the only house with a light on.

It seems there is a deputation of women waiting inside to greet me. The patient's mother, her grandmother (or were they two grandmothers?), two or three aunts, sisters, best friends, a neighbour. Well thank God Mrs Jenkins isn't here this time, I think.

Lurking somewhere in the background of this powerful sisterhood is a solitary male, the origin of all the commotion. I always feel sorry for the men in this situation. They seemed so marginalised.

The noise and the chatter of the women engulfs me like a blanket.

"Hello luvvy, how's yerself? You got 'ere nice an' quick, ven."

"Let's 'ave yer coat and yer 'at."

"Nasty night. Come on in an' get warm, ven."

"How about a nice cup o' tea? That'll warm the cockles, eh, luvvy?"

"She's upstairs, where you left 'er. Pains about every five minutes. She's been asleep since you left, just afore midnight. Then she woke up, about two-ish, pains gettin' worse, an' faster, so we reckons as 'ow we ought 'a call the midwife, eh, Mum?"

Mum agrees, and bustles forth authoritatively.

"We got the water hot, an' a load o' nice clean towels, an' got the fire goin', so it's all nice an' warm for the new baby."

I have never been able to talk much, and in this situation I don't need to. I give them my coat and hat, but decline their tea, as experience has taught me that, in general, Poplar tea is revolting: strong enough to creosote a fence, stewed for hours, and laced with sticky sweet condensed milk.

I am glad that I shaved Muriel earlier in the day when the light was good enough to do it without risk of cutting her. I also gave the required enema at the same time. It's a job I hate, so thankfully it is over; besides which, who would want to give a two-pint soap-and-water enema (especially if there was no lavatory in the house), with all the resultant mess and smell, at two-thirty in the morning?

I go upstairs to Muriel, a buxom girl of twenty-five who is having her fourth baby. The gaslight sheds a soft warm glow over the room. The fire blazes fiercely, and the heat is almost suffocating. A quick glance tells me that Muriel is nearing the second stage of labour – the sweating, the slight panting, the curious in-turned look that a woman has at this time as she concentrates every ounce of her mental and physical strength on her body, and on the miracle she is about to bring forth. She doesn't say anything, just squeezes my hand and gives a preoccupied smile. I left her three hours earlier, in the first stage of labour. She had been niggling in false labour all day and was very tired, so I gave chloral hydrate at about 10 p.m., in the hope that she would sleep all night and wake in the morning refreshed. It hasn't worked. Does labour ever go the way you want it to?

I have to be sure how far on she is, so prepare to do a vaginal examination. As I scrub up, another pain comes on – you can see it building in strength until it seems her poor body will break apart. It has been estimated that, at the height of labour, each uterine contraction exerts the same pressure as the closing of the doors of an underground tube train. I can well believe it as I watch Muriel's labour. Her mother and sister are sitting with her. She clings to them in speechless, gasping agony, a breathless moan escaping her throat until it passes, then sinks back exhausted, to gather her strength for the next contraction.

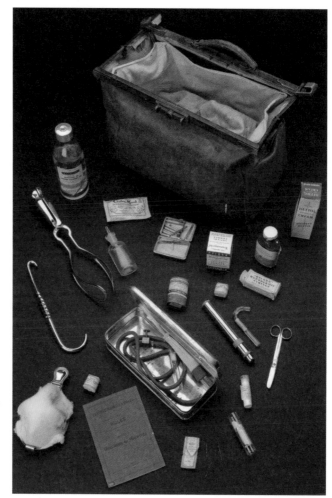

Right. The midwives always carried a bag with them filled with essential equipment, such as scissors, cord clamps, swabs and gauze. This bag is fairly typical of the time.

I put on my gloves and lubricate my hand. I ask Muriel to draw her knees up, as I wanted to examine her. She knows exactly what I am going to do, and why. I put a sterile sheet under her buttocks and slip two fingers into her vagina. The head well down, anterior presentation, only a thin rim of cervix remaining, but waters apparently not yet broken. I listen to the foetal heart, a steady 130. Good. That is all I need to know. I tell her everything is normal, and that she hasn't far to go now. Then another pain starts, and all words and actions have to be suspended in the enormous intensity of labour.

My tray has to be set out. The chest of drawers has been cleared in advance to provide a working surface. I lay out my scissors, cord clamps, cord tape, foetal stethoscope, kidney dishes, gauze and cotton swabs, artery forceps. Not a great deal is necessary, in any case it has to be easily portable, both on a bicycle, and up and down the miles of tenement stairs and balconies.

The bed has been prepared in advance. We supplied a maternity pack, which was collected by the husband a week or two before delivery. It contains maternity pads – "bunnies" we call them – large absorbent sheets, which are disposable, and non-absorbent brown paper. This brown paper looks absurdly old fashioned, but it is entirely effective. It covers the whole bed, all the absorbent pads and sheets can be laid on it and, after delivery, everything can be bundled up into it and burned.

The cot is ready. A good size washing bowl is available, and gallons of hot water are being boiled downstairs. There is no running hot water in the house and I wonder how they used to manage when there was no water at all. It must have been an all night job, going out to collect it and boiling it up. On what? A range in the kitchen that had to be fuelled all the time, with coal if they could afford it, or driftwood if they couldn't.

But I haven't much time to sit and reflect. Often in a labour you can wait all night, but something tells me this one will not go that way. The increasing power and frequency of the pains, coupled with the fact that it is a fourth baby, indicate the second stage is not far away. The pains are coming every three minutes now. How much more can she bear, how much can any woman bear? Suddenly the sac bursts, and water floods the bed. I like to see it that way; I get a bit apprehensive if the waters break early. After the contraction, the mother and I change the soaking sheets as quickly as we can. Muriel can't get up at this stage, so we have to roll her. With the next contraction I see the head. Intense concentration is now necessary.

With animal instinct she begins pushing. If all is well, a multi-gravida can often push the head out in seconds, but you don't want it that way. Every good midwife tries to ensure a slow steady delivery of the head.

"I want you on your left side, Muriel, after this contraction. Try not to push now while you are on your back. That's it, turn over dear, and face the wall. Draw your right leg up towards your chin. Breathe deeply, carry on breathing like that. Just concentrate on breathing deeply. Your sister will help you."

I lean over the low sagging bed. All beds seem to sag in the middle in these parts, I think to myself. Sometimes I have had to deliver a baby on my knees. No time for that now though, another contraction is coming.

"Breathe deeply, push a little; not too hard." The contraction passes and I listen to the foetal heart again: 140 this time. Still quite normal, but the raised heartbeat shows how much a baby goes through in the ordeal of being born. Another contraction.

"Push just a little Muriel, not too hard, we'll soon have your baby born."

She is beside herself with pain, but a sort of frantic elation comes over a woman during the last few moments of labour, and the pain doesn't seem to matter. Another contraction. The head is coming fast, too fast.

"Don't push Muriel, just pant – in, out – quickly, keep panting like that."

I am holding the head back, to prevent it bursting out and splitting the perineum.

It is very important to ease the head out between contractions, and as I hold the head back, I realise I am sweating from the effort required, the concentration, the heat and the intensity of the moment.

The contraction passes, and I relax a little, listening to the foetal heart again – still normal. Delivery is imminent. I place the heel of my right hand behind the dilated anus, and push forward firmly and steadily until the crown is clear of the vulva.

"With the next contraction, Muriel the head will be born. Now I don't want you to push at all. Just let the muscles of your stomach do the job. All you have to do is to try to relax, and just pant like mad."

I steel myself for the next contraction which comes with surprising speed. Muriel is panting continuously. I ease the perineum around the emerging crown, and the head is born.

We all breathe a sigh of relief. Muriel is weak with the effort.

"Well done, Muriel, you are doing wonderfully, it won't be long now. The next pain, and we will know if it's a boy or a girl."

The baby's face is blue and puckered, covered in mucus and blood. I check the heartbeat. Still normal. I observe the restitution of the head through one eighth of a circle. The presenting shoulder can now be delivered from under the pubic arch.

Another contraction.

"This is it Muriel, you can push now – hard."

I ease the presenting shoulder out with a forward and upward sweep.

The other shoulder and arm follow, and the baby's whole body slides out effortlessly.

"It's another little boy," cried the mother. "Thanks be to God. Is he healthy, nurse?"

Muriel was in tears of joy. "Oh, bless him. Here, let me have a look. 'Ow, 'e's loverly."

I am almost as overwhelmed as Muriel, the relief of a safe delivery is so powerful. I clamp the baby's cord in two places, and cut between; I hold him by the ankles upside down to ensure no mucus is inhaled.

He breathes. The baby is now a separate being.

I wrap him in the towels given to me, and hand him to Muriel, who cradles him, coos over him, kisses him, calls him "beautiful, lovely, an angel".

Quite honestly, a baby covered in blood, still slightly blue, eyes screwed up, in the first few minutes after birth, is not an object of beauty. But the mother never sees him that way. To her, he is all perfection. My job is not done, however. The placenta must be delivered, and it must be delivered whole, with no pieces torn off and left behind in the uterus. If there are, the woman will be in serious trouble: infection, ongoing bleeding, perhaps even a massive haemorrhage, which can be fatal. It is perhaps the trickiest part of any delivery, to get the placenta out whole and intact.

The uterine muscles, having succeeded in the massive task of delivering the baby, often seem to want to take a holiday. Frequently there are no further contractions for ten to fifteen minutes. This is nice for the mother, who only wants to lie back and cuddle her baby, indifferent to what is going on down below, but it can be an anxious time for the midwife. When contractions do start, they are frequently very weak. Successful delivery of the placenta is usually a question of careful timing, judgement and, most of all, experience.

They say it takes seven years of practice to make a good midwife. I was only in my first year, alone, in the middle of the night, with this trusting woman and her family, and no telephone in the house.

Please God, don't let me make a mistake, I prayed.

After clearing the worst of the mess from the bed, I lay Muriel on her back, on warm dry maternity pads, and cover her with a blanket. Her pulse and blood pressure are normal, and the baby lies quietly in her arms. All I have to do was to wait.

I sit on a chair beside the bed, with my hand on the fundus in order to feel and assess. Sometimes the third stage can take twenty to thirty minutes.

I muse over the importance of patience, and the possible disasters that can occur from a desire to hasten things. The fundus feels soft and broad, so the placenta is obviously still attached in the upper uterine segment. There are no contractions for a full ten minutes. The cord protrudes from the vagina, and it is my practice to clamp it just below the vulva, so that I can see when the cord lengthens – a sign of the placenta separating and descending into the lower uterine segment. But nothing is happening. It goes through my mind that reports you hear of taxi drivers or bus conductors safely delivering a baby never mention this. Any bus driver can deliver a baby in an emergency, but who would have the faintest idea of how to manage the third stage? I imagine that most uninformed people would want to pull on the cord, thinking that this would help expel the placenta, but it can lead to sheer disaster.

Muriel is cooing and kissing her baby while her mother tidies up. The fire crackles. I sit quietly waiting, pondering.

Why aren't midwives the heroines of society that they should be? Why do they have such a low profile? They ought to be lauded to the skies, by everyone. But they are not. The responsibility they carry is immeasurable. Their skill and knowledge are matchless, yet they are completely taken for granted, and usually overlooked.

All medical students in the 1950s were trained by midwives. They had classroom lectures from an obstetrician, certainly, but without clinical practice lectures are meaningless. So in all teaching hospitals, medical students were attached to a teacher midwife, and would go out with her in the district to learn the skill of practical midwifery. All GPs had been trained by a midwife. But these facts seemed to be barely known.

The fundus tightens and rises a little in the abdomen as a contraction grips the muscles. Perhaps this is it, I think. But no. It doesn't feel right. Too soft after the contraction.

Another wait.

I reflect upon the incredible advance in midwifery practice over the century; the struggle dedicated women have had to obtain a proper training, and to train others. There has been recognised training for less than fifty years. My mother and all her siblings were delivered by an untrained woman, usually called the "goodwife" or the "handywoman". No doctor was present, I was told.

Another contraction coming. The fundus rises under my hand and remains hard. At the same time the forceps that I had clamped to the cord move a little. I test them. Yes, another four to six inches of cord comes out easily. The placenta has separated.

I ask Muriel to hand the baby over to her mother. She knows what I am going to do. I massage the fundus in my hand until it is hard and round and mobile. Then I grasp it firmly, and push downwards and backwards into the pelvis. As I push, the placenta appears at the vulva, and I lift it out with my other hand. The membranes slide out, followed by a gush of fresh blood and some clotted blood.

I feel weak with relief. It is accomplished. I put the kidney dish on the dresser, to await my inspection, and sit beside Muriel for a further ten minutes massaging the fundus, to ensure that it remains hard and round, which will expel residual blood clots.

In later years oxytocics would be routinely given after the birth of the baby, causing immediate and vigorous uterine contraction, so that the placenta is expelled within three to five minutes of the baby's birth. Medical science marches on! But in the 1950s, we had no such aids to delivery.

All that remains is to clean up. While Mrs Hawkin is washing and changing her daughter, I examine the placenta. It seems complete, and the membranes intact. Then I examine the baby, who appears healthy and normal. I bathe and dress him, in clothes that are ridiculously too big, and reflect upon Muriel's joy and happiness, her relaxed easy countenance. She looks tired, I think, but no sign of stress or strain. There never is! There must be an in-built system of total forgetfulness in a woman; some chemical or hormone that immediately enters the memory part of the brain after delivery, so that there is absolutely no recall of the agony that has gone before. If this were not so, no woman would ever have a second baby.

When everything is shipshape, the proud father is permitted to enter. These days, most fathers are with their wives throughout labour, and attend the birth. But this is a recent fashion. Throughout history, as far as I know, it was unheard of. Certainly in the 1950s, everyone would have been profoundly shocked at such an idea. Childbirth was considered to be a woman's business. Even the presence of doctors (all men until the late nineteenth century) was resisted, and it was not until obstetrics became recognised as a medical science that men attended childbirth.

Overleaf. The docks provided essential work for the local men, who were the main breadwinners, enabling their wives to stay at home and look after the children (Millwall Docks, 1955).

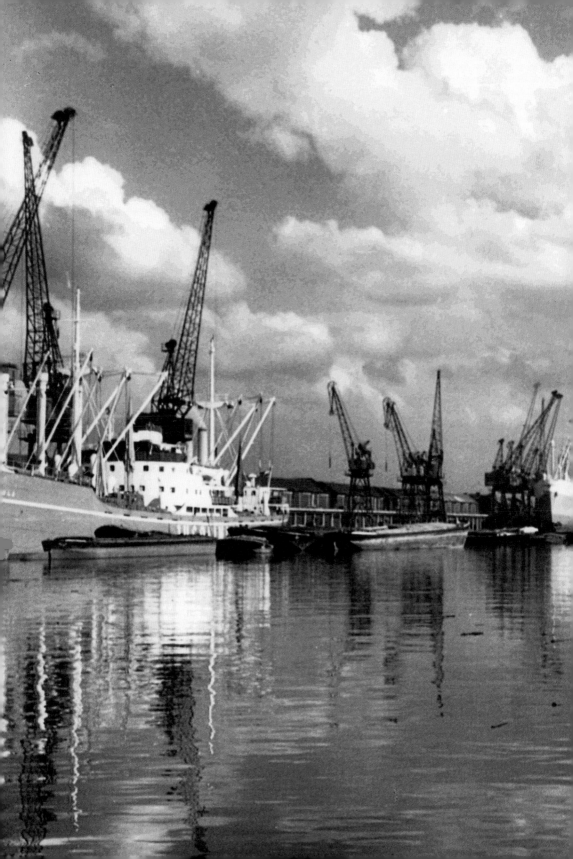

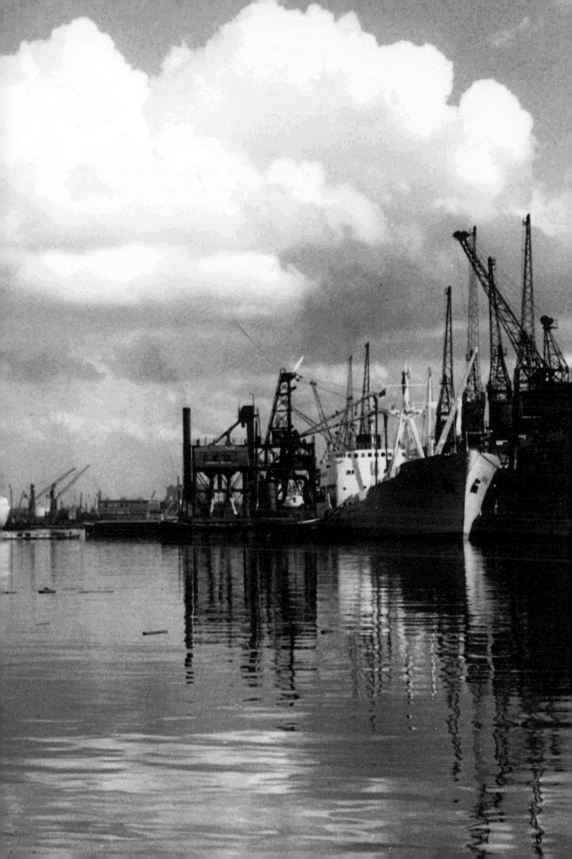

* * *

Jim is a little man, probably less than thirty but he looks nearer forty. He sidles into the room looking sheepish and confused. Probably my presence makes him tongue-tied, but I doubt if he has ever had a great command of the English language. He mutters, "All right then, girl?" and gives Muriel a peck on the cheek. He looks even tinier beside his buxom wife, who could give him a good five stone in weight. Her flushed pink, newly washed skin makes him look even more grey, pinched and dried out. All the result of a sixty-hour working week in the docks, I think to myself.

Then he looks at the baby, hums a bit – he is obviously thinking deeply about a suitable epithet – clears his throat, and says, "Gaw, he ain't 'alf a bit of all right, then." And then he leaves.

I regret that I have not been able to get to know the men of the East End. But it is quite impossible. I belong to the women's world, to the taboo subject of childbirth. The men are polite and respectful to us midwives, but completely withdrawn from any familiarity, let alone friendship. There is a total divide between what is called men's work and women's work. So, like Jane Austen, who in all her writing never recorded a conversation between two men alone, because as a woman she could not know what exclusively male conversation would be like, I cannot record much about the men of Poplar, beyond superficial observation.

I am about ready to leave. It has been a long day and night, but a profound sense of fulfilment and satisfaction lighten my step and lift my heart. Muriel and baby are both asleep as I creep out of the room. The good people downstairs offer me more tea, which again I decline as gracefully as I can, saying that breakfast will be waiting for me at Nonnatus House. I give instructions to call us if there seems to be any cause for worry, but say that I will be back again around lunch time, and again in the evening.

I entered the house in the rain and the dark. There had been a fever of excitement and anticipation, and the anxiety of a woman in labour, on the brink of bringing forth new life. I leave a calm, sleeping household, with the new soul in their midst, and step out into morning sunlight.

I cycled through the dark deserted streets, the silent docks, past the locked gates, the empty ports. Now I cycle through bright early morning, the sun just rising over the river, the gates open or opening, men streaming through the streets, calling to each other; engines beginning to sound, the cranes to move; lorries turning in through the huge gates; the sounds of a ship as it moved. A dockyard is not really a glamorous place, but to a young girl with only three hours sleep on twenty-four hours of work, after the quiet thrill of a safe delivery of a healthy baby, it is intoxicating. I don't even feel tired.

The swing bridge is open now, which means that the road is closed. A great ocean-going cargo boat is slowly and majestically entering the waters, her bows and funnels within inches of the houses on either side. I wait, dreamily watching the pilots and navigators guide her to her berth. I would love to know how they do it. Their skill is immense, taking years to learn, and is passed on from father to son, or uncle to nephew so they say. They are the princes of the docklands, and the casual labourers treat them with the deepest respect.

It takes about fifteen minutes for a boat to go through the bridge. Time to think. Strange how my life has developed, from a childhood disrupted by the war, a passionate love affair when I was only sixteen, and the knowledge three years later that I had to get away. So, for purely pragmatic reasons, my choice was nursing. Do I regret it?

A sharp piercing sound wakes me from my reverie, and the swing bridge begins to close. The road is open again, and the traffic begins to move. I cycle close to the kerb, as the lorries around me are a bit intimidating. A huge man with muscles like steel pulls off his cap and shouts, "Mornin' narse."

I shout back, "Morning, lovely day," and cycle on, exulting in my youth, the morning air, the heady excitement of the docks, but above all in the matchless sensation of having delivered a beautiful baby to a joyful mother.

Why did I ever start? Do I regret it? Never, never, never. I wouldn't swap my job for anything on earth.

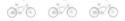

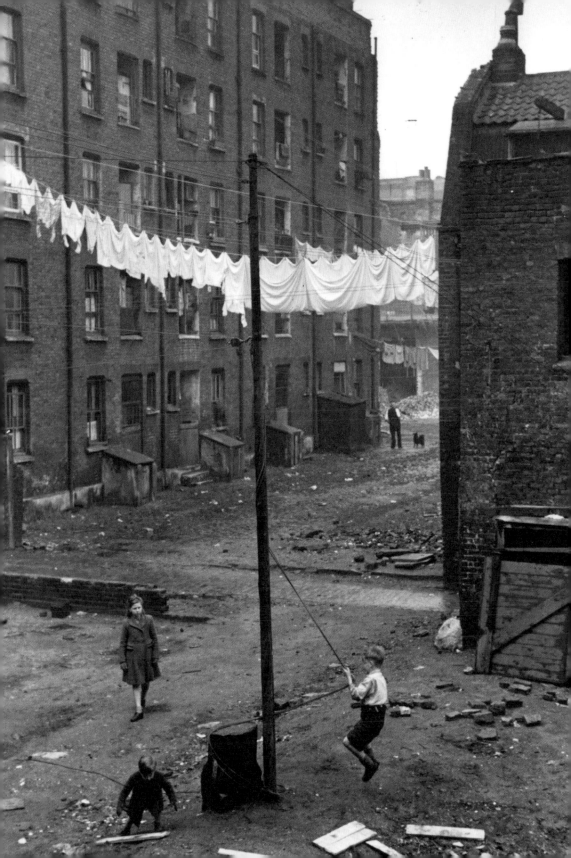

NONNATUS HOUSE

Had anyone told me, two years earlier, that I would be going to a convent for midwifery training, I would have run a mile. I was not that sort of girl. Convents were for Holy Marys, dreary and plain. Not for me. I had thought that Nonnatus House was a small, privately run hospital, of which there were many hundreds in the country at that time.

I arrived with bag and baggage on a damp October evening, having known only the West End of London. The bus from Aldgate brought me to a very different London, with narrow unlit streets, bomb sites, and dirty, grey buildings. With difficulty I found Leyland Street and looked for the hospital. It was not there. Perhaps I had the wrong address.

I stopped a passerby and enquired for the Midwives of St Raymund Nonnatus. The lady put down her string bag and beamed at me cordially, the missing front teeth adding to the geniality of her features. Her metal hair-curlers gleamed in the darkness. She took a cigarette from her mouth and said something that sounded like, "Yer washa nonnatuns arse, eh dearie?"

I stared at her, trying to work it out. I had not mentioned "washing" anything, particularly anyone's arse.

"No. I want the Midwives of St Raymund Nonnatus."

"Yeah. Loike wha' oie sez, duckie. Ve Nonnatuns. Ober dere, dearie. Vat's veir arse."

Opposite: When Jennifer Lee went to work in the East End, the area was still suffering from the effects of heavy bombing during the Second World War. The bombsites became playgrounds for the local children.

19

She patted my arm reassuringly, pointed to a building, stuck the cigarette back in her mouth, and toddled off, her bedroom slippers flapping on the pavement.

At this point in my narrative it would be expedient to mention to the bewildered reader how difficult it is to capture the Cockney dialect in writing. Pure Cockney is, or was, incomprehensible to an outsider, but the ear grows accustomed to the vowels and consonants, the inflexions and idiom, until after a while, it all becomes perfectly obvious. As I write about the Docklands people, I can hear their voices, but the attempt to reproduce the dialect in writing has proved to be something of a challenge!

But I digress.

I looked at the building dubiously; I saw dirty red brick, Victorian arches and turrets, iron railings, no lights, all next to a bomb site. What on earth have I come to? I thought. That's no hospital.

I pulled the bell handle, and a deep clanging came from within. A few moments later there were footsteps. The door was opened by a lady in strange clothes – not quite a nurse, but not quite a nun. She was tall and thin, and very, very old. She looked at me steadily for at least a minute without speaking, then leaned forward and took my hand. She looked all around her, drew me into the hallway, and whispered conspiratorially, "The poles are diverging, my dear."

Astonishment robbed me of speech, but fortunately she had no need of my reply, and continued, with near-breathless excitement, "Yes, and Mars and Venus are in alignment. You know what that means, of course?"

I shook my head.

"Oh, my dear, the static forces, the convergence of the fluid with the solid, the descent of the hexagon as it passes through the ether. This is a unique time to be alive. So exciting. The little angels clap their wings."

She laughed, clapped her bony hands, and did a little skip.

"But come in, come in, my dear. You must have some tea, and some cake. The cake is very good. Do you like cake?"

I nodded.

"So do I. We shall have some together, my dear, and you must give me your opinion on the theory that the depths in space are forever being pulled by the process of gravitation into heavenly bodies."

She turned and walked swiftly down a stone passage, her white veil floating behind her. I was in some doubt about whether to follow, because

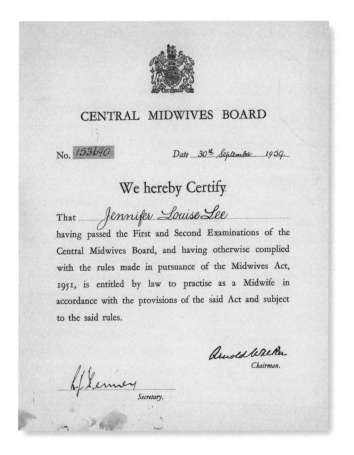

Above: Jennifer Lee was awarded her midwifery certificate in 1959, while she was living and working in the East End.

I thought I must surely have come to the wrong address, but she seemed to expect me to be right behind her, and talked all the while, asking questions to which she clearly did not expect an answer.

She entered a very large Victorian-looking kitchen with a stone floor, stone sink, wooden draining boards, tables and cupboards. The room contained an old-fashioned gas-stove with wooden plate-racks above it, a large Ascot water heater over the sink, and lead pipes attached to the walls. A large coke-burner stood in one corner, the flue running up to the ceiling.

"Now for the cake," said my companion. "Mrs B. made it this morning. I saw her with my own eyes. Where have they put it? You had better look around, dear."

Entering the wrong house is one thing, but poking around in someone else's kitchen is quite another matter. I spoke for the first time. "Is this Nonnatus House?"

The old lady raised her hands in a theatrical gesture and in clear, ringing tones cried out, "Not born, yet born in death. Born to greatness. Born to lead and inspire." She raised her eyes to the ceiling and lowered her voice to a thrilling whisper, "Born to be sanctified!"

Was she mad? I stared at her in dumb stupefaction, then repeated the question, "Yes, but is this Nonnatus House?"

"Oh, my dear, I knew the moment I saw you that you would understand. The cloud rests unbroken. Youth is freely given, the chimes sing of sad indigos, deep vermilions. Let us make what sense of it we can. Put the kettle on, dear. Don't just stand there."

There seemed to be no point in repeating my question, so I filled the kettle. The pipes all around the kitchen rattled and shook with a most alarming noise as I turned on the tap. The old lady poked around, opening cupboards and tins, chatting all the while about cosmic rays and confluent ethers. Suddenly she gave a cry of delight. "The cake! The cake! I knew I would find it."

She turned to me and whispered, with a naughty gleam in her eye, "They think they can hide things from Sister Monica Joan, but they are not smart enough, my dear. Plodding or swift, laughter or despair, none can hide, all will be revealed. Get two plates and a knife, and don't hang around. Where's the tea?"

We sat down at the huge wooden table. I poured the tea, and Sister Monica Joan cut two large slices of cake. She crumbled her slice into tiny pieces, and pushed them around her plate with long, bony fingers. She ate with murmurs of ecstatic delight, and winked at me as she gobbled morsels down.

The cake was excellent, and a fellowship of conspiracy was entered into as we agreed that another slice would be in order.

"They will never know, my dear. They will think that Fred has had it, or that poor fellow who sits on the doorstep eating his sandwiches."

She looked out of the window. "There is a light in the sky. Do you think it is a planet exploding, or an alien landing?"

I thought it was an aeroplane, but I opted for the exploding planet, then said, "How about some more tea?"

"Just what I was about to suggest, and what about another slice of cake? They won't be back before seven o' clock, you know."

She chatted on. I could not make head nor tail of what she was on about, but she was enchanting. The more I looked at her, the more I could see fragile beauty in her high cheekbones, her bright eyes, her wrinkled, pale ivory skin, and the perfect balance of her head on her long, slender neck. The constant movement of her expressive hands, with their long fingers like a ballet of ten dancers, was hypnotic. I felt myself falling under a spell.

We finished the cake with no trouble at all, having agreed that an empty tin would be less conspicuous than a small wedge of cake left on a plate. She winked mischievously, and chuckled.

"That tiresome Sister Evangelina will be the first to notice. You should see her, my dear, when she gets cross. Oh, the hideous baggage. Her red face gets even redder, and her nose drips. Yes, it actually drips! I have seen it." She tossed her head haughtily. "But what can it signify for me? The mystery of the evidence of consciousness is a house in a given time, a function and an event combined, and few are the elite, indeed, who can welcome such a realisation. But hush. What is that? Make haste."

She leaped up, scattering cake crumbs all over the table, the floor, and herself, grabbed the tin and hurried with it to the larder. Then she sat down again, assuming an exaggerated expression of innocence.

Footsteps were heard on the stone floor of the hallway, and female voices. Three nuns entered the kitchen, talking about enemas, constipation, and varicose veins. I concluded that I must, against all expectations, be in the right place.

One of them stopped, and addressed me, "You must be Nurse Lee. We were expecting you. Welcome to Nonnatus House. I am Sister Julienne, the Sister-in-Charge. We will have a little chat together in my office after supper. Have you eaten?"

The face and the voice were so open and honest, and the question so artless, that I could not reply. I felt the cake sitting heavily in the bottom of my stomach. I managed to murmur "yes, thank you" and surreptitiously brushed a crumb off my skirt.

"Well, you will excuse us if we have a small meal. We usually prepare our own supper because we all come in at different times."

The Sisters were bustling about, fetching plates, knives, cheese, biscuits and other things from the larder, and laying them on the kitchen table.

A cry came from behind the door, and a red-faced nun emerged carrying the cake tin.

"It's gone. The tin's empty. Where is Mrs B.'s cake? She made it only this morning."

This must be Sister Evangelina. Her face was getting redder as she glared around.

No one spoke. The three Sisters looked at each other. Sister Monica Joan sat aloof, beyond all reproach, her eyes closed. The cake was doing something nasty to my intestines, and I knew that the enormity of my crime could not be concealed. My voice was husky as I whispered, "I had a little."

The red face and heavy figure advanced toward Sister Monica Joan. "And she's had the rest of it. Look at her, covered in cake crumbs. It's disgusting. Oh, the greedy thing! She can't keep her hands off anything. That cake was for all of us. You … you …"

Sister Evangelina was shaking with rage as she towered over Sister Monica Joan, who remained absolutely immobile, her eyes closed, as though she had not heard a word. She looked fragile and aristocratic. I could not bear it, and found my voice. "No, you've got it wrong. Sister Monica Joan had a slice, and I had the rest."

The three nuns stared at me in astonishment. I felt myself blush all over. Had I been a dog caught stealing the Sunday roast, I would have crept under the table with my tail between my legs. To have entered a strange house, and to have consumed the best part of a cake without the knowledge or consent of the lawful owners, was a solecism worthy of severe retribution. I could only mutter, "I'm sorry. I was hungry. I won't do it again."

Sister Evangelina snorted and banged the tin on the table.

Sister Monica Joan, whose eyes were still closed, head turned away, moved for the first time. She took a handkerchief from her pocket and handed it to Sister Evangelina, holding it by a corner with thumb and forefinger, the other fingers arched fastidiously. "Perhaps it is time for a little mopping up, dear," she said sweetly.

Rage boiled even more fiercely. The redness of Sister Evangelina's features turned to purple, and moisture gathered round her nostrils.

"No thank you, dear. I have one of my own," she spat out through clenched teeth.

Sister Monica Joan gave an affected little jump, brushed her face elegantly with the handkerchief, and murmured, as though to herself, "Methinks 'tis raining. I cannot abide the rain. I will retire. Pray excuse me, Sisters. We will meet at Compline."

She smiled graciously at the three Sisters, then turned to me, and gave me the biggest, naughtiest wink I had ever seen in my life. Haughtily, she sailed out of the kitchen.

I felt myself squirm with embarrassment as the door closed and I was left alone with the three nuns. I just wanted to sink through the floor, or run away. Sister Julienne told me to take my case to the top floor, where I would find a room with my name on the door. I had expected a heavy silence and three pairs of eyes following me as I left the kitchen, but Sister Julienne started talking about an old lady she had just visited, whose cat appeared to be stuck up the chimney. They all laughed, and to my intense relief the atmosphere lightened at once.

In the hallway, I seriously wondered whether or not to cut and run. The fact that I was in something like a convent, and not a hospital, was ridiculous, and the whole saga of the cake, humiliating. I could have just picked up my case and vanished into the darkness. It was tempting. In fact I might have done so had the front door not opened at that moment and two laughing young girls appeared. Their faces were pink and freshened by the night air, their hair untidy from the wind. A few spots of rain glistened on their long gaberdine raincoats. They were about my age, and looked happy and full of life.

"Hello!" said a deep, slow voice. "You must be Jenny Lee. How nice. You'll like it here. There are not too many of us. I'm Cynthia, and this is Trixie."

But Trixie had already disappeared down the passage towards the kitchen with the words: "I'm famished. See you later."

Cynthia's voice was astonishing – soft, low, and slightly husky. She also spoke extremely slowly, and with just a touch of laughter in her tone. In another type of girl, it would have been the cultivated, sexy voice of allure. I had met plenty of that type in four years of nursing, but Cynthia was not one of their number. Her voice was completely natural, and she could speak no other way. My discomfort and uncertainty left me, and we grinned at each other, friends already. I decided I would stay.

Later that evening I was called to Sister Julienne's office. I went filled with dread, expecting a severe dressing-down about the cake. Having endured four years of tyranny from hospital nursing hierarchies, I expected the worst, and ground my teeth in anticipation. Sister Julienne was small and plump. She must have worked about fifteen or sixteen hours that day, but she looked as fresh as a daisy. Her radiant smile reassured me and dispelled my fears. Her first words were, "We will say nothing more about the cake."

I gave a great sigh of relief and sister Julienne burst out laughing, "Strange things happen to us all in the company of Sister Monica Joan. But I assure you, no one will mention it again. Not even Sister Evangelina."

She said the last words with special emphasis, and I found myself laughing also. I was completely won over, and glad I had not been so rash as to run away.

Her next words were unexpected. "What is your religion, nurse?"

"Well … er … none … er … that is, Methodist – I think."

The question seemed astonishing, irrelevant, even slightly silly. To ask about my education, my training and experience in nursing, my plans for the future – all that would have been anticipated and acceptable. But religion? What had religion to do with anything?

She looked very grave, and said gently, "Jesus Christ is our strength and our guidance here. Perhaps you will join us sometimes at Church on a Sunday?"

Sister then went on to explain the training I would receive, and the routine of Nonnatus House. I would be under the supervision of a trained midwife for all visits for about three weeks, and then go out alone for ante- and post-natal work. All deliveries would be supervised by another midwife. Classroom lectures were held once a week in the evening, after work. All study would be done in our spare time. She sat quietly explaining other details, most of which went over my head. I was not really listening, but wondering about her, and why I felt so comfortable and happy in her company. A bell rang. She smiled.

"It is time for Compline. I must go. We will meet in the morning. I hope you have a restful night."

The impact Sister Julienne made upon me – and, I discovered, most people – was out of all proportion to her words or her appearance. She was not imposing or commanding, nor arresting in any way. She was not even particularly clever. But something radiated from her and, ponder as I might, I could not understand it. It did not occur to me at the time that her radiance had a spiritual dimension, owing nothing to the values of the temporal world.

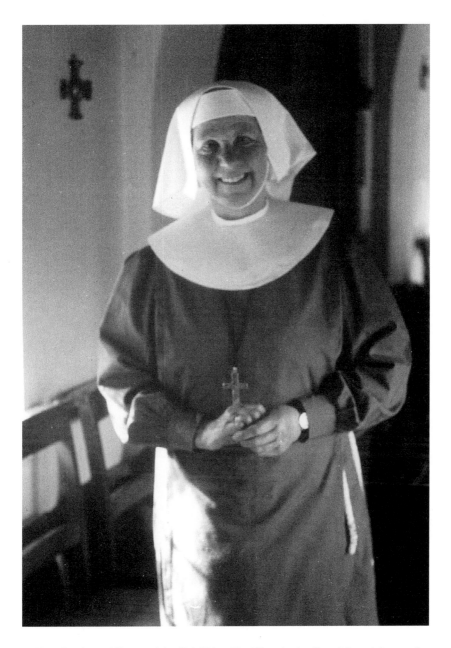

Above: Based on real-life nun and Jennifer's lifelong friend Sister Jocelyn, Sister Julienne is just one of the characters in the *Call the Midwife* trilogy whose name has been changed.

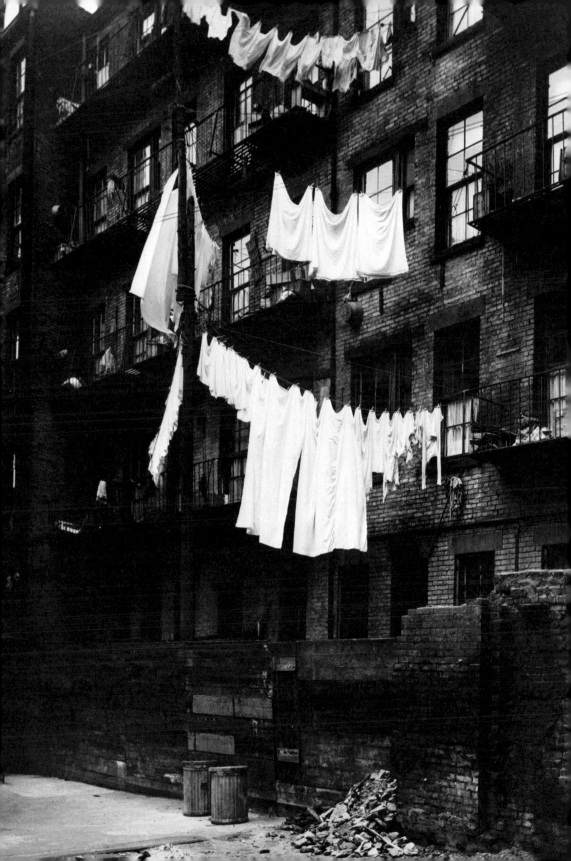

MORNING VISITS

It was about 6 a.m. when I arrived back at Nonnatus House after Muriel's delivery, and I was ravenous. A night's work, and a six to eight mile cycle ride can sharpen a young appetite like nothing else. The house was quiet when I entered. The nuns were in Chapel, and the lay staff not yet up. I was tired, but I knew that I had to clean my delivery bag, wash and sterilise my instruments, complete my notes and leave them on the office desk before I could eat.

Breakfast was laid out in the dining room, and I would take mine first, then go to bed for a few hours. I raided the larder. A pot of tea, boiled eggs, toast, home-made gooseberry jam, cornflakes, home-made yoghurt and scones. Heaven! Nuns always have a lot of home-made food, I had discovered. The preserves came from the many church bazaars and sales that seemed to go on throughout the year. The delicious cakes and biscuits and crunchy bread were made either by the nuns or by the many local women who came in to work at Nonnatus House. Any staff who had missed a meal through being called out had a free run of the larder. I was deeply grateful for this liberality, which was so unlike hospitals, where you had to plead for a bit of food if you had missed a meal for any reason.

It was a royal feast. I left a note asking to be called at about 11.30 a.m., and persuaded my tired legs to carry me up to my bedroom. I slept like a

Opposite: Many people lived in overcrowded tenements and the sight of lines of laundry hanging from the balconies would have been a common one to Jennifer and her fellow midwives (c. 1930s).

baby, and when someone roused me with a cup of tea, I couldn't remember where I was. The tea reminded me. Only the kind Sisters would send a cup of tea up to a nurse who had been working all night. In hospital it would be a bang on the door, and that would be that.

Downstairs I looked at the daybook. Only three calls before lunch. One to Muriel, and two visits to patients in the tenements that I would pass on the way. Four hours of sleep had refreshed me completely, and I got out the bike and cycled off in high spirits in the sunshine.

The tenements were always grim looking, whatever the weather. They were constructed as a four-sided building with an opening on one side, all the flats faced inwards. The buildings were about six storeys high, and sunlight seldom reached the inner courtyard, which was the social centre for the tenement dwellers. The courtyard contained all the washing lines and as there were literally hundreds of flats in each block, they were never without loads of washing flapping in the wind. The dustbins were also in the courtyard.

In the times I am writing about, the 1950s, there was a lavatory and running cold water in each flat. Before the introduction of these facilities, the lavatories and water were in the courtyard, and everyone had to go down to use them. Some of the tenements still retained the lavatory sheds, which were now used to house bikes or motor cycles. There did not seem many of them – perhaps three dozen at the most, and I wondered how there could have been enough lavatories for the occupants of about five hundred flats.

I threaded my way through the washing, and reached the stairway that I wanted. All the stairways were external, made of stone steps, and led up to a balcony, facing inwards, which ran the length of the building, going round all the corners, continuously. Each of the flats led off this balcony. Whereas the inner courtyard was the centre of social life, the balconies were the lanes, teeming with life and gossip. The balconies for the tenement women were equivalent to the streets of the terraced house dwellers. So close was the living space, that I doubt if anyone could get away with anything without all the neighbours knowing. The outside world held very little interest for the East Enders, and so other peoples' business was the primary topic of conversation – for most it was the only interest, the only amusement or diversion. It is not surprising that savage fighting frequently broke out in the tenements.

The tenements looked unusually cheerful in the noonday sun when I arrived that day. I picked my way through the litter and dustbins and washing in the courtyard. Small children crowded around. The midwife's delivery bag was an object of intense interest – they thought we carried the baby in it.

I found my entry, and climbed the five storeys to the flat I wanted.

All the flats were more or less the same: two or three rooms leading off each other. A stone sink in one corner of the main room; a gas stove and a cupboard constituting the kitchen. The lavatories, when they were introduced, had to be installed near the water supply, so they were situated in a corner, near to the sink. The installation of lavatories in each flat had been a great leap forward in public hygiene, because it improved the conditions in the courtyard. It also avoided the necessity of chamber pots in every flat which had to be emptied daily, the women carrying them downstairs to the emptying troughs. The ordure in the courtyards used to be disgusting, I was told.

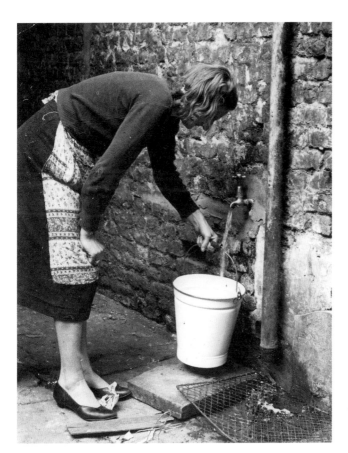

Right. In the 1950s, although many tenement flats had inside lavatories and running water, some of the older buildings still had lavatory sheds and communal taps. In such cases, water had to be brought in from outside for the midwife's use.

The tenements of London's East End were built around the 1850s, mainly to house the dock workers and their families. In their day, they were probably considered to be adequate housing, quite sufficient for any family. They were certainly an improvement on the mud-floor hovels that they replaced, which barely protected a family from the elements. The tenements were brick built with a slate roof. Rain did not penetrate and they were dry inside. I have no doubt that 150 years ago, they were considered to be luxurious. A large family of ten to twelve people in two or three rooms would not have been judged as overcrowding. After all, the vast majority of mankind has lived in such conditions throughout history.

But times change, and by the 1950s the tenements were considered to be slum areas. The rents were a lot cheaper than the terraced houses, and consequently only the poorest families, those least able to cope, entered the tenements. Social law seems to suggest that the poorest families are often the ones that produce the greatest number of children, and the tenements were always teeming with them. Infectious diseases ran through the buildings like wildfire. So did the pests: fleas, body lice, ticks, scabies, crabs, mice, rats, and cockroaches. The pest control men from the council were always busy. The tenements were deemed unfit for human habitation and evacuated in the 1960s, and stood empty for over a decade. They were finally demolished in 1982.

Edith was small and stringy, and as tough as old boots. She looked a good deal older than forty years. She had brought up six children. During the war they had been bombed out of a terraced house, but it had not been a direct hit, and the family had survived. The children were then evacuated. Her husband was a dock labourer, and she was a munitions worker. After the bombing, she and her husband had moved into the tenements, which were cheaper to rent. They both lived there throughout the entire Blitz, and miraculously the tenements, which were the most densely populated dwellings, were not hit. Edith did not see her children for five years, but they were reunited in 1945. The family continued to live in the tenements, because of the rent, and because they had become used to the life. How anyone could manage in two rooms with six growing children was always beyond my understanding. But they did, and thought nothing of it.

She had not been pleased to fall pregnant again, in fact she was furious, but like most women who have a baby late in life, she was besotted with the little thing when he arrived, and cooed over him all the time. The flat was hung with nappies all over the place – there were no disposable nappies in those days – and a pram further reduced the living space in the crowded room.

Edith was up and doing. It was her tenth day after delivery. We kept mothers in bed for a long time after delivery in those days – ten to fourteen days known as the "lying-in" period. Medically speaking, this was not good practice, as it is far better for a woman to get moving as soon as possible, thus reducing the risk of complications such as thrombosis. But this was not known back then, and it had been traditional to keep women in bed after a birth. The great advantage was that it gave the woman a proper, and well-earned, rest. Other people had to do all the household chores, and for a brief period, she could lead a life of idleness. She needed to gather her strength, because once she was on her feet again, everything would devolve to her. When you consider the physical effort required to carry all the shopping up those stairs: coal and wood in the winter, paraffin for stoves, or rubbish carried down to the dustbins in the courtyard; if you consider the fact that to take the baby out, the pram had to be bumped down the stairs, one step at a time, and then bumped up again to get home, often loaded with groceries, as well as the baby, you might begin to understand how tough those women had to be. Almost every time you entered the tenements, you would see a woman bumping a big pram up or down. If they lived at the top, this would mean about seventy steps each way. The prams had big wheels, which made it possible, and were well sprung, which bounced the baby around. The babies loved it, and laughed and shrieked with glee. It was also dangerous if the steps were slippery, because the whole weight of the pram had to be controlled by the handle, and if the mother missed her footing or something happened and she let go, the pram and baby would go cascading down the length of the steps. I always helped when I saw a woman with a pram by taking the other end, therefore half the weight, which was considerable. The whole weight, for a woman alone, must have been tremendous.

Edith was in a grubby dressing gown, down-trodden slippers and hair curlers. She was simultaneously feeding her baby and smoking. The radio was blaring out pop music. She looked perfectly happy. In fact she looked a better colour, and younger than she had a couple of months earlier. The rest had obviously done her good.

"Hello, luvvy. Come on in. How about a nice cup of tea?"

I explained that I had other calls to make and declined the tea. I was able to see how feeding was going. The baby was sucking voraciously, but it struck me that Edith's thin little breasts probably did not contain much milk. However, it was far better for her to continue than to put the baby on to formula milk straight away, so I said nothing. If the baby fails to gain weight, or shows real signs of hunger, we can talk about it then, I thought. It was our practice to visit each day post-natally for a minimum of fourteen days, so we saw a lot of each patient.

It became the fashion about that time to put babies on to formula milk, and to suggest to the mother that this would be best for the baby. The Midwives of St Raymund Nonnatus did not go down this path, however, and all our patients were advised and helped to breastfeed for as long as possible. A fortnight of rest in bed helped to facilitate this, as the mother was not tiring herself by rushing around, and all her physical resources could go into producing milk for the baby.

As I glanced around the crowded room, the minimal kitchen area, and the general lack of facilities, it flashed through my mind that bottle-feeding would be the worst thing for the baby. Where on earth would Edith keep bottles, and tins of formula milk? How would she sterilise them? Would she bother to? Or even bother to keep them clean, never mind sterilising? There was no refrigerator, and I could well imagine bottles of half-consumed milk left lying around the place, to be given a second or third time to the baby, with no thought to the fact that bacteria quickly builds up in milk that has been left to go cold, and then warmed up again. No, breastfeeding would be much safer, even if there was not quite enough milk.

I remember lectures during my Part I midwifery training about the advantages of bottle-feeding, which sounded very convincing. When I first came to work with the Nonnatus Midwives, I thought them very old fashioned in always recommending breastfeeding. I had not taken into account the social conditions in which the Sisters worked. The lecturers were not dealing with real life. They were dealing with classroom situations and ideal young mothers who existed only in the imagination, from educated middle-class backgrounds, women who would remember all the rules, and do everything they were told to do. These classroom pundits were remote from silly young girls who would get the formula mixed up, get the measurements wrong, fail to boil the water, be unable to sterilise the bottles or the teats, fail to wash the bottles. Such theorists could not even imagine a half-empty bottle being left for twenty-four hours, then given to the baby, nor envisage a bottle rolling across the floor, picking up cat hairs, or any other dirt. Our lecturers never mentioned to us the possibility of anything else being added to the formula, such as sugar, honey, rice, treacle, condensed milk, semolina, alcohol, aspirin, Horlicks, Ovaltine. Perhaps such a possibility had never come the way of the writers of these textbooks. But they had been encountered often enough by the Nonnatus nuns.

Edith and her baby looked quite happy, so I did not disturb them, but said we would call the next day to weigh the baby, and to examine her.

I had another visit to make, to Molly Pearce, a girl of nineteen who was expecting her third baby and who had not turned up at the antenatal clinic for the last three months. As she was very near to full term, we needed to assess her.

There was noise coming from inside the door as I approached. It sounded like a row. I've always hated any sort of row or scene, and instinctively shrank away. But I had a job to do, so I knocked on the door. Instantly there was silence inside. It lasted a couple of minutes, and the silence seemed more menacing than the noise.

I knocked again. Still silence, then a bolt pulled back, and a key turned – it was one of the few times I had known a door to be locked in the East End.

The unshaven face of a surly looking man stared suspiciously at me through a crack in the door. Then he swore obscenely, and spat on the floor at my feet, and made off down the balcony towards the staircase. The girl came towards me. She looked hot and flushed, and was panting slightly. "Good riddance," she shouted down the balcony, and kicked the doorpost.

She looked about nine months pregnant, and it occurred to me that rows of that sort could put her into labour, especially if violence was involved. But I had no evidence of that, as yet. I asked if I could examine her, as she had not been to antenatal clinic. She reluctantly agreed, and let me into the flat.

The stench inside was overpowering. It was a foul mixture of sweat, urine, faeces, cigarettes, alcohol, paraffin, stale food, sour milk, and unwashed clothes. Obviously Molly was a real slattern. The vast majority of women

Overleaf: Poverty and ignorance often contributed to the bad diets that some young pregnant women in the East End suffered from. This public health poster (1948), produced by the Ministry of Information, encourages pregnant women to eat a healthy diet and gives examples of the types of food they should be eating.

EXPECTANT MOTHERS

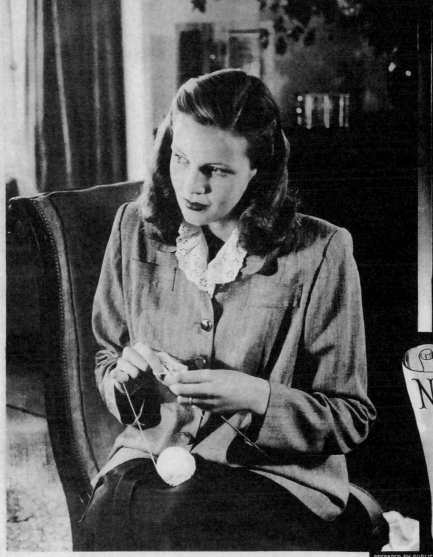

C
BI

OATM
FRUIT
WITH

FISH
TOMA
BAKE

OATC

BUTT

MARM
HONE

WEA
MILK

AN

Now y
We
First
An

FAST	DINNER	TEA
ORRIDGE, EAL	MEAT, CHEESE, FISH, RABBIT, OFFAL, SAUSAGE.	CHEESE, EGG, MEAT, FRESH OR TINNED FISH, THICK SOUP, PEAS OR BEANS.
BACON &	GRAVY, SAUCE.	
NS.		SALAD OR RAW FRUIT.
	RAW SALAD, GREENS.	BREAD, BISCUIT,
TOAST.	ROOT VEGETABLE, PEAS, BEANS	CAKE.
RGARINE	POTATO	BUTTER, MARGARINE, JAM.
E, JAM,	STEAMED BAKED PUDDING, CUSTARD, MILK PUDDING & FRUIT,	COCOA, WEAK TEA OR COFFEE,
COFFEE.	BREAD, CHEESE.	MILK.
	ORANGE DRINK.	

NOT FORGET YOUR EXTRA RATION BOOK!

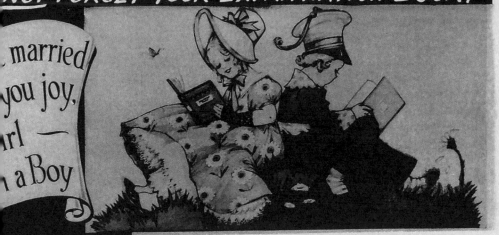

married
you joy,
rl —
a Boy

SCIENTIFIC ADVISER'S DIVISION — MAY. 1948

that I met had a true pride in themselves and their homes, and worked desperately hard. But not Molly. She had no such home-making instincts.

She led me into the bedroom, which was dark. The bed was filthy. There was no bed linen, just the bare mattress and pillows. Some grey army surplus blankets lay on the bed and a wooden cot stood in the corner. This is no place for a delivery, I thought to myself. It had been assessed as adequate by a midwife some months earlier, but quite obviously the domestic conditions had deteriorated since that time. I would have to report back to the Sisters.

I asked Molly to loosen her clothes and lie down. As she did so, I noticed a great black bruise on her chest. I enquired how it had happened. She snarled and tossed her head. "'Im," she said, and spat on the floor. She offered no other information, and lay down. Perhaps my unexpected arrival has saved her from another blow, I thought.

I examined her. The baby's head was well down, the position seemed to be normal, and I could feel movement. I listened for the foetal heart, which was a steady 126 per minute. She and the baby seemed quite normal and healthy, in spite of everything.

It was only then that I noticed the children. I heard something in the corner of the dark bedroom, and nearly jumped out of my skin. I thought it was a rat. I focused my eyes in that direction, and saw two little faces peering round from behind a chair. Molly heard my gasp, and said, "It's all right. Tom, come 'ere."

But, of course, there must be young children around, I thought. This was her third pregnancy, and she was only nineteen, so they would be under school age. Why hadn't I noticed them before?

Two little boys of about two or three years old came out from behind the chair. They were absolutely silent. Boys of that age usually rush around, making no end of noise, but not these two. Their silence was unnatural. They had big eyes, full of fear, and they took a step or two forward, then clung to each other as though for mutual protection and retreated behind the chair again.

"That's all right, kids, it's only the nurse. She won't hurt you. Come 'ere."

They came out again, two dirty little boys, with snot and tear marks staining their faces. They were wearing only jumpers, a practice I had seen a lot in Poplar, and for some reason I found it particularly repellent. A toddler was dressed only at the top, and left naked from the waist down. It seemed to be especially prevalent among little boys. I was told that the women saved on washing this way. The child, before he was toilet trained, could then just urinate anywhere, and there would be no nappies or clothes to wash. Children would run around the tenement balconies and courtyards all day like this.

Tom and his little brother crept out from the corner, and ran to their mother. They seemed to be losing their fear. She put out an arm affectionately and they cuddled up to her. Well at least she's got some mothering instincts, I thought. I wondered how much time those little children spent behind the chair when their father was at home.

But I was not a health visitor, nor a social worker, and there was no point in speculating on that sort of thing. I resolved to report my observations to the Sisters, and told Molly that we would come back later that week, to ascertain that everything was available for a home delivery.

I still had Muriel to visit, and it was with great relief that I left the foul atmosphere of that flat.

The bright cold air outside and the cycle ride down to the Isle of Dogs refreshed my spirits, and I sped along.

"Hello, luvvy, how's yourself?" was the greeting shouted at me by several women, known and unknown to me. This was always the greeting called out from the pavement.

"Lovely, thanks, ah's yerself?" I always replied. It was difficult not to slip into the cockney lingo.

I don't believe it, I said to myself, as I turned into Muriel's street, she can't be here already. Sure enough, Mrs Jenkins was there with her stick and her string bag, her head scarf over her curlers, and the same old long mildew-encrusted coat that she wore summer and winter. She was talking to a woman in the street, hanging intently on to to every word. She saw me slow down and came up to me and grabbed my sleeve with her filthy, long nailed hands.

"How is she, and the little one?" she rasped.

I was impatient, and pulled my arm away. Mrs Jenkins turned up at every delivery. No matter how far the distance, how bad the weather, how early or late in the day, Mrs Jenkins would always be seen hanging around the street. No one knew where she lived, or how she got her information, or how she managed to walk, sometimes three or four miles, to a house where a baby had been born. But she always did. I was irritated and passed her without speaking. I regarded her as a nosy old busybody. I was young, too young to understand. Too young to see the pain in her eyes, or to hear the tortured urgency in her voice. "'Ow is she? An' ve li'l one. 'Ow's ve li'l one?"

I went directly into the house without even knocking, and Muriel's mother immediately came forward, busy and smiling. These older generation mothers knew that they were absolutely indispensable at times like these, and it gave them a great sense of fulfilment, an ongoing purpose in life. She was all bustle and information. "She's been asleep since you left. She's been to the toilet and passed water. She's had some tea and now I'm getting her a nice bit of fish. Baby's been to the breast, I've seen to that, but she ain't got no milk yet."

I thanked her and went up to the room. It looked clean, fresh and bright, with flowers on the chest of drawers. Compared to the filth and squalor of Molly's flat, it looked like paradise.

Muriel was awake but sleepy. Her first words to me were, "I don't want no fish. Can't you tell mum that? I don't feel like it, but she won't listen to me. She might listen to you."

Clearly there was a difference of opinion between mother and daughter. I did not want to be involved. I checked her pulse and blood pressure – normal. Her vaginal discharge was not excessive; the uterus felt normal too. I checked her breasts. A little colostrum was coming out but no milk, as her mother had said. I wanted to try to get the baby to feed, in fact that was the main purpose of my visit.

In the cot the baby was sleeping soundly. Gone was the puckered appearance, the discoloration of the skin from the stress and trauma of birth, the cries of alarm and fear at entering this world. He was relaxed and warm and peaceful. Nearly everyone will say that seeing a newborn baby has an effect on them, ranging from awe to astonishment. The helplessness of the newborn human infant has always made an impression on me. All other mammals have a certain amount of autonomy at birth. Many animals, within an hour or two of birth, are up on their feet and running. Others, at the very least, can find the nipple and suck. But the human baby can't even do that. If the nipple or teat is not actually placed in the baby's mouth and sucking encouraged, the baby would die of starvation. I have a theory that all human babies are born prematurely. Given the human life span – three score years and ten – to be comparable with other animals of similar longevity, human gestation should be about two years. But the human head is so big by the age of two that no woman could deliver it. So our babies are born prematurely, in a state of utter helplessness.

I lifted the tiny creature from his cot and brought him to Muriel. She knew what to do, and had started squeezing a little colostrum from the nipple. We tried brushing a little of this over the baby's lips. He was not interested, only squirmed and turned his head away. We tried again, with the same reaction. It took at least a quarter of an hour of patiently trying to encourage the baby, but eventually, we persuaded him to open his mouth sufficiently to insert the nipple. He took about three sucks, and went off to sleep again. Sound asleep, as though exhausted from all his efforts. Muriel and I laughed.

"You would think he'd been doing all the hard work," she said, "not you and me, eh, nurse?"

We agreed to leave it for the time being. I would be back again in the evening, and she could try again during the afternoon, if she wanted to.

As I went downstairs, I smelt cooking. It may not have been to Muriel's liking, but it certainly got my gastric juices going. I was starving, and a delicious lunch awaited me at Nonnatus House. I bade them goodbye, and made for my bicycle. Mrs Jenkins was standing over it, as though she were keeping guard. How am I going to get rid of her? I thought. I didn't want to talk. I just wanted to get back to my lunch, but she was hanging on to the saddle. Clearly she was not going to let me go without some information.

"'Ow is she? An' ve li'l one. 'Ow's ve li'l one?" she hissed at me, her eyes unblinking.

There is something about obsessive behaviour that is off-putting. Mrs Jenkins was more than that. She was repellent. About seventy, she was tiny and bent, and her black eyes penetrated me, shattering any pleasant thoughts of lunch. She was toothless and ugly, in my arrogant opinion, and her filthy claw-like hands were creeping down my sleeve, getting unpleasantly close to my wrists. I pulled myself to my full height, which was nearly twice hers, and said in a cold professional voice, "Mrs Smith has been safely delivered of a little boy. Mother and baby are both well. Now, if you will excuse me, I must go."

"Fank Gawd," she said, and released my coat sleeve and my bicycle. She said nothing else. Crazy old thing, I thought crossly as I rode off. She ought not to be allowed out.

It was not until about a year later, when I was a general district nurse, that I learned more about Mrs Jenkins … and learned a little humility.

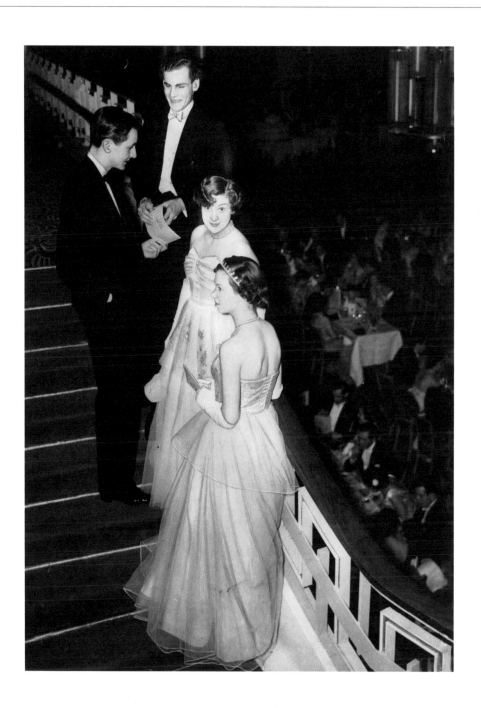

CHUMMY

The first time I saw Camilla Fortescue-Cholmeley-Browne ("just call me Chummy"), I thought it was a bloke in drag. Six foot two inches tall, with shoulders like a front-row forward and size eleven feet, her parents had spent a fortune trying to make her more feminine, but to no effect.

Chummy and I were new together, and she arrived the morning after the memorable evening when Sister Monica Joan and I had polished off a cake intended for twelve. Cynthia, Trixie and I were leaving the kitchen after breakfast when the front doorbell rang, and this giant in skirts entered. She blinked short-sightedly down at us from behind thick, steel-rimmed glasses, and said, in the plummiest voice imaginable, "Is this Nonnatus House?"

Trixie, who had a waspish tongue, looked out of the door into the street. "Is there anyone there?" she called, and came back into the hallway, bumping into the stranger.

"Oh, sorry, I didn't notice you," she said, and made off for the clinical room.

Cynthia stepped forward, and greeted the woman with the same exquisite warmth and friendliness that had chased away my thoughts of bolting the night before. "You must be Camilla."

"Oh, just call me Chummy."

Opposite: Like these debutantes at the Queen Charlotte's Ball (Grosvenor House, 1950), Chummy would have attended many formal parties and social events after making her debut.

"All right then Chummy, come in and we will find Sister Julienne. Have you had breakfast? I'm sure Mrs B. can fix you up with something."

Chummy picked up her case, took two steps, and tripped over the doormat. "Oh lawks, clumsy me," she said with a girlish giggle. She bent down to straighten the mat and collided with the hallstand, knocking two coats and three hats on to the floor.

"Frightfully sorry. I'll soon get them," but Cynthia had already picked them up, fearing the worst.

"Oh thanks, old bean," said Chummy, with a "haw-haw".

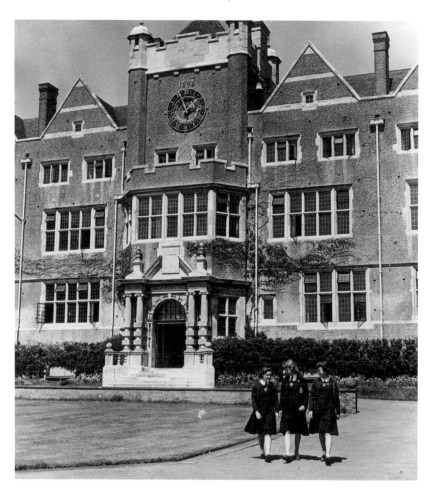

Above: The front entrance to Roedean School, based near Brighton in Sussex. The daughters of many wealthy families attended the school, which was designed by architect John W. Simpson.

Can this be real, or is she putting it on? I thought. But the voice was entirely real, and never changed, nor did the language. It was always "good show", or "good egg", or "what-ho", and, strangely enough, for all her massive size, her voice was soft and sweet. In fact, during the time that I knew her, I realised that everything about Chummy was soft and sweet. Despite her appearance, there was nothing butch about her. She had the nature of a gentle, artless young girl, diffident and shy. She was also pathetically eager to be liked.

The Fortescue-Cholmeley-Brownes were top drawer County types. Her great-great-grandfather had entered the Indian Civil Service in the 1820s, and the tradition had progressed through the generations. Her father was Governor of Rajasthan (an area the size of Wales), which he still, even in the 1950s, traversed on horseback. All this we learned from the collection of photographs on display in Chummy's room. She was the only girl amongst six brothers. All of them were tall, but unfortunately she was about an inch taller than the rest of the family.

All the children had been educated in England, the boys going to Eton, and Chummy to Roedean. They were placed in the care of guardians in this country, as the mother remained in India with her husband. Apparently Chummy had been at boarding school since she was six years of age, and knew no other life. She clung to her collection of family photographs with touching fervour – perhaps they were the closest she ever got to her family – and particularly loved one taken with her mother when she was about fourteen.

"That was the holiday I had with Mater," she said proudly, completely unaware of the pathos of her remark.

After Roedean came finishing school in Switzerland, then back to London to the Lucy Clayton Charm School to prepare her for presentation at Court. Those were the days of debutantes, when the daughters of the "best" families had to "come out", an expression meaning something quite different today. At that time it meant being presented formally to the monarch at Buckingham Palace. Chummy was presented and two photographs were proof of the event. In the first, an unmistakable Chummy in a ridiculous lacey ball gown, with ribbons and flowers, stood amongst a group of pretty young girls similarly attired, her huge, bony shoulders towering above their heads. The second photo was of her presentation to King George VI. Her great size and angular shape emphasised the petite charm of the Queen and the exquisite beauty of the two princesses, Elizabeth and Margaret. I wondered if Chummy was aware of how absurd she looked in the photos, which she was so pleased and so happy to display.

After the debutante bit came a year at a cordon-bleu school which took a small number of select young ladies on a residential basis. Chummy learned all the arts of the perfect hostess – the perfect hors d'oeuvre, the perfect pâté de foie gras – but remained ungainly, awkward, oversized, and generally unsuited to hostessing in any society. So a course of study at the best needlework school in London was deemed to be the right thing for her. For two years Chummy crocheted, embroidered and tatted, made lace and quilting and broderie anglaise. For two years she machined and set shoulders and double hemmed. All to no avail. While the other girls herringboned and feather-stitched and chatted happily, or sadly, of their boyfriends and lovers, Chummy, liked by all but loved by none, remained silent, always the odd chum out.

She never knew how it happened, but suddenly, unsought, she found her vocation: nursing and God. Chummy was going to be a missionary.

In a fever pitch of excitement, she enrolled at the Nightingale School of Nursing at St Thomas's Hospital in London. She was an instant success, and won the Nightingale Prize three years in succession. She adored the work on the wards, feeling for the first time in her life confident and competent, knowing that she was where she should be. Patients loved her, senior staff respected her, junior staff admired her. In spite of her great size she was gentle, with an intuitive understanding of patients, especially the very old, very sick, or dying. Even her clumsiness – a hallmark of earlier years – left her. On the wards she never dropped or broke a thing, never moved awkwardly or crashed into things. All these traits seemed to beset and torment her only in social life, for which she remained wholly ill-adapted.

Of course, young doctors and medical students, 90 per cent of whom were male and always on the look out for a pretty nurse, made fun of her and passed crude jokes about the difficulty of mounting a carthorse, and which of them had the organ of a stallion suited to the job. Freshmen were told of the ravishingly lovely nurse on North Ward, with whom it would be possible to fix a blind date, but they fled in horror when the blindness was given sight, vowing vengeance upon the jokers. Fortunately, such stories or pranks never reached Chummy's ears and passed straight over her head unnoticed. Had she been informed, it is very likely that she would just not have understood, and would have beamed amiably at her tormentors, shaming them with her innocence.

Chummy's entry into midwifery was less successful, but no less spectacular. It was some days before she could go out on the district. In the first place, no uniform would fit her. "Never mind, I'll make it," she said cheerfully. Sister Julienne doubted if there was a pattern available. "Not to worry, actually I can make it out of newspaper." To everyone's astonishment, she did. Material was obtained, and, in no time at all, a couple of dresses were made.

The bicycle was not so easy. For all the genteel education and ladylike accomplishments, no one had thought it necessary to teach her to ride a bicycle. A horse yes, but a bicycle, no.

"Never mind, I can learn," she said cheerfully. Sister Julienne said it was hard for an adult to acquire the skill. "Not to worry. I can practise," was her equally exuberant response.

Cynthia, Trixie and I went with her to the bicycle shed, and selected the largest – a huge old Raleigh, of about 1910 vintage, made of solid iron with a scooped-out front and high handlebars. The solid tyres were about three inches thick, and there were no gears. The whole contraption weighed about half a ton, and for this reason no one rode it. Trixie oiled the chain and we were ready for the off.

The time was just after lunch. We agreed to push Chummy up and down Leyland Street until she found her balance, after which we would travel in convoy to where the roads were quiet and flat. Most people who have tried to ride a bicycle in adult life for the first time will tell you that it is a terrifying experience. Many will say that it is impossible, and give up. But Chummy was made of sterner stuff. The Makers of the Empire were her forebears, and their blood flowed in her veins. Besides which, she was going to be a missionary, for which it was necessary that she should be a midwife. If she had to ride a bicycle to achieve this, so be it – she would ride the thing.

We pushed her, huge and shaking, shouting "pedal, pedal, up, down, up, down" until we were exhausted. She weighed about twelve stone of solid bone and muscle, and the bike another six stone, but we kept on pushing. At four o'clock the local school ended, and children came pouring out. About ten of them took over, giving us girls a well-earned rest as they ran along beside and behind, pushing and shouting encouragement.

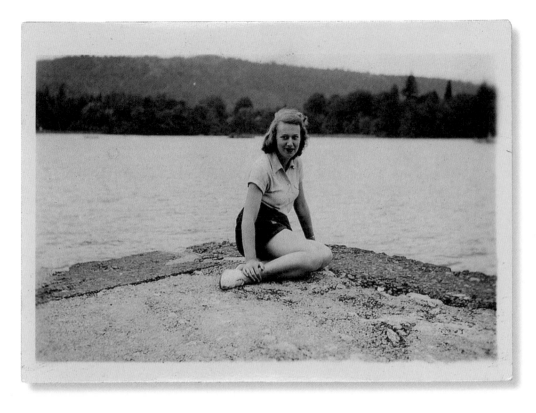

Above: Cynthia, pictured above in 1950, is one of the few real-life characters whose name did not change in the books. Cynthia and Jennifer remained friends until Cynthia's death in 2006.

Several times Chummy fell heavily to the ground. She hit her head on the kerb, and said, "Not to worry – no brains to hurt." She cut her leg, and murmured, "Just a scratch." She fell heavily on to one arm, and proclaimed, "I have another." She was indomitable. We began to respect her. Even the Cockney children, who had seen her as a comic turn, changed their tune. A tough-looking cookie of about twelve, who had been openly jeering at first, now looked solemnly at her with admiration.

The time had come to venture further than Leyland Street. Chummy could balance and she could pedal, so we agreed to half an hour cycling together around the streets. Trixie was in front, Cynthia and I on either side of Chummy, the children running behind, shouting.

We got to the top of Leyland Street and no further. It had not occurred to us to show Chummy how to turn a corner. Trixie turned left, calling "just follow me", and rode off. Cynthia and I turned left, but Chummy kept going straight ahead. I saw her fixed expression as she came straight for me, and after that all was confusion. Apparently a policeman had been in the act of crossing the street when the two of us hurtled into him. We came to rest on the opposite pavement. Seeing a representative of the law hit full frontal by a couple of midwives was joy for the children. They screamed with delight, and doors opened all down the street, emitting even more children and curious adults.

I was lying on my back in the gutter, not knowing what had happened. From this position I heard a groan, and then the policeman sat up with the words, "What fool did that?" I saw Chummy sit up. She had lost her glasses, and peered round. Maybe this could account for her next action or maybe she was dazed. She slapped the man heavily on the back with her huge hand and said, "No whingeing, now. Cheer up, old bean. Stiff upper lip and all that, what?" Clearly she was unaware that he was a policeman.

He was a big man, but not as big as Chummy. He fell forward at the blow, his face hitting one of the bicycles, and he cut his lip. Chummy merely said, "Oh, just a little scratch. Nothing to make a fuss about, old sport," and slapped him on the back again.

The policeman was outraged. He took out his notebook, and licked his pencil. The children vanished. The street cleared. He looked at Chummy with menace. "I'll take your name and address. Assaulting a policeman is a serious offence, I'll have you know."

I swear it was Cynthia's sexy voice that got us off. Without her, we would have been up before the magistrate the next day. I never knew how she did it, and she was quite unconscious of her charm. She said little, but the man's anger quickly vanished, and he was eating out of her hand in no time at all. He picked up the bicycles and escorted us down the street to Nonnatus House. He left us with the words, "Nice meeting you young ladies. I hope we meet again sometime."

Chummy had to spend three days in bed. The doctor said she had delayed shock and mild concussion. She slept for the first thirty-six hours, her temperature raised and pulse erratic. On the fourth day she was able to sit up, and asked what had happened. She was horrified when we told here, and deeply remorseful. As soon as she could go out, her first visit was to the police station to find the constable she had injured. She took with her a box of chocolates and a bottle of whisky.

Don't be afraid
of SOAP
and WATER

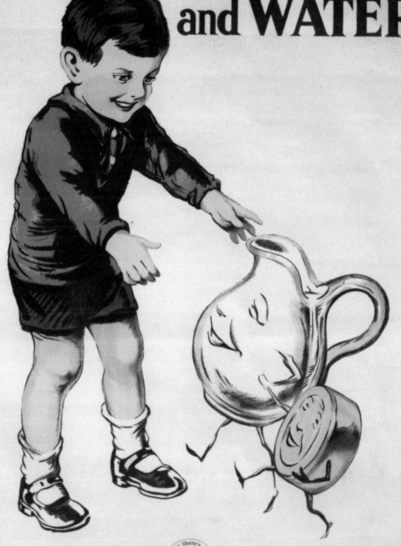

ISSUED BY HEALTH & CLEANLINESS COUNCIL. ALDWYCH HOUSE, LONDON, W.C.2.

MOLLY

When I called at the Canada Buildings to reassess Molly for a home confinement, she was out. It took three calls before I found her in. On the second attempt, I thought I heard movement in the flat, and knocked several times. There certainly was someone inside, but the door was locked, and no one came to open it.

On the third visit, Molly answered the door. She looked dreadful. She was only nineteen, but she looked pale and haggard. Lank greasy hair hung down her dirty face, and the two filthy little boys clung to her skirt. A week had passed since the first visit when I had interrupted a fight and a glance around the room told me that the domestic situation was worse, not better. I told her that we were reassessing her flat for a home confinement, and that perhaps it would be better if she went into hospital for the delivery. She shrugged, seeming indifferent. I pointed out that she had been to no antenatal clinics, and that this could be dangerous. She shrugged again. I was getting nowhere.

I said, "How is it that four months ago, the Midwives assessed your place as satisfactory for a home confinement, and now it is not?".

She said, "Well, me mum come in, and cleaned up, din't she?"

At last some communication. There was a mother on the scene. I asked for her mother's address. It was in the next block. Good.

Opposite: This Health and Cleanliness Council poster states "Don't be afraid of Soap and Water". Poor hygiene and cleanliness contributed to the spread of disease, particularly among the poor in the postwar period.

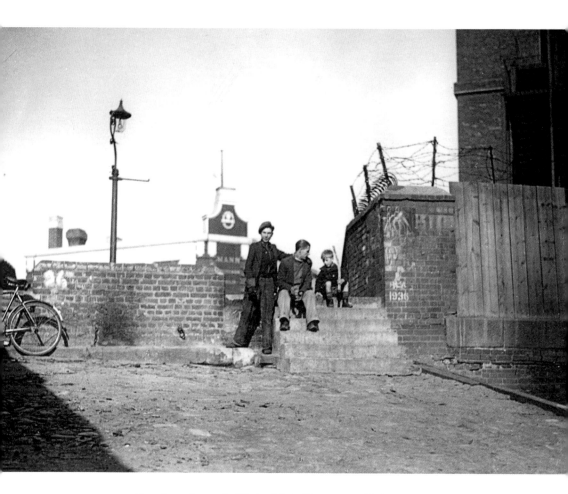

Above: A rare photograph of Blackwall Stairs (the entrance to Blackwall Way, c.1938).

A hospital confinement had to be booked in advance by the expectant mother concerned through her doctor. I was not at all sure that Molly would do this; she seemed too slovenly and apathetic to bother about anything. If she won't go to antenatal clinic, she won't bother to change the arrangements for delivery, I thought, and I could imagine a midnight call to Nonnatus House in two or three weeks' time to which we would have to respond. I resolved to see her mother, and report to her doctor.

The Canada Buildings, named Ontario, Baffin, Hudson, Ottawa and so on, were six blocks of densely populated tenements lying between Blackwall Tunnel and Blackwall Stairs. They were about six storeys high, and very primitive, with a tap and a lavatory at the end of each balcony. It was beyond me how anyone could live there, and maintain cleanliness or self-respect. It was said that there five thousand people living in the Canada Buildings.

I found her mother Marjorie's address in the Ontario Buildings, and knocked. A cheery voice called "Come on in luvvy". The usual invitation of an East Ender, whoever you were. The door was unlocked, so I stepped straight into the main room. Marjorie turned round as I entered with a bright smile. The smile vanished as soon as she saw me and her hands dropped to her sides.

"Oh no. No. Not again. You've come about our Moll, 'aven't you?" She sat down on a chair, buried her face in her hands, and sobbed.

I was embarrassed. I didn't know what to do or say. Some people are good at dealing with the problems of others, but not me. In fact, the more emotional people get, the less I am able to cope. I put my bag on a chair and sat down beside her, saying nothing. It gave me the chance to look around the room.

Having seen Molly's squalor, I had expected to see her mother's place in the same sort of condition, but nothing could have been more dissimilar. The room was clean and tidy, and smelt nice. Pretty curtains hung at clean windows. The mats were clean, well brushed and shaken. A kettle was bubbling on the gas stove. Marjorie was wearing a clean dress and pinafore, her hair was brushed and looked nice.

The kettle gave me an idea, and as the sobs lessened I said, "How about making a nice cup of tea for us both? I'm parched."

She brightened up and said, with typical cockney courtesy, "Sorry nurse. Don't mind me. I gets that worked up about Moll, I do."

She got up and made the tea. The activity helped her, and she sniffed away the tears. Over the next twenty minutes, it all came out, her hopes and her heartache.

Molly was the last of five children. She had never known her father, who had been killed at Arnhem during the war. The whole family had been evacuated to Gloucestershire.

Marjorie said, "I don't know if that upset her, or what, but the others turned out all right, they did."

Overleaf. In the early 20th century, many East End families lived in slums, in very poor conditions, struggling to make ends meet (c.1912).

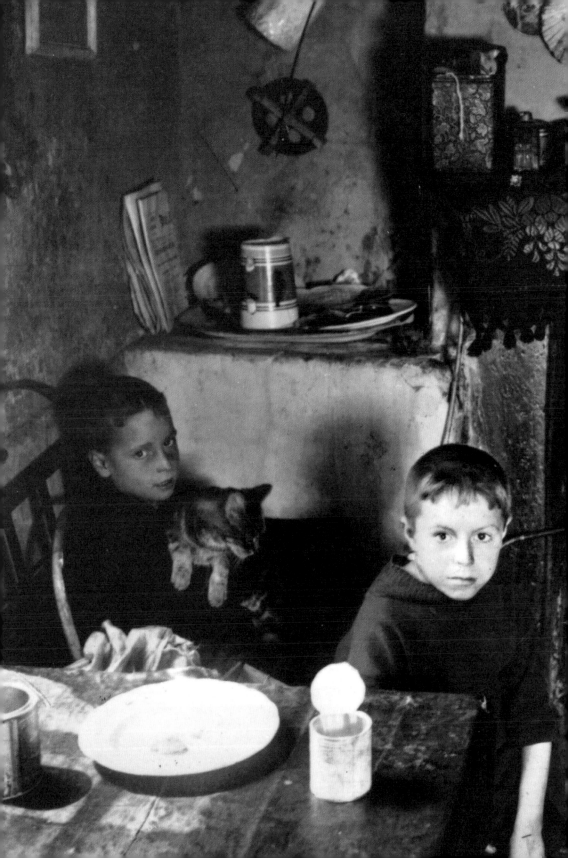

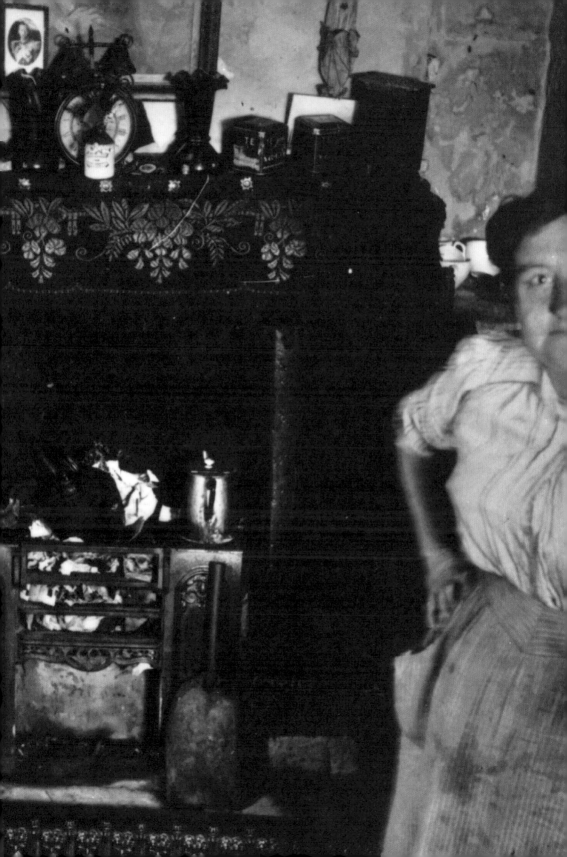

The family returned to London, and settled in Ontario Buildings. Molly seemed to adapt to the new surroundings and her new school, and was reported to be doing well.

"She was that bright," Marjorie said. "Always top o' the class. She could've been a secitary an' worked in an orfice up West, she could. Oh, it breaks my heart, it do, when I thinks on it."

She sniffed and pulled out her handkerchief. "She was about fourteen when she met that turd. His name's Richard, an' I calls 'im Richard the Turd." She giggled at her little joke. "Then she was stopping out late, saying she was down the Youth Club, but I reckoned as how she was telling me lies, so I asks the Rector, an' he tells me Moll wasn't even a member. Then she was stoppin' out all night. Oh, nurse, you can't even know what that does to a mother."

Quiet sobs came from the neat little figure in the flowered apron.

"Night after night I walked the streets, looking for 'er, but I never found 'er. 'Course I never. She'd come home in the morning, an' tell me a pack of lies, as though I was daft, an' go off to school. When she was sixteen, she said she was going to marry her Dick. I reckoned as how she was pregnant anyhow, so I says, 'That's the best thing you can do, my luvvy.'"

They married, and took two rooms in Baffin Buildings. From the start, Molly never did any housework. Marjorie went in and tried to show her daughter how to keep her rooms clean and tidy, but it was no use. The next time she went, the place was as dirty as ever.

"I don't know where she gets her lazy ways from," Marjorie said.

At first Dick and Molly seemed fairly happy, and although Dick did not appear to be in any regular job, Marjorie hoped for the best for her daughter. Their first baby was born, and Molly seemed happy, but quite soon, things began to get worse. Marjorie noticed bruises on her daughter's neck and arms, a cut above her eye, a limp on one occasion. Each time Molly said she had fallen down. Marjorie began to have her suspicions, but relations between her and Dick, never cordial, were breaking down.

"He hates me," she said "and won't never let me come near her or the boys. There's not nuffink I can do. I don't know what's worse, knowing he hits me daughter, or knowing he hits the kids. The best time was when he done six months inside. Then I knew as how they was safe."

She started crying again, and I asked her if social services could do anything to help.

"No, no. She won't say a word against him, she won't. He's got such a hold on her, I don't think she's got a mind of her own any more."

I felt deeply sorry for this poor woman, and her silly daughter. But most of all I felt sorry for the two little boys, whom I had seen in a pitiful state on the occasion when I had interrupted a fight. And now a third child was coming.

I said, "My main reason for coming to see you is about the new baby. Molly is booked for a home confinement, but that, I believe, is only because you had cleaned the place up before our assessment." She nodded. "We think now that a hospital delivery would be best, but she has got to book it, and she must go to antenatal clinics. I don't think she will do either. Can you help?"

Majorie burst into tears again. "I'll do anything in the world for her and the kiddies, but the Turd, he won't let me go near them. What can I do?"

She bit her fingernails and blew her nose.

It was a tricky situation. I thought perhaps we would simply have to refuse a home delivery, and inform the doctors. Molly would then be told that she must go into hospital when labour started. If she refused antenatal treatment, that would be entirely her own fault.

I left poor Marjorie to her sad thoughts, and reported back to the Sisters. A hospital confinement was in fact arranged without Molly's active consent, and I thought that would be the last we heard of her.

It was not to be. About three weeks later the Midwives received a phone call from Poplar Hospital asking if we could arrange post-natal visits for Molly, who had discharged herself and the baby on the third day after delivery.

This was almost unprecedented. In those days it was accepted by everyone, medical and lay people alike, that a new mother should stay in bed for two weeks. Apparently Molly had walked home, carrying the baby and this was considered to be very dangerous. Sister Bernadette went straight round to Baffin Buildings.

She reported back that Molly was there, looking a good deal cleaner, but as sullen as ever. Dick was not at home. He was supposed to have been looking after the children whilst Molly was in hospital, but whether he had or not was anyone's guess. Majorie had offered to take care of them, but Dick had refused, saying they were his kids, and he wasn't going to let that interfering old bag poke her nose into his family.

There had been no food in the flat. Perhaps Molly had anticipated this, and that was why she'd discharged herself. She had no money on her, but on the way home with the baby, had called in the cooked meat shop, and begged a couple of meat pies on tick. As the butcher knew and respected her mother, he let Molly have them. The two little boys, dressed only in filthy jumpers, were sitting on the floor devouring the pies ravenously when Sister Bernadette had arrived.

Molly hardly spoke, Sister told us. She had submitted to being examined, and the baby, a little girl, to examination, but remained morosely silent all the while. Sister had said she was going to tell Marjorie that her daughter was home.

"Please yerself," was all the reply she got.

Marjorie had had no idea of the turn of events, and ran round to Baffin Buildings straight away. Unfortunately Dick chose the same moment to return, and they met on the landing. He lunged at her drunkenly, and Marjorie ducked. Had he hit her, she would have fallen down the stone staircase. After that, all the poor woman dared to do was to buy food and leave it on the landing outside her daughter's door.

Our custom was to visit twice a day for fourteen days after delivery. Molly and baby were satisfactory, from a purely medical point of view, but the domestic situation was as bad as ever. Sometimes Dick was at home, sometimes not. Poor Marjorie was never seen there. She would have made all the difference in the world to Molly and the little boys. Her cheerfulness alone would have lightened the atmosphere, but she was never allowed in. She had to content herself with coming round to Nonnatus House to ask the Sisters how her daughter and grandchildren were getting on. One day she gave us a bag of baby clothes to take on our next visit. She said she didn't like to leave them on the landing, in case they got damp.

Over the next few days several nurses visited Molly, all reporting the same disquieting condition. One nurse said that she was very nearly sick in the room, and had to rush outside into the fresh air in order to control her stomach. On the eighth evening I called, and there was no reply to my knock. The door was locked, so I knocked again – no response. I thought Molly might be busy with the baby and unable to answer. As it was only 5 p.m., I continued my visits, intending to return later.

It was about 8 p.m. when I got back to Baffin Buildings. I was tired, and it seemed a long climb up to the fifth floor. I was almost tempted to skip it.

After all, Molly and baby were medically satisfactory, which was our remit. But something prompted me not to miss this visit, so I wearily climbed the stairs.

I knocked, and there was no reply again. I knocked again, louder – she can't still be busy, I thought. A door opened just down the balcony, and a woman appeared.

"She's out," she said, her fag drooping off her lower lip.

"Out! You can't mean it. She's only just had a baby."

"Well, she's out, I tells yer. Saw 'er go, I did. Tarted up an' all, she was."

"Well where's she gone to?" It flashed through my mind that she had gone to her mother's. "Has she taken the three children?"

The woman uttered a shriek of laughter, and the fag dropped to the floor. She stooped to pick it up, and her hair curlers clacked together as she bent.

"What! Three kids! You must be joking. Three kids wouldn't do her much good, would it now?"

I didn't like the woman. There was something about the knowing way she grinned at me that was most unpleasant. I turned my back on her, knocked again, and called through the letterbox. "Would you let me in, please, it's the nurse."

There was definitely a movement inside, I heard it quite distinctly. Self-conscious, because I knew that woman was sneering at me, I kneeled down and looked through the letterbox.

Two eyes, close to mine, met my gaze. They were a child's eyes, and they stared at me unblinking for about ten seconds, then vanished. This enabled me to see into the room.

A faint greenish-blue light came from an unguarded paraffin stove. A pram stood nearby, in which I presumed the baby was sleeping. I saw one little boy running across the room. The other was sitting in a corner.

I caught my breath sharply. The woman must have heard it. She said, "Well, do you believe me now? I told you she was out, din't I?"

I felt I must take this woman into my confidence. She might be able to help. "We can't leave the three children alone with that paraffin heater. If one of them knocks it over, they will be burned to death. If Molly's out, where's the father?"

The woman drew closer. She clearly enjoyed being the bearer of bad news. "He's a bad lot, that Dick, he is. You mark my words. You don't wants to 'ave nuffink to do with 'im. He's no good to her, and she's no better than she should be. Oh, it's a shame, I says to our Bette, it's a shame, I says. Them poor little kids. They didn't ask to be born, did they, now? I always says it's a ..."

I cut her short. "That paraffin heater is a death-trap. I'm going to inform the police. We've got to get in there."

Her eyes gleamed, and she sucked her teeth. She clutched my arm and said: "You going to call the police, then? Cor!"

She dashed off down the balcony and knocked on another door. I imagined her bearing the news all around Baffin Buildings, even if it took her the entire night. Tiredness had left me, and I sped down the stairs to street level, and just about ran to the nearest phone box. The police listened with concern to my story and said they would come at once. Marjorie had to be informed, I decided, so my next call was Ontario Buildings.

Poor woman. When I told her she crumpled, as though I had hit her in the stomach.

"Oh no, I can't bear any more," she moaned. "I guessed as much. She's gone on the game, then."

So innocent was I, that I didn't know what she meant.

"What game?" I said, thinking she meant darts or billiards or gambling in a local pub.

Marjorie looked at me compassionately. "Never you mind, ducky. You don't need to know about that sort of thing. I must go and see after them kiddies."

We went together in silence. The police were already at the door working on the lock. I had thought that they would bring a locksmith with them, but no – most policemen are expert at picking locks. Do they learn it in College? I wondered.

A crowd had gathered on the balcony. No one wanted to miss a thing. Marjorie stepped forward saying that she was the grandmother, and when the door was opened she was the first to enter. The police and I followed.

The room was suffocatingly hot, and the stench putrid. The children were not to be seen, apart from the baby, who was blissfully asleep. I went over to her, and she looked surprisingly well cared for, clean and well fed. The rest of the room was indescribable. It was full of flies to begin with, and a heap of excrement and dirty nappies in a corner was crawling with maggots.

Marjorie went into the bedroom, gently calling the boys' names. They were behind the chair. She took them in her arms, tears streaming down her face.

"Never mind, my luvvies. Nanna's got you."

The police were taking notes, and I thought perhaps I should leave, as the grandmother would now take charge. But at that moment, there was a commotion outside, and Dick appeared in the doorway. Obviously he had not known that the police were in his flat. As soon as he saw them he turned to run, but his path was barred by the onlookers. They had let him in, but they were not going to let him out again. Perhaps there were several scores to be settled between Dick and his neighbours. He was told that he would be cautioned about the neglect of three children under the age of five.

He swore, spat, and said, "What's wrong with 'em? Kids are all right. Nothing wrong, far as I can see."

"It's a very good thing for you that there is nothing wrong. Leaving them alone with a paraffin heater alight and unguarded would have caused a fire if one of the children had knocked it over."

Dick started to whine. "That's not my fault. I didn't put the heater on. The missus did. I didn't know she'd gone out and left it. The lazy slut. I'll give her what for when I sees her."

The policeman said: "Where is your wife?"

"'Ow should I know?"

Marjorie shouted at him. "Yer villain. Yer know where she is. An' you made her go, didn't you. Yer swine."

Dick was all innocence. "What's the old cow on about now?"

Marjorie was about to scream a reply, but the policeman stopped her. "You can settle your differences when we have gone. We have put it on record that you have been cautioned about leaving your children unattended, and in a dangerous situation. If it occurs again, you will be charged."

Dick was all wheedling charm. "You can take it from me, this will not occur again, officer. I apologise, and will see it never happens again."

The police prepared to leave. Dick said, pointing to Marjorie, "And you can take her with you, and all."

She gave an anguished cry, and held the two little boys closer to her. She appealed to the policemen, "I can't leave them here, the baby, the boys. Can't you see? I can't leave them like this."

Dick said in a soothing, cheery voice, "Don't you worry, old lady. I can look after me kids. There's nuffink to worry about." Then, to the policeman: "Yer can leave 'em safe wiv me. You got my word for it."

Neither of the policemen were fools and they were not taken in for a moment by this display of paternal devotion. But they had no power to do anything but caution him.

One of them turned to Marjorie, "You can only stay here if you are invited, and you certainly cannot take the children away without the father's consent."

Dick was triumphant. "You heard. You've got to have the father's consent. And I'm the father, and I don't consent, see? Now get out."

I spoke for the first time. "Well what about the baby? She is only eight days old, and she is being breastfed. She will wake up hungry soon. Where is Molly?"

I don't think he had noticed me before. He turned, and ogled me up and down. I almost felt him undressing me with his eyes. He was a nauseating specimen, but no doubt he thought he was God's gift to women. He came over to me.

"Don't you worry, nursey. My missus will feed her when she gets back. She's just popped out for a minute."

He took my hand in both of his own, and stroked my wrist. I pulled it sharply away. I wanted to smack his leering face, which he was pushing so close to my own, I could smell his foul breath. I turned my head away in disgust. He drew even closer, his eyes gleaming with mocking interest. He dropped his voice so that no one else could hear,

"Hoity-toity eh? I know how to take you down a peg or two, Miss Hoity-Toity."

I knew how to deal with men like that. Height is a great leveller, and we were level. I didn't need to say a word. I turned my head slowly to look him straight in the eyes, and held his gaze. Slowly his smirk faded, and he turned away. Few men can withstand a woman's look of utter contempt.

Marjorie was kneeling on the floor crying uncontrollably, and hugging the two little boys. The policeman went over to her, took her elbow to help her to her feet, and said gently: "Come on mother, you can't stay here."

Marjorie got up, and the children retreated silently towards the chair in the bedroom. She gave a despairing moan, and allowed the policeman to lead her to the door. She stumbled out, a broken woman, looking twenty years older than when she had entered. She was led through the crowd at the door, and there were many sympathetic voices.

"Oh poor soul."

"Oh it's a shame."

"Don' yer jus' feel for 'er, poor soul."

"'e's a bad'un, an' all."

"It's a shame, oi sez."

She was escorted back to Ontario Buildings, and I returned to Nonnatus House, with much to think about that night.

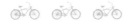

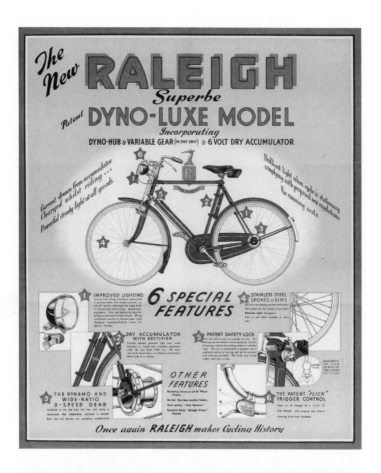

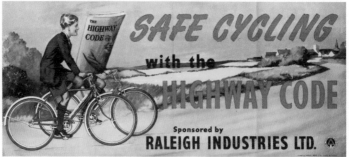

THE BICYCLE

The hidden steel of a Fortescue-Cholmeley-Browne was revealed to us over the next few weeks as Chummy mastered the skills of riding a bicycle. After the accident Sister Julienne was seriously in doubt as to whether it would be possible, but Chummy was adamant. She could and would learn.

Every spare minute of her time was spent practising. All her district work had to be done on foot in the meantime, and this took far longer than it would have taken on a bicycle. Consequently she had less spare time than anyone else. But she utilised each and every minute of freedom. She would push the old Raleigh up Leyland Street, a slight incline, and then free wheel down; up and down hundreds of times until she acquired her balance. She got up a couple of hours early each morning, and went out every evening from about 8 to 10 p.m., coming back exhausted and breathless. "Well, actually, there's no point in just learning to ride in the daylight," she argued gaily, with irrefutable logic.

These rides in the dark were usually accompanied by crowds of cheering or jeering children. This might have been a menace, had Chummy not gained the respect of an older lad who had joined us on the first day when Cynthia, Trixie and I had been trying to teach her. Jack was a particularly tough specimen of about thirteen, accustomed to fighting for his rights. He soon dispersed the little kids; a few blows, a few kicks, and they were gone. Then he presented himself in front of the bicycle, her champion.

"You gets any more trouble from that lot, Miss, jes' call me. Jack. I'll take care of 'em."

"Oh, that's frightfully good of you, Jack. Actually, I'm most awfully grateful. This old machine's a lively little filly, what?"

Chummy's posh voice must have been as incomprehensible to Jack as his Cockney accent was to her, but nevertheless, they struck a friendship then and there.

After that Chummy learned rapidly. Jack was out early and late, running, pushing, helping her in every way. He developed a particularly ingenious way of teaching her to steer the bike and turn corners; he pedalled whilst she steered! Chummy controlled the handlebars, sitting on the saddle, her legs trailing, whilst he stood on the pedals, doing all the hard work. To propel her twelve stone weight must have been hard work, but Jack was no puny thirteen-year-old, and took pride in his manliness. Early and late he could be heard shouting: "Turn left, Miss; NO, LEF', yer dafty. Easy does it. Not too sharp, now. Aim for that phone box, and keep yer eyes on it."

Neither of them saw defeat as a possibility, and within three weeks they were riding all the way from Bow to the Isle of Dogs in the dark November mornings.

Jack did not own a bicycle, and reluctantly he had to admit that the time had come for Chummy to try on her own. He pushed her off, and she pedalled confidently down the street and round the corner. Sadly he waved as she turned out of sight. He had been useful, and now the fun was all over. He kicked a stone, and slouched off homewards, hands in pockets, one foot in the gutter, the other on the kerb.

But Chummy was not one to let a friendship die, still less to allow kindness and help to pass unnoticed. She discussed it with us at lunch, and we agreed that a gift of some sort would be appropriate. Various were the suggestions – a jar of sweets, a football, a penknife – but Chummy was not happy with any of these ideas. Sister Julienne, ever practical and wise, pointed out that the time, effort and commitment on Jack's part had been very great, so therefore her debt to him was great.

Opposite: The cost of a bicycle probably would have been out of the reach of most working-class families and Chummy's present to Jack would have been greatly appreciated.

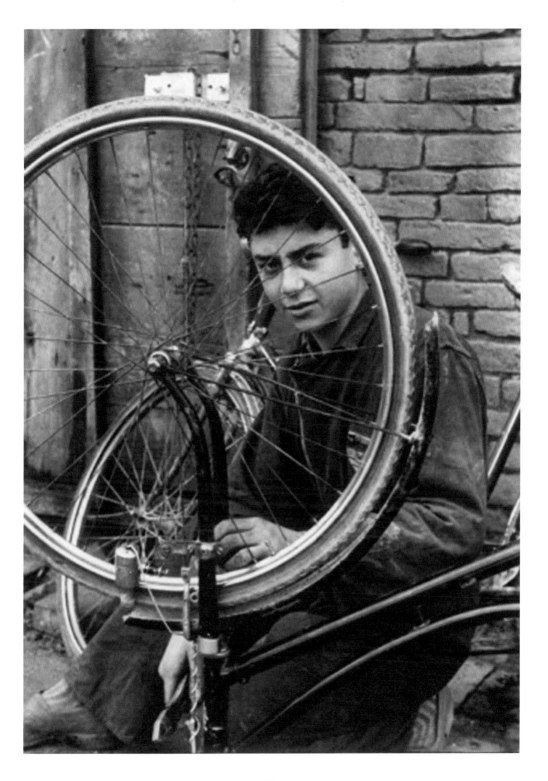

"I don't think the boy should be fobbed off with a trivial token. I feel he should receive something that he really wants and would value. On the other hand, it depends entirely upon what you, the giver, can afford, and only you can know this."

Chummy brightened, and a huge smile lit her features. "Actually, I know what Jack wants more than anything else – a bicycle! And I'm pretty sure Pater would buy one for him if I explained the circumstances, what? He's a sporting old stick, and always coughs up for a good cause. I'll write to him tonight."

Of course Pater coughed up, happy to see his only daughter fulfilled at last. He could no more understand her determination to become a missionary than he could understand her passion for midwifery, but he would support it to the end.

A new bicycle meant a new life for Jack. Very few boys had such a possession in those days. For him, it meant more than status. It meant freedom. He was an adventurous boy, and went miles beyond the East End on his bike. He joined the Dagenham Cycling Club and competed in time trials and road races. He went camping alone in the Essex countryside. He went as far as the coast, and saw the sea for the first time.

Chummy was delighted, and his continued friendship was her greatest joy. He seemed to feel she needed his protection, and so every day after school Jack would turn up at Nonnatus House to escort her on her evening visits. His instinct that the children of the Docks would tease and torment her were right, because on the whole the cockneys did not take to Chummy, and made fun of her behind her back. Her huge size, pedalling steadily along the streets on an ancient solid-wheeled bicycle, brought crowds of children to a standstill, and they lined the pavement shouting things like "what-ho" and "jolly good show, actually" or "steady on, old bean" amid loud-mouthed guffaws. And, to rub salt into the wound, they called her "The Hippo".

Poor Chummy treated it with good humour, but we all knew how deeply it hurt her. But when tough, pugnacious, street-wise Jack was with her, the children kept their distance. We all saw him on different occasions, standing in the street or the tenement courtyards, holding two bicycles, his lower jaw thrust forward, his stocky legs slightly apart, coolly looking around him, confident that a look was all that was needed to to protect "Miss".

Twenty-five years later, a shy young girl called Lady Diana Spencer became engaged to marry Prince Charles, heir to the throne. I saw several film clips of her arriving at various engagements. Each time when the car stopped, the front nearside door would open, and her bodyguard would step out and open the rear door for Lady Diana. Then he would stand, jaw thrust forward, legs slightly apart, and look coolly around him at the crowds, a mature Jack, still practising the skills he had acquired in childhood, looking after his lady.

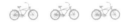

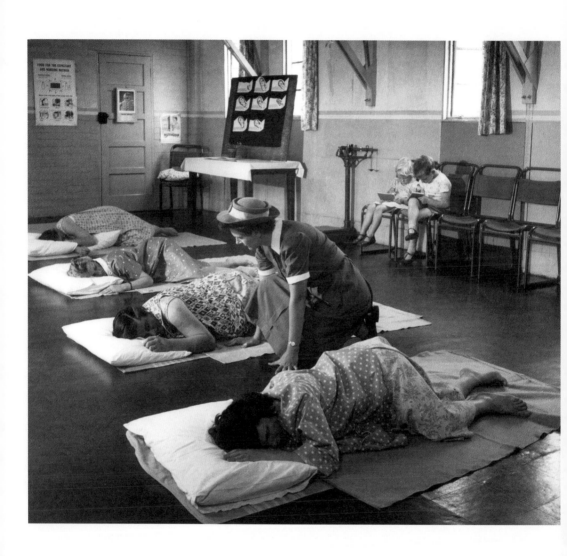

ANTENATAL CLINIC

There must be aspects of every job that are disliked. I did not like antenatal work. In fact I would go so far as to say that I hated antenatal clinic, and dreaded the arrival of each Tuesday afternoon. It was not just the hard work – though that was hard enough. The midwives tried to organise the day-book so that we could finish our morning visits by twelve noon. We had an early lunch, and at one-thirty we started to set up the clinic in order to open the doors at 2 p.m. Then we worked through until we were finished, often as late as 6 or 7 p.m. After that, our evening visits began.

That did not bother me – hard work never did. What really got me, I think, was the sheer concentration of unwashed female flesh, the pulsating warmth and humidity, the endless chatter, and above all the smell. However much I bathed and changed afterwards, it was always a couple of days before I could get rid of the nauseating smells of vaginal discharge, urine, stale sweat, unwashed clothes. It all mingled into a hot, clinging vapour that penetrated my clothes, hair, skin – everything. Many times, during the routine antenatal clinics, I had to go out into the fresh air and lean over the rail by the door, heaving, forcing down the urge to be sick.

Yet we are all different, and I did not meet any other midwife who was affected in this way. If I mentioned it, the reaction was one of genuine surprise. "What smell?" or "Well, perhaps it got a bit hot." So I didn't

Opposite: Midwives often provided vital information to expectant mothers. Here a midwife gives a birthing class.

make any further comments about my own reaction. I had to remind myself continuously of the huge importance of antenatal work, which had contributed so greatly to the drop in maternal deaths. Memory of the history of midwifery, and the endless sufferings of women in childbirth, kept me going when I was thinking, I just cannot bring myself to examine another woman.

Total neglect of women in pregnancy and childbirth had been the norm. Among many primitive societies, women menstruating or with child, or in labour or suckling the child, were regarded as unclean, polluted. The woman was isolated and frequently could not be touched, even by another woman. She had to go through the whole ordeal alone. Consequently only the fittest survived, and by the processes of mutation and adaptation, inherited abnormalities, such as disproportion in the size of the pelvis and the foetal head, died out of the race, particularly in remote parts of the world, and labour became easier.

In Western society, which we call civilisation, this did not occur, and a dozen or more complications, some of them deadly, were superimposed on the natural hazards: overcrowding, staphylococcal and streptococcal infection; infectious diseases such as cholera, scarlet fever, typhoid and tuberculosis; venereal disease; rickets; multiple and frequent childbirth; the dangers from infected water. If you add to all this the attitude of indifference and neglect that often surrounded childbirth it is not hard to understand how childbirth came to be known as "the curse of Eve", and how women could often expect to die in order to bring forth new life.

The Midwives of St Raymund Nonnatus held their clinic in a church hall. The idea today of conducting a full-scale antenatal clinic in a converted old church hall is horrifying, and sanitary inspectors, public health inspectors, every inspector you can think of would be there condemning it. But in the 1950s it was by no means condemned, in fact the nuns were highly praised for the initiative and ingenuity they had shown in the conversion. No structural changes had been made, apart from the installation of a lavatory and running cold water. Hot water was obtained from an Ascot water heater fixed to the wall near the tap.

Heating was provided by a large coke fire in the middle of the hall. It was a black cast iron construction which had to be lit earlier in the morning by Fred, the boilerman. Such coke fires were very common in those days,

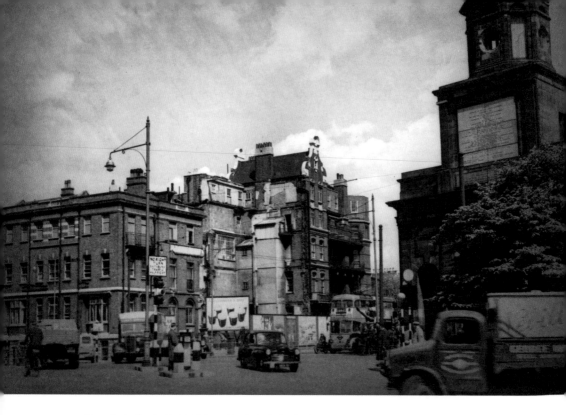

Above: Poplar Hospital (c. 1950). A small underfunded and under-resourced maternity unit operated here from 1948. It relied on the "knowledge, skill and experience of the midwife".

and I have seen them even in hospital wards. (I recall one ward where it was the practice to sterilise our syringes and needles by boiling them in a saucepan placed on the stove). These stoves were very solid, flat topped, and you had to fill them by opening the circular lid and tipping the coke in from a coke-hod. It required quite a bit of muscle power. The stove was situated in the middle of the space, so that heat was radiated all around. The flue went straight up the middle, to the roof.

A few examination couches were available, with movable screens to provide privacy, and wooden desks with chairs, where we wrote up our notes. A long marble-topped surface stood near the sink, upon which we placed our instruments and other equipment. A gas jet stood on this surface, with a box of matches beside it. This single jet of flame was used continuously for boiling up the urine. I can smell it now, more than fifty years later!

The clinic, and those like it all over the country, may sound primitive today but it had saved countless thousands of lives of both mothers and babies. The Midwives' clinic was the only one in the area until 1948, when a small maternity unit of eight beds was opened in Poplar Hospital. Prior to that, the hospital had no maternity unit even though Poplar was said to have a population of fifty thousand people per square mile. When the decision was taken after the war to open a hospital unit, no special provision was made. Quite simply, two small wards were allocated for maternity – one for lying-in, and the other for delivery, doubling-up as an antenatal clinic. This was inadequate, but it was better than nothing at all. Accommodation, equipment, technology, were not really important. What was important was the knowledge, skill and experience of the midwife.

Clinical examination was what I shrank from the most. It can't be as bad as last week, I thought as we prepared to open the doors. I shuddered as I remembered it. Thank God I was wearing gloves, I thought. What would have happened if I had not?

She had been in my mind on and off for the whole of the past week. She had flounced into the clinic at about 6 p.m. in her hair curlers and slippers, a fag hanging from her lower lip, and with her were five children under seven. Her appointment had been for 3 p.m. I was clearing up after a not too stressful afternoon. Two of the other student midwives had left, and the third was still with her last patient. Of the Sisters, only Novice Ruth remained, (a "novice" in the religious life, not in midwifery). She asked me to see Lil Hoskin.

It was Lil's first antenatal visit, even though she had had no periods for five months. This is going to take another half an hour, I sighed to myself as I got out the notes. I scanned through them: thirteenth pregnancy, ten live births; no history of infectious disease; no rheumatic fever or heart disease; no history of tuberculosis; some cystitis but no evidence of nephritis; mastitis after the third and seventh babies, but otherwise all babies breastfed.

Her previous notes gave me most of her obstetric history, but I needed to ask some questions about the present pregnancy.

"Have you had any bleeding?"

"Nope."

"Any vaginal discharge?"

"A bit."

What colour?"

"Mos'ly yellowish."

"Any swelling of the ankles?"

"Nope."

"Any breathlessness?"

"Nope."

"Any vomiting?"

"A bit. Not much though."

"Constipated?"

"Yep, not 'alf!"

"Are you sure you are pregnant? You haven't been examined or tested."

"I should know," she said meaningfully, with a shriek of laughter.

The children by now were rushing around all over the place. The hall, being large and virtually empty, was like a great play area for them. I didn't mind – no healthy child can resist a wide open space, and the urge to run is powerful if you are only five years old. But Lil thought she must exercise some show of authority. She grabbed a passing child by the arm and dragged him to her. She gave him a great blow across the side of the face and ear with a heavy hand, and screamed.

"Shut up and behave yourself, you li'l bleeder. And that goes for the lot of you and all."

The child squealed with pain and the injustice of the blow. He retreated about ten yards from his mother, and screamed and stamped, until he could scarcely breathe. Then he paused, took a deep breath, and started all over again. The other children had stopped running around, and a couple started whimpering. A happy but noisy scene with five little children had been turned in an instant into a battlefield by this stupid woman. I hated her from that moment.

Novice Ruth came up to the child, and tried to comfort him, but he pushed her away, and lay on the floor kicking and screaming. Lil grinned and said to me: "Don't mind him, he'll get over it." Then louder, to the child: "Shu' yer face or yer'll get another."

I couldn't bear it, so to prevent her doing any more harm, I told her that I must examine her urine, gave her a gallipot, and asked her to go into the lavatory to supply a sample for me. After that, I said, I would want to examine her, and would need her undressed below the waist, and lying on one of the couches.

Her slippers slapped across the wooden floor as she went. She came back giggling, and gave me the specimen, then flopped over to one of the couches. I ground my teeth. What has she got to giggle about, I thought. The child was still lying on the floor, but not screaming so much. The other children looked sullen, making no attempt to play.

I went to the work surface to test the urine. The litmus paper turned red, showing normal acidity. The urine was cloudy, and the specific gravity high. I wanted to test for sugar, and lit the gas jet. I half filled a test tube with urine, and added a couple of drops of Fehlings solution, and boiled the contents. No sugar was present. Lastly, I had to test for albumen by refilling the test tube with fresh urine, and boiling the upper half only. It did not turn white or thick, indicating that albumen urea was not present.

This took about five minutes to complete, during which time the child had stopped crying. He was sitting up and Novice Ruth was playing with him with a couple of balls, pushing them back and forth. Her refined, delicate features were offset by her white muslin veil which fell down as she leaned over. The child grabbed it and pulled. The other children laughed. They seemed happy again. No thanks to their rough and brutal mother, I thought as I went over to Lil, who was now lying on the couch.

She was fat, and her flabby skin was dirty and moist with perspiration. A dank, unwashed smell rose from her body. Have I got to touch her? I thought as I approached. I tried to remind myself that she and her husband and all the children probably lived in two or three rooms with no bath, or even hot water, but it did not dispel my feeling of revulsion. Had she not hit her child in that heartless manner, my feelings might have softened towards her.

I put on my surgical gloves, and covered her lower half with a sheet, because I wanted to examine her breasts. I asked her to pull up her jumper. She giggled, and wobbled around, pulling it up. The smell intensified as her armpits were exposed. Two large pendulous breasts flopped down either side of her, prominent veins coursing towards huge, near-black nipples. These veins were a reliable sign of pregnancy. A little fluid could be squeezed from the nipples. Just about diagnostic, I thought. I told her this.

She shrieked with laughter. "Told you so, didn't I?"

I took her blood pressure at that point, and it was fairly high. She will need more rest, I thought, but I doubt if she will get it. The children had recovered their spirits, and were racing about once again.

I pulled her jumper down and uncovered her abdomen, which was large, the skin simply covered with stretch marks. The slightest pressure from my hand showed a fundus above the umbilicus.

"When was your last period?"

"Search me. Las' year, I reckons." She giggled, and her tummy flopped up and down.

"Have you felt any movements yet?"

"Nope."

"I am going to listen for the baby's heart beat."

I reached for the pinard foetal stethoscope. This was a small metal, trumpet-shaped instrument, used by placing the larger end over the abdomen, and then pressing the ear against the flattened smaller end. Normally the steady thud of the heartbeat could be heard quite clearly. I listened at several points, but could hear nothing. I called Novice Ruth, as I felt I needed confirmation, and also an assessment of the duration of pregnancy. She couldn't hear a heartbeat either, but thought that other signs indicated pregnancy. She asked me to do an internal examination to confirm it.

I had been expecting this, and dreading it. I asked Lil to draw her knees upwards and part her legs. As she did so, the odour of stale urine, vaginal discharge, and sweat wafted up to greet me. I struggled to control the nausea. I mustn't be sick, was all I could think of at that moment. Tufts of pubic hair stuck up in clumps, matted together by sticky moisture and dirt. She might have crabs, I thought. Novice Ruth was watching me. Maybe she understood how I was feeling – the nuns were very sensitive, but they spoke little. I dampened a swab with which to clean the moist bluish vulva, and it was whilst I was cleaning her that I noticed that one side was very oedematous, swollen with fluid, whilst the other was not. I started to part the vulva with two fingers, and it was then that my finger encountered a hard, small lump on the oedematous side. I rubbed my finger over it several times. It was easily palpable; hard lumps in soft places make one think of cancer.

I could feel Novice Ruth watching me very closely all the time. I raised my eyes, and looked at her questioningly. She said, "I'll get a pair of gloves. Do not proceed just yet, nurse."

She returned a couple of seconds later, and took my place. She did not say a word until she withdrew her hand, and covered Lil again with the blanket.

"You can put your legs down now, Lil, but stay where you are, please, because we will want to examine you again in a minute. Come with me to the desk, will you, nurse?"

At the desk, which was at the other end of the room, she said to me very quietly: "I think the lump is a syphilitic chancre. I am going to ring Dr Turner straight away and ask him if he can come to examine her while she is still here. If we send her away with instructions to go to a doctor, there is a high chance that she will not go. The spirochaeta pallida of syphilis can cross the placenta and infect the foetus. However, the chancre is the first stage of syphilis, and with early diagnosis and treatment there is a good chance of cure, and the baby will be spared."

I nearly fainted, in fact I remember having to grip the table before I could sit down. I had been touching her – the revolting creature – and her syphilitic chancre. I couldn't speak, but Novice Ruth said to me kindly, "Don't worry. You were wearing gloves. You won't have caught anything."

She left to go to Nonnatus House to ring the doctor. I couldn't move. I sat at the table for a full five minutes, fighting down wave after wave of nausea, and shuddering. The children were playing all around me, perfectly happy. There was no movement from behind the screen, until the low, steady sound of contented snoring penetrated my ears. Lil was asleep.

The doctor arrived about fifteen minutes later, and Novice Ruth asked me to accompany him. I must have looked pale, because she asked, "Are you all right? Will you manage?"

I nodded dumbly. I couldn't say no. After all, I was a trained nurse, accustomed to all sorts of frightful situations. Yet even after five years of hospital work – casualty, theatre, cancer patients, amputations, dying, death – nothing and no one had caused such profound revulsion in me as that woman Lil.

The doctor examined her and took a scrape of tissue from the chancre for the pathology lab. He also took a sample of blood for a Wassermann's test. Then he said to Lil, "I think you have a very early infection of venereal disease. We …"

Before he had finished speaking she gave a great baying laugh. "Oh Gawd! Not again! That's a laugh, that is!"

The doctor's face was stony. He said, "We have caught it early. I am going to give you penicillin now, and you must have another injection each day for ten days. We must protect your baby."

"Please yourself," she giggled, "I'm easy," and winked at him.

His face was expressionless as he drew up a massive dose of penicillin and injected it into her thigh. We left her to get dressed, and went over to the desk.

"We will get the results from pathology on the blood and serum," he said to Novice Ruth, "but I don't think there is any doubt about diagnosis. Would you Sisters arrange to visit daily for the injections? I think if we ask her to come to surgery she won't bother, or will forget. If the foetus is still alive, we must do our best."

It was well after seven o'clock. Lil was dressed, and yelling to the children to come with her. She lit another fag, and called out gaily, "Well, tara all."

She looked knowingly at Novice Ruth, and said, with a leer – "Be good" – and shrieked with laughter.

I told her that we would call each day to give her another injection. "Please yerself," she said with a shrug, and left.

I still had all my cleaning up to do. I felt so tired my legs could hardly move. The moral and emotional shock must have contributed to the fatigue.

Novice Ruth grinned at me kindly. "You have to get used to all sorts in this life. Now, do you have any evening visits?"

I nodded. "Three post-natal. One of them up in Bow."

"Then you go and do them. I will clean up here."

As I left the clinic, I thanked her from the bottom of my heart. The fresh air revived me, and the cycle ride dispelled my fatigue.

The following morning, when I looked at the day book, I saw that I had to administer the penicillin injection to Lil Hoskin, Peabody Buildings. I groaned inwardly. I had known it would have to be me. The instruction was that it should be my last call before lunch, and that the syringe and needle should be kept separate from the midwifery case, also, that I should wear gloves. I didn't need telling.

The Peabody Buildings in Stepney were notorious. They had been condemned for demolition about fifteen years before, but were still standing and still housing families. They were the worst type of tenements, because the only water came from a single tap at the end of each balcony, where the only lavatory was situated. There were no facilities in the flats. My attitude towards Lil softened. Perhaps I would be like her if I had to live in such conditions.

The door was open, but I knocked.

"Come on in, luvvy. I'm expecting you. I've got some water ready for you."

How kind. She must have gone to a lot of trouble to get water and heat it up. The flat was filthy and stinking. Hardly a square inch of floor space

Overleaf: Poverty and inadequate housing resulted in some families living in shocking conditions in the 1950s. Jennifer considered many of the women she came across "heroines". Despite their circumstances, they didn't complain and managed to keep their families together and themselves and their children happy.

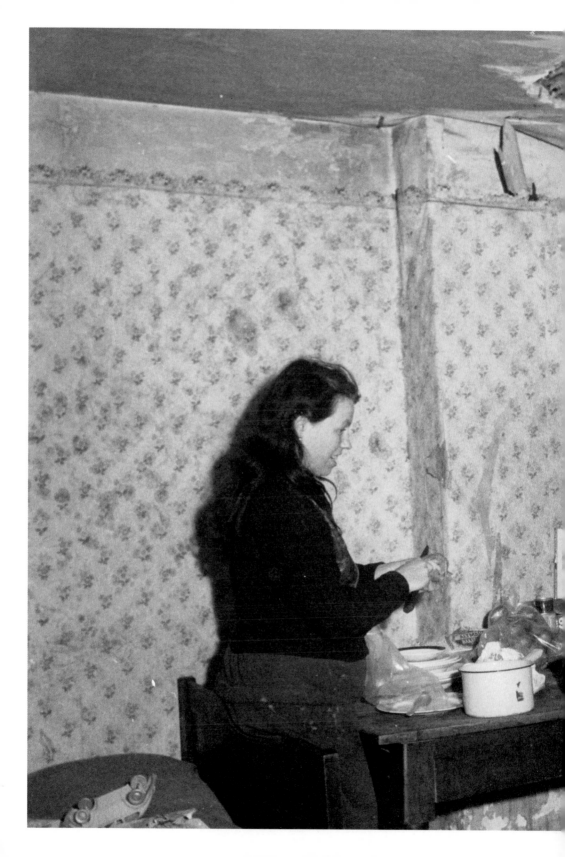

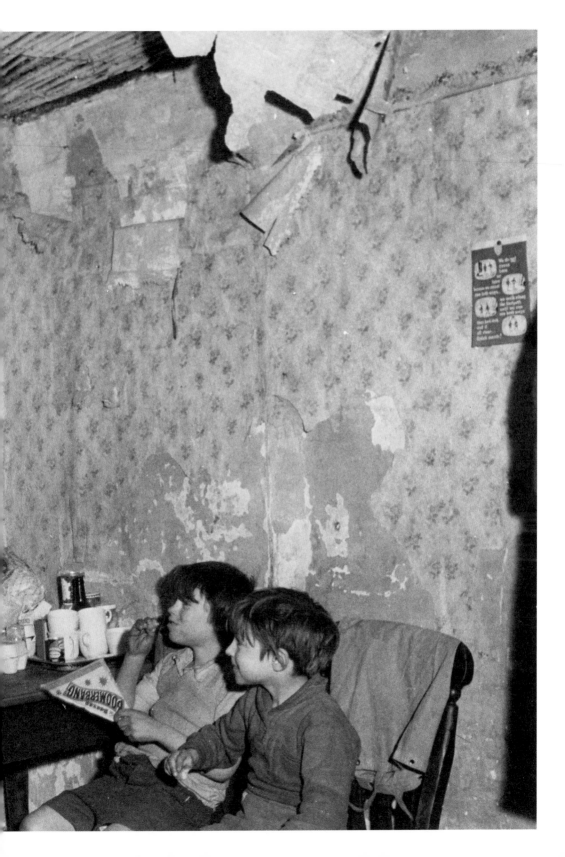

could be seen, and small children, naked from the waist down, tumbled around all over the place.

Lil seemed different in her own surroundings. Maybe the clinic had intimidated her in some way, so that she had felt the need to assert herself by showing off. She did not seem so loud and brash in her own home. The irritating giggle, I realised, was no more than constant and irrepressible good humour. She pushed the children around, but not unkindly.

"Get out of it, yer li'l bleeder. The nurse can't get in." She turned to me. "Here you are. You can put your things down here."

She had gone to the trouble of clearing a small space on the table, and had put a washing bowl beside it, with soap and a grubby towel.

"Thought you'd need a nice, clean towel, eh ducky?"

Everything is relative.

I put my bag on the table, but took out only the syringe, needle, ampoule, gloves and cotton swab soaked in spirit. The children were fascinated.

"Get back, or I'll clip your ear," Lil said gaily. Then to me, "Do you wants me leg or me arse?"

"Doesn't matter. Whichever you prefer."

She lifted her skirts and bent over. The huge round backside looked like a positive affirmation of solidarity. The children gawped, and crowded in closer. With a shrill scream of laughter Lil kicked backwards, like a horse.

"Garn. Ain't you seen this before?"

She roared with laughter, and the bottom wobbled so much it was impossible to inject it.

"Look, hold on to the chair and keep still for a second, will you?" I was laughing now.

She did, and the injection was over in less than a minute. I rubbed the area hard to disperse the fluid, as it was a large dose. I put everything into a brown paper bag to keep it separate. Then I washed my hands and dried them on her towel, just to please her. We carried our own towel, but I thought that to use it would be a conspicuous snub.

She came to the door with me, and out onto the balcony, all the children following. "See you tomorrow, then. I'll look forward to yer comin. I'll 'ave a nice cup of tea for yer."

I cycled off with much to think about. In her own surroundings, Lil was not a disgusting old bag, she was a heroine. She kept the family together, in appalling conditions, and the children looked happy. She was cheerful and uncomplaining. How she had come to pick up syphilis was none of my business. I was there to treat the condition, not to judge.

The next day when I called, I was so pre-occupied with wondering how I could decline the offer of a cup of tea, that when the door opened, I stood staring awkwardly, stupidly, at Lil, who was not Lil. She looked a bit shorter and fatter, the same slippers, the same hair curlers, the same fag – but different.

A familiar screech of laughter revealed toothless gums. She poked me in the stomach. "Yer thinks I'm Lil, don' yer? They all thinks that. I'm 'er mum. We looks like two peas, we does. Lil's had a mis an' gorn to 'ospital. Good riddance, I sez. She's got enough with ten o' them, an' him in an' out all the time."

A few questions elicited the facts. Lil had felt ill shortly after I had left the previous day, and was later sick. She had lain down on the bed, and sent one of the children to fetch Gran. Contractions had started, and she was sick again. Then she must have become unconscious.

Gran said to me, "I'll cope with a mis any time, but not a dead woman. No, sir."

She'd called a doctor, and Lil was taken straight to The London Hospital. We later learned that a macerated foetus was extracted. It had probably been dead for three or four days.

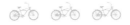

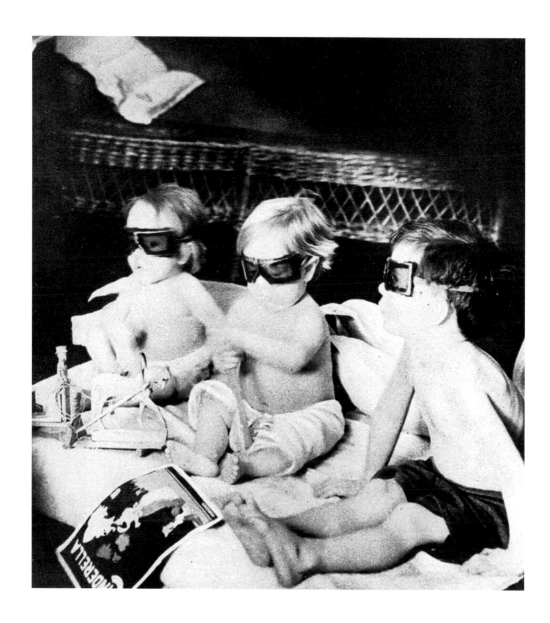

RICKETS

It is hard to imagine today that until the last century no woman had any specialist obstetric care during pregnancy. The first time a woman would see a doctor or midwife was when she went into labour. Therefore, death and disaster, either for mother or child, or both, were commonplace. Such tragedies were looked upon as the will of God, whereas, in fact, they were the inevitable result of neglect and ignorance. Society ladies would have a doctor visiting them during pregnancy, but such visits were not antenatal care and would probably be more like social calls than anything else, because no doctor was trained in antenatal care.

The pioneer in this branch of obstetrics was a Dr J. W. Ballantyne of Edinburgh University. (Indeed some of the greatest discoveries and advances made in medicine seem to come from Edinburgh.) Ballantyne wrote a paper in 1900 deploring the abysmal state of antenatal pathology, and urging that a pre-maternity hospital was necessary. An anonymous gift of £1,000 allowed the first ever bed for antenatal care to be inaugurated, in 1901, at the Simpson Memorial Hospital. (Simpson, another Scot, developed anaesthetics.)

This was the first such bed in the civilised world. It is an incredible thought. Medicine was developing rapidly. The staphylococcus had been isolated; so had the tuberculous bacillus. The heart and circulation were understood. The functions of liver, kidneys, and lungs had been ascertained. Anaesthetics and surgery were advancing apace. But no one, it seems, thought that pre-maternity care might be necessary for the life and safety of a pregnant woman and her child.

It was ten years later, in 1911, before the first antenatal clinic was opened in Boston, USA. Another opened in Sydney, Australia, in 1912. Dr Ballantyne had to wait until 1915, fifteen years after his seminal paper, before he saw an antenatal clinic open in Edinburgh. He, and other far-sighted obstetricians, were faced with bitter opposition from colleagues and politicians who regarded antenatal care as a needless expenditure of public money and medical time.

At the same time the struggle by visionary and dedicated women was in progress to gain properly regulated training in the art of midwifery. If Dr Ballantyne was having a hard time, these women found it harder. You have to imagine what it was like to be on the receiving end of vicious antagonism: sneering, contempt, ridicule, slights about one's intelligence, integrity and motives.

In those days, women even ran the risk of dismissal for their opinions. And this treatment came from other women, as well as men. In fact, "in-fighting" between various schools of nurses who had some sort of training in midwifery was particularly nasty. One eminent lady – the matron of St Bartholomew's Hospital – branded the aspiring midwives as "anachronisms, who would in the future be regarded as historical curiosities".

The medical opposition seems to have arisen mainly from the fact that "women are striving to interfere too much in every department of life".* Obstetricians also doubted the female intellectual capacity to grasp the anatomy and physiology of childbirth, and suggested that they could not therefore be trained. But the root fear was – guess what? – you've got it, but no prizes for quickness: money. Most doctors charged a routine one guinea for a delivery. The word got around that trained midwives would undercut them by delivering babies for half a guinea! The knives were out.

In the 1860s the Council of Obstetrics estimated that, out of around 1,250,000 births annually in Britain, about 10 per cent were attended by a doctor. Some researchers put the figure as low as 3 per cent. Therefore, all

---

* From *Behind the Blue Door in A History of the Royal College of Midwives*, Hansard, p. 23. This is a quote from the proposed Bill for the Registration of Midwives, 1890, from a speech made by Charles Bradlaugh MP.

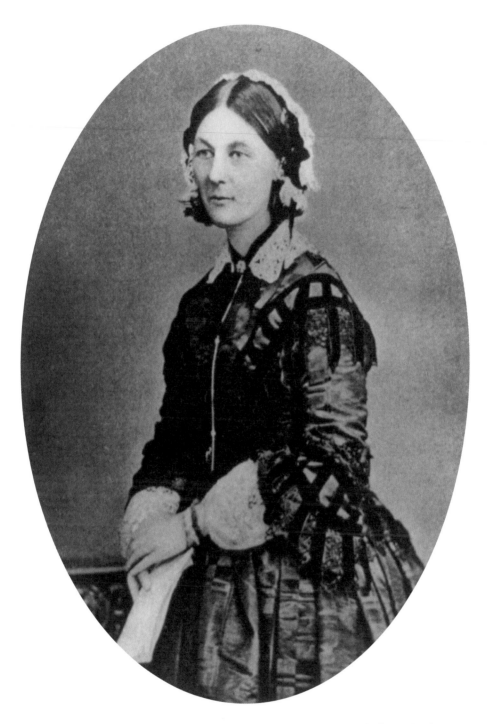

Above: Florence Nightingale was among the people who criticised the lack of training for midwives in England, calling it little more than "women-slaughter to practise as we do".

the rest – well over one million women annually – were attended by women with no training, or by no one at all, other than a friend or relative.

In the 1870s Florence Nightingale wrote *Notes on Lying-in Infirmaries*, drawing attention to "the utter absence of any *means* of training in any existing institution", saying "it is a farce or mockery to call women who attend childbirth, midwives. In France, Germany, and even Russia they consider it woman-slaughter to practice as we do. In these countries everything is regulated by Government – with us, by private enterprise." The guinea earned by doctors for a delivery was a significant part of their income. The threat of being undercut by trained midwives had to be resisted. The fact that thousands of women and babies were dying annually for want of proper attention did not come into it.

However, the courageous, hard-working, dedicated women eventually won. In 1902 the Midwives Act was passed, and in 1903 the Central Midwives Board issued their first certificate to a trained midwife. Fifty years later I was proud to be a successor of these wonderful women, and to be able to offer my trained skills to the long-suffering, cheerful, resilient women of the London Docklands.

At the church hall, the antenatal clinic had been set up again. It was mid-winter, and the coke-stove was burning fiercely. It was well guarded on all four sides for the protection of the numerous little children running around. Lil had been in my mind on and off during the past fortnight – a curious mixture of revulsion and admiration. Whilst I admired the way she coped, I hoped I would not have to meet her again, at least not in the intimate patient/midwife relationship.

The pile of notes on the desk told me it would be a busy afternoon – no time to brood about Lil and her syphilis. There were seven piles of notes, with about ten folders in each pile. Another seven o'clock finish, if we were lucky.

I glanced at the top of the first pile, and saw the name Brenda, a woman of forty-six with rickets. She would be admitted to hospital for a Caesarean, and she was booked with the London Hospital in Whitechapel, but we were looking after her antenatally. At that moment she hobbled in, punctual to the minute for her two o'clock appointment. As I was at the desk, and the other staff were not available, I took her for examination and check-up.

Opposite: The terrible body deformation caused by rickets (c.1870).

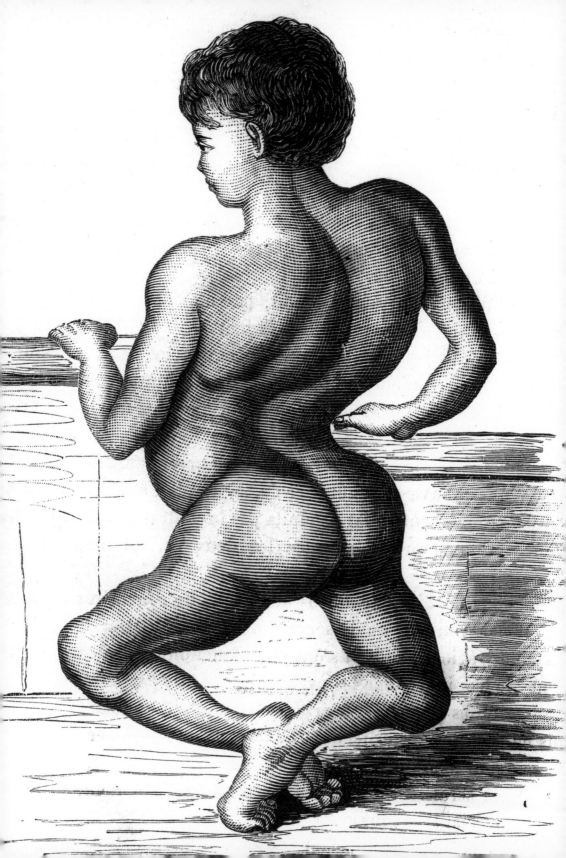

My heart went out to little Brenda. Rickets showed itself in malformation of the bones. For centuries it was not known what caused the condition. It was thought, perhaps, to be inherited. The child was thought to be "puny" or "sickly" or even just lazy, as rachitic children always stand and walk very late. The bones are shortened and thickened at the ends, and bend under pressure. The spine is deformed, as many vertebrae are crushed. The sternum is bent, and therefore the ribcage is barrelled and frequently twisted in shape. The head is large and square shaped, with a jutting, flattened lower jaw. Frequently, the teeth drop out. As if these deformities were not enough, rachitic children always had a lower immunity to infection, and bronchitis, pneumonia and gastro-enteritis constantly occurred.

The condition was common throughout Northern Europe, especially in cities, and no one knew what caused it, until in the 1930s it was found to be due to the simplest of causes: a lack of Vitamin D in the diet causing deficiency of calcium in the bone.

Such a simple reason for so much suffering! Vitamin D is found abundantly in milk,meat, eggs and especially in meat fat and fish oils. You would think most children would have had an adequate diet of these items, wouldn't you? But no, not poor children from deprived backgrounds. Vitamin D can also be made spontaneously in the body by the effect of ultra-violet rays on the skin. You might think there should be enough sun in Northern Europe to balance things. But no, the sun was not for poor children in industrial cities where the density of buildings virtually blocked out the natural light, and where children had to work long hours in factories and workshops or workhouses.

So these children grew up crippled. All the bones of their bodies were deformed, and the long bones of the legs buckled and bent under the weight of the upper body. During adolescence, when growing ceased, the bones ossified into that position.

Even today, in the twenty-first century, you can still see a few very old people hobbling around who are very short, with legs that bow outwards. These are the brave survivors who have spent a lifetime struggling to overcome the effects of the poverty and deprivation of childhood nearly a century ago.

Brenda beamed at me. Her strange face, with an oddly shaped lower jaw, was alight with eager anticipation. She knew she would have to have a

Caesarean section, but that did not bother her. She was going to have a baby, and this time it would live. That was all that mattered to her, and she was intensely grateful to the Sisters, the hospital, the doctors – everyone – but above all to the National Health Service, and the wonderful people who had arranged that everything should be free, that she wouldn't have to pay.

Brenda's obstetric history was tragic. She had married young, and in the 1930s had had four pregnancies. Every baby had died. The tragedy for a woman with rickets is that, along with all the other bones, the pelvis is also deformed, and a flat, or rachitic pelvis develops. The baby therefore cannot be delivered, or at any rate can only be delivered with great difficulty. Brenda had had four long, obstructed labours, and each time the baby had died. She was lucky not to have died herself, as countless numbers of women did in earlier decades all over Europe.

The incidence of rickets had always been slightly higher among little girls than among boys. The reason for this was probably social, and not physiological. Poor mothers of large families tended often (and still do!) to favour the sons, so the boys got more food. Boys have always been more mobile, and go outside to play more.

In Poplar, it was always the boys who were down at the water's edge, or in the wharfs or the bomb sites. So they were getting sunlight on their bodies, whilst their sisters were kept at home. Also, many holiday projects were organised by socially aware philanthropists. Summer camps, which took poor boys to the country for a month under canvas, were quite common, and these camps were lifesavers for thousands of boys. But I have yet to hear of summer camps for girls one hundred years ago. Perhaps it was not considered suitable to take girls away from home and put them under canvas. Or perhaps the needs of girls were simply overlooked. Anyway, one way or another, they missed out. The life-giving sun was withheld from them each summer, and rickety little girls grew up to become deformed women who could conceive and carry a child for nine months, but could not deliver the baby.

It will never be known how many women died of exhaustion in the agony of obstructed labour: the poor were expendable, and their numbers not counted. Where was it I had read, in some ancient manual for the *Instruction of Women attending the Lying-in*: "If a woman is in labour for more than ten or twelve days, you should seek a doctor's aid"? Ten or twelve days of obstructed labour, in the hands of an untrained woman! Dear heaven – was there no mercy, no understanding? I had to shut such agonising thoughts out of my mind, and quietly thank God that obstetric practice had moved on. Yet even in my training days, the most up-to-date textbooks taught that a woman with a rachitic pelvis should have a "trial labour of eight to twelve hours to test the endurance of both mother and foetus".

Brenda had been subjected to four such trial labours in the 1930s. Why on earth, after the first disaster, it had not been agreed that she should have a Caesarean section for the delivery of subsequent babies, I could not imagine. Possibly she could not afford to pay for it, because, before 1948, all medical treatment had to be paid for.

Brenda's husband had been killed on active service in the war in 1940, so she had not had any more pregnancies. However, at the age of forty-three she had married again, and now she was pregnant once more.

Her joy and excitement at the prospect of a living baby seemed to fill the antenatal clinic, and throw everything else into shadow. She called out: "'Allo, sis, ah's yerself?" to everyone in sight, and to queries about her health, she responded, "I'm wonderful. Never bin better. On top 'o the world all the time."

I followed her over to the couch, and it stabbed my heart to see her little bow legs struggling to carry her. With each step the right leg in particular bent outwards, and her left hip swung precariously in the opposite direction. I had to arrange two stools and a chair before she could climb on to the couch, but she managed it, with awkward movements. It was painful to see. She was panting, and beaming in triumph when she got up. It seemed that every difficulty in life was a challenge to her, and every one successfully overcome was an occasion for rejoicing. She was not, by any stretch of the imagination, a good-looking woman, but I was not at all surprised that she had found a second husband who, I had no doubt, loved her. Brenda was only six months pregnant, but her abdomen looked abnormally large, due to her tiny stature, and also to the inward curving of the spine, which pushed the uterus forward and upwards. She could feel movements, and I could hear the foetal heartbeat. Her pulse and blood pressure were normal, but her breathing was laboured. I remarked on it.

"Don't mind me. That's nothing much," she said cheerfully.

I did not feel confident about examining Brenda's misshapen body, so I asked Sister Bernadette to confirm, which she did. Brenda was as healthy as could be expected, and was carrying a healthy foetus.

We saw her every week for the next six weeks, and she struggled on with increasing difficulty, using two sticks to help her get about. Her happiness never left her and she never complained. At thirty-seven weeks she was admitted to The London Hospital for bed rest, and a Caesarean section was successfully carried out at thirty-nine weeks.

A fine healthy daughter was delivered, whom she called Grace Miracle.

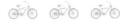

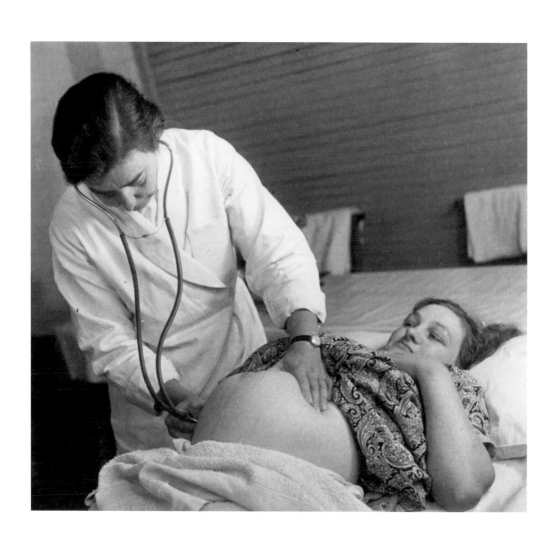

ECLAMPSIA

Throughout history, and until after the end of the Second World War in 1945, most babies were born at home. Then the drive for hospital delivery started, and it was so successful that by 1975 only one per cent of babies were born at home. The district midwife became very nearly an extinct species.

The fashion, or trend, is reversing slightly today, and the home birth rate is around two per cent. Perhaps this is because hospital delivery presents new and totally unexpected risks for mother and baby, and people are getting wise to this fact.

Sally came to us because she believed her mother more than she believed the doctor, who had advised hospital for her first baby.

Her mother had said, "Nark 'im. You go to the Nonnatuns, luvvy. They'll see yer right."

Gran had stepped in, too, with a wealth of ancient folklore, and hair-raising stories about the lying-in infirmaries, which used to be feared more than death itself by women.

In vain the doctor tried to convince Sally that modern hospitals were not like the old infirmaries, but he was no match for Mum and Gran, so he retired from the ring, and Sally booked with the Midwives of St Raymund Nonnatus.

Opposite: A midwife listens to an unborn baby's heart (c. 1946). Regular examinations were important to safeguard the health of both mother and baby.

We saw patients antenatally once a month for the first six months, then fortnightly for six weeks, followed by weekly check-ups for the last six weeks of pregnancy. All went well with Sally for the first seven months. She was a pretty little twenty-year-old, and she and her husband occupied two rooms in her mother's house. She was a telephonist, and her mum, who attended every antenatal visit, was proud of her.

I sat down with her, and went through her notes. Her blood pressure had been quite normal for the first six months. On the previous visit it had been slightly raised. I was concerned to find the BP even higher when I took it. I asked her to go to the scales, and found that she had gained five pounds weight in a fortnight. Warning bells were beginning to ring in my head.

I told Sally that I would like to examine her, and followed her over to the couch. By so doing, I was able to see that her ankles were swollen. A diagnosis was taking shape in my mind. She lay on the couch and I was able to feel, quite certainly, pitting oedema up to the knees – not very pronounced, but palpable to experienced fingers. Water retention – that would account for the weight gain. I examined the rest of her body for oedema, but could find none.

"Are you still getting any sickness?" I asked.

"No."

"Any stomach pains?"

"No."

"Any headaches?"

"Well, yes, now that you mention it, I have. But I puts it down to working on the phones."

"When do you give up work?"

"I gave up las' week."

"And are you still getting headaches?"

"Well, yes, I am that, but Mum says not to worry. It's normal."

I glanced sideways at the mother, Enid, who was beaming and nodding wisely. Thank God the girl had come to antenatal clinic. Mum is not always right!

"Stay there, would you, Sally? I want to test your urine. Have you brought a specimen?"

She had, and Enid produced it after rummaging around in her voluminous handbag.

I went over to the Bunsen burner, which was on the marble slab, and lit it. The urine was quite clear and looked normal as I poured a little into the test tube. I held the upper half of the glass vial over the flame. As it heated the urine turned white, whilst the urine in the lower half of the tube, which was unheated, remained clear.

Albumen urea. A diagnosis of pre-eclampsia. I stood quite still for a moment, thinking.

It is strange how you forget things, even momentous things in life. I had forgotten Margaret, but as I stood by the sink looking at that test tube, Margaret and the whole of my first and only horrifying experience of eclampsia flooded into my mind.

Margaret was twenty, and must have been very beautiful, though I never saw her beauty. I saw dozens of photographs of her though, which her adoring and heartbroken husband, David, showed me. All photographs were black and white in those days. They had a particular charm, created by the effects of light and shadow. In some of the photos, Margaret's intelligence and sensitivity claimed your attention, in others her laughing, puckish humour made you want to share the joke. In others, her huge, clear eyes looked fearlessly into the future, and in all of the snaps, her soft brown hair hung curling over her shoulders. One memorable photo was of a laughing young girl standing in a swimsuit beside the sea in Devon, with the spray from the waves leaping up the cliff face, and the wind blowing through her hair. The balance of her body on her long, slim legs and the angle of the shadows from the setting sun made an exquisite photo, by any standards. She looked like the sort of girl I would want to know – but I never did, except through David. She was a musician, a violinist, but I never heard her play.

All these photos David showed me during the two days of watching. When I first met him I'd assumed he must be her father. But no, he was her husband and lover, and worshipped the very ground beneath her feet. He was a scientist, and looked a very reserved, controlled, unapproachable sort of man, perhaps even cold and unemotional. But still waters run deep, and over those two long days the intensity of his passion and pain nearly split the hospital apart. Sometimes he was talking to her, sometimes to himself, occasionally to the staff. Sometimes he muttered prayers, or a few words forced out through sobbing tears. From these fragments, and the case history, I pieced together their story. There was nothing of the cold remote scientist about David.

They had met at a music club, at which Margaret was performing. He couldn't take his eyes off her. All through the interval, and the social afterwards, he followed her every movement with his eyes. He thought he might speak to her, but stammered and couldn't get the words out. He couldn't understand why; he was an articulate man. He did not know what was happening to him. She continued laughing and talking with other people while he retreated to a corner, scarcely able to breathe for the beating of his heart.

In the following days and weeks, he couldn't get her out of his head. Still he didn't understand. He thought it was the music that had affected him so deeply. He felt restless and ill at ease and his comfortable bachelor habits afforded him no comfort. Then he bumped into her in a Lyons Corner House, and amazingly she remembered him, though he couldn't think why. They had lunch together, and this time, far from being tongue-tied, he couldn't stop talking. In fact they talked for hours. They had a thousand things to say to each other, and he had never felt so relaxed and happy with anyone in all his forty-nine years of fairly solitary life. He thought, She can't possibly be interested in a dried-up old fogey like me, smelling of formaldehyde and surgical spirits. But she was. Perhaps she saw the integrity, the spiritual strength and the depths of untapped emotion in that quiet man. She was his first and only love, and he lavished on her all the passion of youth, with the tenderness and consideration of maturity.

Afterwards he said to me, "I am just thankful that I knew her at all. If we had not met, or if we had met and just passed each other by, all the great literature of the world, all the poets, all the great love stories would have been meaningless to me. You cannot understand what you have not experienced."

They had been married for six months, and she was six months pregnant, when she was admitted to the antenatal ward of the City of London Maternity Hospital where I was working. According to her antenatal records, Margaret had been in perfect health throughout the pregnancy. She had been seen at the clinic two days earlier, and everything had been quite normal – weight, pulse, blood pressure, urine sample, no sickness – nothing that would indicate what was to come.

On the day of admission she had awoken early, and was sick, which was unusual as morning sickness had passed about eight weeks earlier. She returned to the bedroom, saying there were spots in front of her eyes.

David was concerned, but she said she would lie down again. It was a bit of a headache, and would go if she had another sleep. So off he went to work, saying he would telephone at eleven o'clock, to see how she felt. The telephone rang and rang. He imagined he could hear it echoing through the empty house. She might be out, of course, having woken up refreshed, but a premonition told him to go home.

He found her unconscious on the bedroom floor, with blood smeared all around her mouth, across her cheek, and in her hair. His first thought was that there had been a burglary, during which she had been attacked, but the total absence of any signs of a break-in, and the apparent depth of unconsciousness, the stertorous breathing, the bounding heartbeat that he could feel through her night dress, told him that something serious had happened.

The hospital sent an ambulance straight away, in response to his frantic phone call. A doctor came also, as the implications of David's description were very grave. Margaret was sedated with morphine before the ambulance men were allowed to move her.

We were told to prepare a side-ward to receive a possible case of eclampsia. It was during my first six months of midwifery training, and the ward sister showed me and another student how this should be done. The bed was pushed against the wall, with pillows stuffed down the crack. The head of the bed was padded with more pillows and secured tightly with sheets. Oxygen was brought in: a mouth wedge and airway tube were in readiness, also suction apparatus. The window was covered with a dark cloth to black out most of the light.

Margaret was deeply unconscious on admission. Her blood pressure was so high that the systolic was over 200 and diastolic 190. Her temperature was 104 degrees Fahrenheit and her pulse was 140. A catheter specimen of urine was obtained and tested. So heavy was the deposit of albumen that upon boiling the urine turned solid like the white of an egg. There was no doubt of the diagnosis.

Eclampsia was, and still is, a rare and mysterious condition of pregnancy, with no known cause. Usually there are warning signs before onset known as pre-eclampsia, which responds to treatment, but if untreated may progress to eclampsia. Rarely, very rarely, it occurs with no warning in a perfectly

Overleaf. The London Hospital (c. 1920s), where Jennifer Lee first came across Margaret.

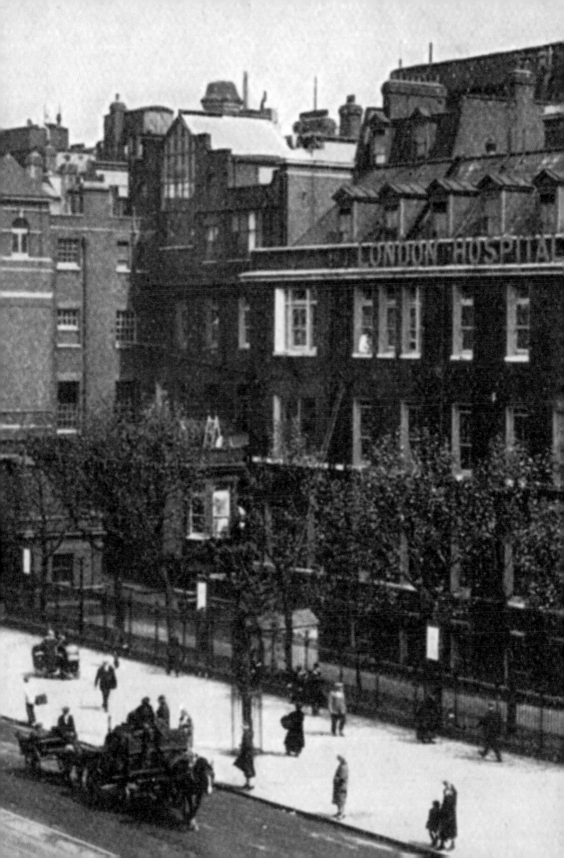

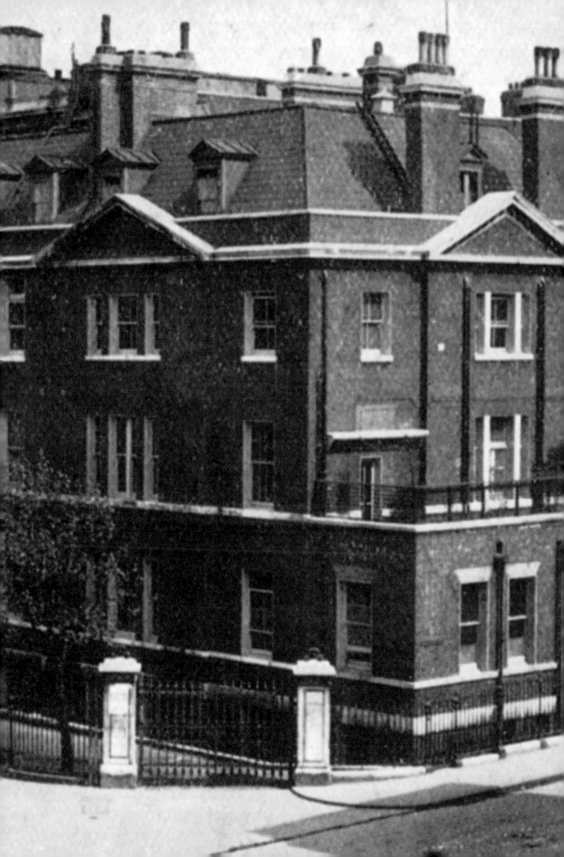

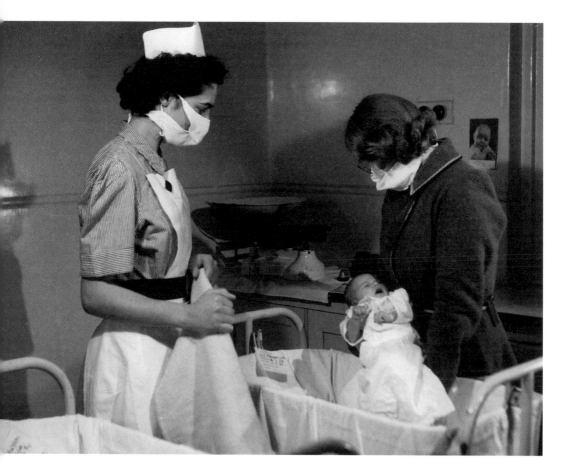

Above: Midwives did far more than deliver babies; they also gave vital ante- and post-natal care, providing essential advice and information to mothers.

healthy woman, and in the space of a few hours it can develop to convulsion stage. When this stage is reached, the pregnancy is unstable, and the foetus unlikely to survive. The only treatment is immediate delivery of the baby by Caesarean section.

Theatre had been alerted and was ready to receive Margaret. The baby was dead on delivery, and Margaret returned to the ward. She never regained consciousness. She was kept under heavy sedation in a darkened room, but even then she had repeated convulsions that were terrifying to see. A slight twitching was followed by vigorous contractions of all the muscles of the body. Her whole body became rigid, and the muscular spasm bent her body backwards, so that for about twenty seconds only her head and heels rested on the bed. Respiration ceased, and she became blue with asphyxia. Quite quickly, the rigidity passed, followed by violent convulsive movements and spasms of all her limbs. It was hard to keep her from hurling herself on to the floor, and quite impossible to keep a tongue wedge in place. With the violent movements of the jaw she bit her tongue to pieces. She salivated profusely, and foamed at the mouth, which mingled with the blood from her lacerated tongue. Her face was congested and horribly distorted. Then the convulsion subsided, and a deep coma would follow, lasting for an hour or so and followed by another convulsion.

These terrible fits occured repeatedly for a little over thirty-six hours, and on the evening of the second day, she died in her husband's arms.

All this flooded into my mind in the few seconds that I stood at the sink, looking at the sample of Sally's urine. David. What had happened to that poor man? He had staggered out of the hospital half blind, half mad, dumb with shock and grief. Sadly, in nursing, and particularly in hospital nursing, you meet people during some of the most profound moments in their lives, and then they are gone from you for ever. There was no way that David would be hanging around the maternity hospital where his wife had died, just to reassure the nurses. And equally, hospital staff could not go chasing after him to find out how he was coping. I remembered with gratitude what he said to me just after she died, and the words of some great writer (I cannot recall who), came to mind:

> *He who loves knows it. He who loves not, knows it not.*
> *I pity him, and make him no answer.*

There was no time to mope. I had to see Sister and report on Sally's condition.

Sister Bernadette was in charge on that day. She listened to my report, looked at the urine sample, and said, "There may be contamination from a vaginal discharge, so we will take a catheter specimen of urine. Could you just get things ready for catheterisation, please, while I go over to Sally and examine her."

When I took the tray over to the couch Sister had already made a full examination, and confirmed everything I had reported.

She said to Sally, "We are going to insert a small tube into your bladder to drain off some urine for testing in path. lab."

Sally protested, but eventually submitted, and I catheterised her. Then Sister said to her, "We think there is a problem with this pregnancy that requires absolute rest, and a special diet, and certain drugs to be administered daily. For this, you must go to hospital."

Sally and her mother were alarmed.

"What's up? I feels all right. Just a bit of a headache, that's all."

Her mother butted in, "If there's anything wrong with our Sal I can look after 'er. She can take it easy at home, like."

Sister was very firm. "It's not just a question of taking it easy and staying in bed some of the time. Sally has to have absolute bed rest, twenty-four hours a day, for the next four to six weeks. She will have to have a special no-salt diet, with low fluid intake. She will need to have certain sedative drugs four times a day. She will need to be watched carefully, and her pulse, temperature and blood pressure will have to be taken several times every day. The baby's progress will also have to be checked daily. You cannot possibly do all this at home. Sally needs immediate hospital treatment, and if she does not get it, the baby will be at risk, and also the health of the mother."

This was a very long speech for Sister Bernadette, who was usually very quiet. It was absolutely effective, though, for it silenced Sally's mum, who gave a squeak, and said nothing.

"I am going now to ring the doctor, to ask him if he can find a bed for you immediately at one of the maternity hospitals. I want you to stay where you are, lying quietly on the couch. I don't want you to go home."

Then she said to Enid: "Perhaps you would go home and get some things for Sally in hospital – nightdresses, toothbrush, things like that, and bring them back here."

Enid scurried off, glad of something to do.

Sally had a couple of hours to wait before an ambulance came, and she was taken into this in a wheel chair. I think she was bewildered by all the fuss and the attention she was getting, especially as she didn't feel ill, had walked to the clinic, and was quite capable of walking out.

Sally was taken to The London Hospital in Mile End Road. She was admitted to the antenatal ward, where there were ten to twelve other young women in just the same stage and condition of pregnancy as herself. She received complete bed-rest, even to the extent of being pushed to the toilet in a wheel chair. She was sedated, and given a specific diet and low fluid intake. Over the next four weeks her blood pressure gradually came down, the oedema subsided, and the headache passed. At thirty-eight weeks of pregnancy, labour was induced. Sally's blood pressure began to rise during the labour, so as soon as she was fully dilated, she was given a light anaesthetic, and a fine healthy baby was delivered by forceps.

Mother and baby both remained well during the post-natal period.

Eclampsia is as much a mystery today as it was fifty years ago. It was, and still is, thought to be caused by some defect in the placenta. But nothing has been proven, even though thousands of placentas must have been examined by researchers attempting to isolate this supposed "defect".

Sally's case was typical of pre-eclampsia. Had she not been diagnosed, and received prompt and expert treatment, her condition could have led to eclampsia. But the simple treatment that I have described – total rest and sedation – may have averted its development.

Margaret, who died in that ghastly way, had a very rare onset of sudden, violent eclampsia, with no warning signs, and no pre-eclamptic phase. I have never seen another such case, but they do still occur occasionally.

Pre-eclampsia and eclampsia are still leading causes of maternal and perinatal mortality in the UK, in spite of modern antenatal care. What befell the women with pre-eclampsia when there was no antenatal care? It does not take a great deal of imagination to answer that one. Yet doctors who advocated the study of and provision for proper antenatal care were regarded, one hundred years ago, as eccentrics and time-wasters. The same attitude poured scorn on the idea of a structured and regulated training for midwives.

Let those of us who have borne children thank God that those days are now past.

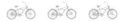

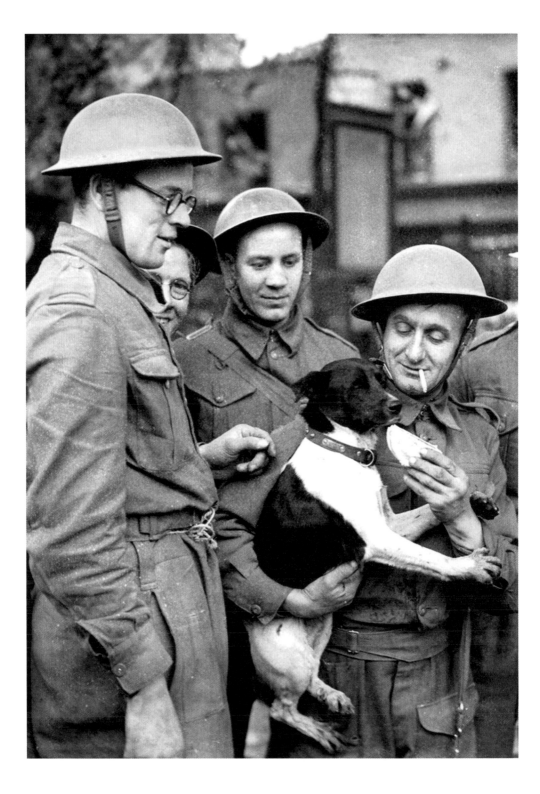

FRED

A convent is essentially a female establishment. However, of necessity, the male of the species cannot be excluded entirely. Fred was the boiler-man and odd-jobber of Nonnatus House. He was typical of the Cockney of his day and age. Stunted growth, short bowed legs, powerful hairy arms, pugnacious, obstinate, resourceful; all these attributes were combined with endless chat and irrepressible good humour. His most striking characteristic was a spectacular squint. One eye was permanently directed north-east, whilst the other roved in a south-westerly direction. If you add to this the single yellow tooth jutting from his upper jaw, which he generally held over his lower lip and sucked, you would not say he was a beautiful specimen of manhood. However, so delightful was his optimism, good humour and artless self-confidence that the Sisters held him in great affection, and leaned on him heavily for all practical matters. Sister Julienne had a particularly strong line in helpless feminine appeal, "Oh Fred, the window in the upper bathroom won't close. I've tried and tried, but it's no use. Do you think ...? If you can find time, that is ...?"

Of course Fred could find time. For Sister Julienne he would have found time to move the Albert Docks. Sister Julienne was deeply grateful, and praised his skill and expertise. The fact that the window in the upstairs bathroom was fixed permanently closed from that time onwards was no inconvenience, and not mentioned by anyone.

Opposite: Members of the Pioneer Corps feed Spot, the dog (Stepney, 1940). Fred had been consigned to the unit during the Second World War.

The only person who did not respond with delight to Fred's particular brand of Cockney charm was Mrs B., who was a Cockney herself, had seen it all before, and was not impressed. Mrs B. was Queen of the Kitchen. She worked from 8 a.m. to 2 p.m. each day, and produced superb food for us. She was an expert in steak and kidney pies, thick stews, savoury mince, toad-in-the-hole, treacle puddings, jam roly-poly, macaroni puddings and so on, as well as baking the best bread and cakes you could find anywhere. She was a large lady with formidable frontage, and a particular glare as she growled, "Nah then – don' chew mess up my kitchen." As the kitchen was the meeting-point for all staff when we came in, often tired and hungry, this remark was frequently heard. We girls were very docile and respectful, especially as we had learned from experience that flattery usually resulted in a tart or a wedge of cake straight from the oven.

Fred, however, was not so easily tamed. For one thing, the orientation of his eyes being what it was, he genuinely could not see the mess he was making; for another, Fred was not going to kowtow to anyone. He would grin at Mrs B. wickedly, suck his tooth, slap her ample bottom, and chuckle, "Come off it, old girl." Mrs B.'s glare would turn into a shout, "You ge' out of my kitchen you ugly mug, and stay ou'." Unfortunately Fred couldn't stay out, and she knew it. The coke stove was in the kitchen, and he was responsible for stoking it, raking it out, opening and shutting the flues, and generally keeping it in good order. As Mrs B. did much of her cooking, and all of her baking, on that stove, she knew that she was dependent on him. So a strained truce prevailed between them. Only occasionally – about twice a week – a shouting match erupted. I noticed with interest that during these altercations neither of them swore – no doubt this was out of respect for the nuns. Had they been in any other environment, I felt sure the air would have been blue with obscenities.

Fred's duties were morning and evening for boiler stoking and extra time by arrangement for odd jobs. He came in seven days a week for the boiler, and the job suited him very well. It was a steady job, but it also allowed him plenty of time to pursue the other activities he had built up over the years.

Fred lived with his unmarried daughter Dolly in the lower two rooms of a small house backing on to the docks. He had been called up during the war but, due to his eyesight, had been unable to enter the armed services. He was therefore consigned to the Pioneer Corps, where, if Fred is to be believed, he spent six years serving King and Country by cleaning out latrines.

Compassionate leave was granted to him in 1942, when his wife and three of their six children were killed by a direct hit. He was able to spend a little time with his three living children, who were shocked and traumatised, in a hostel in North London before they were evacuated to Somerset, and he was ordered back to the latrines.

After the war, he took two cheap rooms and brought up the remains of his family single-handed. It was never easy for him to find a regular job, because his eyesight was erratic, and because he would not commit himself to be away from home for long hours – he knew that his children needed him. So he had developed a wide range of money-making activities, some of which were legal.

Whilst we, the lay staff, took our breakfast in the kitchen, Fred was generally attending to his boiler, so there was plenty of opportunity to press him for stories, which we did unashamedly, being young and inquisitive. For his part Fred would always oblige, as he clearly loved spinning his yarns, often prefaced by, "You're never going to believe this one." A laughing audience of four young girls was music to his ears. Young girls will laugh at anything!

One of his regular jobs, and the best paid he assured us, as it was highly skilled, was that of a cooper's barrel bottom knocker for Whitbreads the brewer. Trixie, the sceptic, snapped, "I'll knock your bottom for you", but Chummy swallowed it whole and said gravely, "Actually, it sounds frightfully interesting. Do tell us more." Fred liked Chummy, and called her "Lofty".

"Well, these here beer barrels, like, they've gotta be sound, like, and the only way of testin' 'em is by knockin' the bottoms and listening. If it comes up wiv one note, it's sound. If it comes up wiv anover, it's faul'y. See? Easy, bu' I can tell you, it takes years of experience."

We had seen Fred in the market selling onions, but did not know that he grew them. Having the ground floor of a small house gave him a small garden, which was given over to onions. He had tried potatoes – "no money in spuds" – but onions proved to be a money-maker. He also kept chickens and sold the eggs, and the birds as well. He wouldn't sell to a butcher, "I'm not 'aving no one take 'alf the profits", but sold directly to the market. He wouldn't take a stall either, "I'm not paying no bleedin' rent to the council", and laid a blanket on the floor in any space available, selling his onions, eggs and chickens from there.

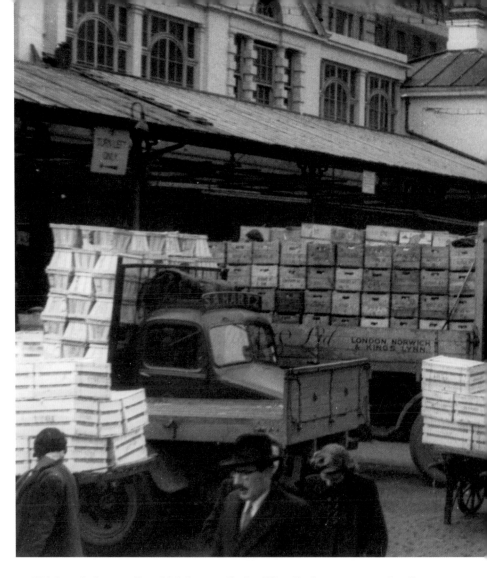

Chickens led to quails, which he supplied to West End restaurants. Quails are delicate birds, requiring warmth, so he kept them in the house. Being small, they do not need much space, so he bred and reared them in boxes which he kept under the bed. He slaughtered and plucked them in the kitchen.

Chummy, always eager, said, "You know, I think that's frightfully clever, actually. But wouldn't it be a bit whiffy, what?"

Trixi cut her short. "Oh, shut up. We're having our breakfast," and reached for the cornflakes.

Fred's enthusiasm for drains was enough to put anyone off their breakfast. Cleaning out drains was obviously a passion, and his north-east

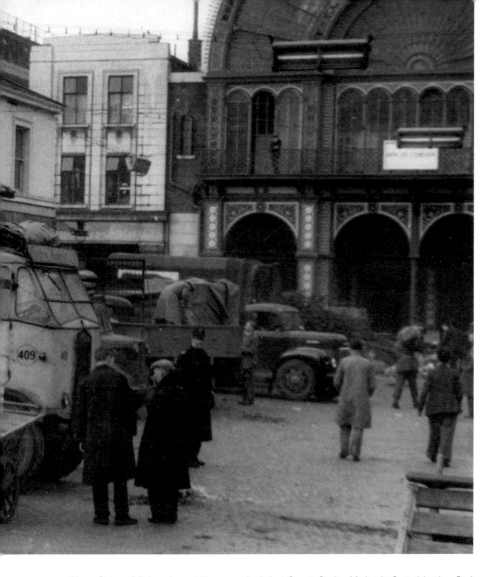

Above: Crates of fruit and vegetables are unloaded at Covent Garden Market in Central London. Fred purchased crates of cheap apples from here for his toffee apples.

eye gleamed as he poured out the effluvial details. Trixie said, "I'll stuff you down a drain, if you don't watch it," and made for the door, toast in hand. But Fred, a poet with rod and suction, was not to be discouraged. "The best job I ever had was up in Hampstead, see? One of them posh houses. Lady's real la-di-da, toffee-nosed. I lifts up the man'ole cover an' there it is, like, fillin' the whole chamber: a frenchy – a rubber, you know – caught at the inflow end, an' blown up with muck an' water. Huge, it was, huge."

His eyes rolled expressively at their different angles as he expanded his arms. Chummy shared his enthusiasm, but not his meaning.

"You never seen nuffink like it, a yard long, an' a foot wide, strike me dead. Ve lady, ever so posh like, looks at it an' says 'oh dear, whatever can it be?' an' I says 'well if you don't know, lady, you musta bin asleep' an' she says 'don't you be saucy, my good fellow'. Well, I gets the thing out, an' charges her double, an' she pays up like a lamb."

He grinned impishly, rubbed his hands together, and sucked his tooth.

"Oh, jolly well done, Fred, good for you. It was frightfully clever getting double the fee, actually."

Fred's best line, with the highest profit margin, had been fireworks. His unit of the Pioneer Corps had been attached to the Royal Engineers in North Africa for a time. Explosives had been in daily use. Anyone, however humble, working with the REs, is bound to learn something about explosives and Fred had picked up enough to give him confidence to embark on fireworks manufacture in the kitchen of his little house after the war.

"S'easy. You just need a load of the right kind of fertiliser, an' a touch of this an mix it wiv a bi' of that an' bingo, you've got yer bang."

Chummy said, wide-eyed with apprehension: "But isn't it frightfully dangerous, actually, Fred?"

"Nah, nah, not if you knows what you is a-doin', like what I does. Sold like nobody's business, they did, all over Poplar. Everyone was wantin' 'em. I could've made a fortune if they'd left me alone, the bleeders, beggin' yer pardon, miss."

"Who? What happened?"

"Rozzers, police, got 'old of some of me fireworks an' tested 'em, an' sez they was dangerous, an' I was endangering 'uman life. I asks you – I asks you. Would I do anyfing like that, now? Would I?" He looked up from his position on the floor, and spread out his ash-covered hands in innocent appeal.

"Of course not Fred," we all chorused. "What happened?"

"Well, they charged me, din't they, but the magistrate, he lets me off wiv a fine, like, because I 'ad three kids. He was a good bloke, he was, the magistrate, but he says I would go to prison if I does it again, kids or no kids. So I never done it no more."

His most recent economic adventure had been in toffee apples, and very successful it was, too. Dolly made the toffee mixture in the little kitchen, while Fred purchased crates of cheap apples from Covent Garden. All that was needed was a stick to put the apple on, dip it in the toffee, and in no time at all rows of toffee apples were lined up on the draining board. Fred couldn't imagine why he hadn't thought of it before. It was a winner. One-hundred per cent profit margin and assured sales with the large number of children around. He foresaw a rosy future with unlimited sales and profits.

A week or two later, it was clear that something had gone wrong from the silence of the small figure crouched down by the stove, manipulating the flue. No cheerful greeting, no chat, no tuneless whistle – just a heavy silence. He wouldn't even respond to our questions.

Eventually Chummy left the table and went over to him.

"Come on, Fred. What's up? Perhaps we can help. And even if we can't, you will feel better if you tell us." She touched his shoulder with her huge hand.

Fred turned and looked up. His north-east eye drooped, and a little moisture glinted in the south-west. His voice was husky as he spoke.

"Fevvers. Quail's fevvers. Tha's wha's up. Someone complained fevvers was stuck to me toffee apples. So food safety boffins come an' examined 'em an' said fevvers an' bits of fevvers was stuck to all me toffee apples, an' I was endangerin' public 'ealth."

Apparently the health inspector had asked at once to see where the toffee apples were made, and when shown the kitchen, in which the quails were regularly slaughtered and plucked, had immediately ordered that both occupations be discontinued, on pain of prosecution. So great was the disaster to Fred's economy that it seemed nothing could be said to comfort him. Chummy was so kind, and assured him that something else would turn up, something better, but he was not reassured, and it was a glum breakfast that morning. He had lost face, and it hurt.

But Fred's triumph was yet to come.

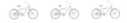

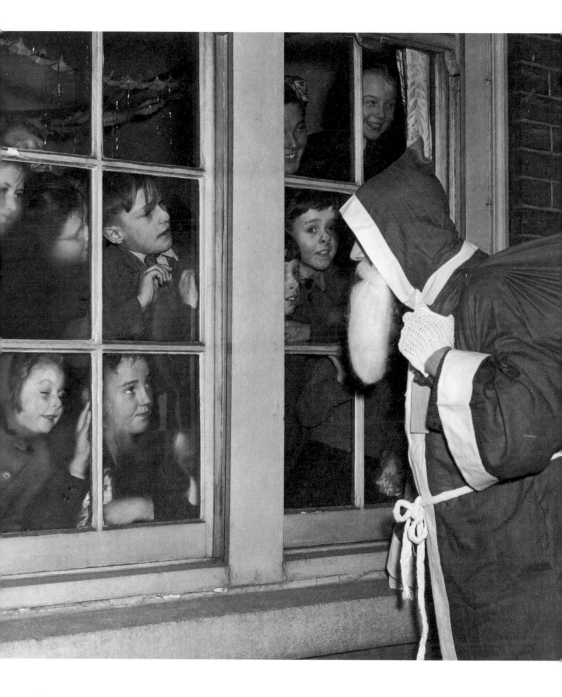

A CHRISTMAS BABY

Betty Smith's baby was due in early February. As she dashed happily around all December, preparing Christmas for her husband and six children, her parents and in-laws, grandparents on both sides, brothers, sisters and their children, uncles and aunts, and a very ancient great-grandmother, none of the family dreamed that the baby would be born on Christmas Day.

Dave was a wharf manager in the West India Docks. He was in his thirties, clever, competent and he knew his job inside out. He was greatly valued by the Port of London Authority, and he earned a good wage. In consequence, the family was able to live in one of the large Victorian houses just off Commercial Road. Betty never ceased to thank her lucky stars that she had married Dave just after the war, and was able to leave the tenements, with the cramped living conditions and minimal sanitation. She loved her big, roomy house, and that is why she had always been glad to have the family descend on her for Christmas. The children loved it. With about twenty-five little cousins coming from all over Poplar, Stepney, Bow, and Canning Town, they were going to have a high old time.

Uncle Alf was Father Christmas. The house was at the bottom of an incline, and Uncle Alf had a home-made sleigh on wheels. This was taken to the top of the street, loaded with a sack of presents, and at a given signal, pushed off. The children did not know how it was done. All that they saw was Father Christmas trundling gently towards them, with no

Opposite: Children peer out of the window at Father Christmas, bearing a large sack of gifts (1950).

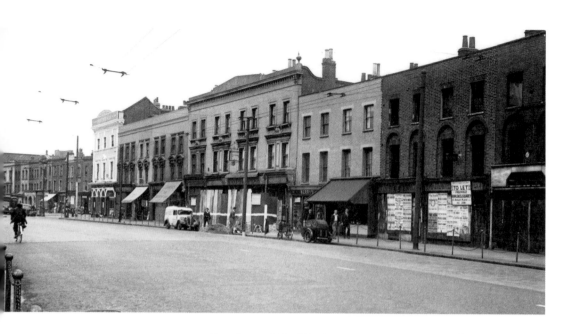

Above: Commercial Road, East London, in 1952.

apparent means of propulsion, and stopping at their house. They were in an ecstasy of delight.

But this year, things were to be rather different. Instead of Father Christmas on a sleigh, a midwife arrived on a bicycle. Instead of a sack full of presents, a baby came, naked and crying.

My Christmas was also very different. For the first time in my life I began to understand that Christmas is a religious festival, and not just an occasion for overeating and drinking. It had all begun in late November with something that I was told was Advent. This meant nothing to me, but for the nuns it meant a time of preparation. Most people prepare for Christmas as Betty had done, buying food, drinks, presents and treats. The nuns prepared rather differently, with prayer and meditation.

The religious life is a hidden life, so I would not see or hear what was going on, but as the four weeks of Advent progressed, I began to feel intuitively that something was in the air. I couldn't put my finger on it, but as children pick up a feeling of excitement from their parents, so I "caught" from the Sisters a real feeling of calm, peace and joyful expectancy, which I found to be strangely disturbing and unwelcome.

It came to a head on Christmas Eve when I returned late from my evening visits. Sister Julienne was around, and said to me, "Come with me to the Chapel, Jennifer, we put up the crib today."

Not wishing to be rude by saying I would rather not, I followed her. The chapel was unlit, except for two candles placed by the crib. Sister Julienne kneeled at the altar rail to pray. Then she said to me, "Our blessed Saviour was born on this day."

I remember looking at the small plaster figures and the straw and things, and thinking, how on earth can an intelligent and well-informed woman take all this seriously? Is she trying to be funny?

I think I murmured something polite about it being very peaceful, and we parted. However, I was not at peace within myself. Something was nagging at me that I was trying to resist. Was it then or was it later that the thought came to me: if God really does exist, and is not just a myth, it must have consequence for the whole of life. It was not a comfortable thought.

For many years I had attended a Christmas midnight Mass somewhere, not for religious reasons, but for the drama and beauty of the ceremony. I was not fussy about denomination. When I was living in Paris, I had been in the habit of attending the Russian Orthodox Church in Rue Darue, for the beauty of the singing. The Christmas mass from 11 p.m. to about 2 a.m. counts as one of the greatest musical experiences of my life. The liturgy, sung by the Russian bass voice of the cantor, rising in quarter-tones, has never left my inner ear, even though more than fifty years have passed.

The Sisters and lay staff attended All Saints Church, East India Dock Road for midnight Mass. I was astonished to find the church absolutely packed. Strong, tough dockers, hard-bitten casual labourers, giggling teenagers in their winkle-pickers, whole families carrying babies, small children, all were there. The crowd was enormous. All Saints is a large Victorian church, and it must have held five hundred people that night. The service was as I had expected – impressive, beautiful, dramatic, but devoid of any spiritual content as far as I was concerned. I wondered why. Why was it the whole meaning of life for these good Sisters, yet just a piece of well executed theatre for me?

We were having lunch around the big table on Christmas Day when the telephone rang. Everyone groaned. We had hoped for a day of rest. The nurse who answered it came back to say that Dave Smith was reporting that his wife seemed to be in labour. The groan turned into a gasp of anxiety.

Sister Bernadette jumped up with the words, "I'll go and talk to him." She came back a few minutes later, and said, "It sounds as though it is labour. At thirty-four weeks this is unfortunate. I have informed Dr Turner, and he will come at once if we need him. Who is on call today?" I was.

We prepared to go out together. I was a student at the time, and was always accompanied by a trained midwife. From the first moment I had watched Sister Bernadette at work, I knew that she was a gifted midwife. Her knowledge and skill were balanced by her intuition and sensitivity. I would have entrusted my life to her hands, without the slightest hesitation.

Together we left the cosy warmth of an excellent Christmas dinner, and fetched a delivery pack and our midwifery bags from the sterilising room. The pack was a large box, containing pads, sheets, waterproof paper, and so on, which was usually taken to the house a week before the expected delivery. The blue bag contained our instruments and drugs. We fitted them both to our bicycles, and pushed out into a cold windless day.

I had never known London to be so quiet. Nothing seemed to stir, except for two midwives cycling silently along the deserted road. Normally the East India Dock Road is dense with heavy goods lorries going to and from the docks, but on that day the broad thoroughfare looked majestic and beautiful in its solitary silence. Nothing moved on the river or in the docks. Not a sound, but the occasional cry of a seagull. The stillness of the great heart of London was unforgettable.

We arrived at the house, and Dave let us in. Through the window we had seen a big Christmas tree, a fire, and a room crowded with people. About a dozen little faces of curious children were pressed to the window pane as we arrived.

Dave said, "Betty's upstairs. I didn't see no cause to send them home, and she don't want it. She likes a bit of noise, says it will help her."

The sound of lusty singing "Old MacDonald Had a Farm" came from the front room, accompanied by an out-of-tune piano. Full vocal justice was given to the animal noises by various uncles, expert in being the horse, the pig, the cow, the duck. The children screamed with laughter, and shouted for more.

We went upstairs to Betty's room, where the peace and silence contrasted with the noise and clamour below. A fire had been lit and was burning brightly. Hardly any time had been given to Betty's mother to prepare a delivery room, but she had worked miracles. Surfaces had been cleaned, extra linen provided, hot water was available, even the cot had been prepared.

Betty's first words were, "This is a turn up for the books, eh, Sister?"

She was a cheerful, down-to-earth sort of woman, who took everything in her stride. No doubt she had the same confidence in Sister Bernadette that I had. I opened the delivery pack, and covered the bed with brown waterproof paper, then the draw sheets and maternity pads. We gowned and scrubbed up, and Sister examined her. The waters had broken an hour earlier. I saw intense concentration on Sister's face, and then a look of grave concern. She said nothing for a few moments as she slowly took off her gloves, then said gently:

"Betty, your baby seems to be a breech presentation. That means the bottom is coming first, instead of the head. This is a perfectly normal way for the baby to lie until about thirty-five weeks, but then the baby usually turns, and the head is presented first. Your baby has not turned. Now, whilst thousands of babies are born quite safely in breech, there is a greater risk than a head presentation. Perhaps you should consider a hospital delivery."

Betty's reaction was immediate and dogmatic. "No. No hospital. I'll be OK with you, Sister. All me babies have been delivered by the Nonnatuns and born in this room, and I don't want nothing else. What do you say, mum?"

Her mother agreed, and recalled that her ninth had been a breech, and that her neighbour Glad had had no less than four, arse first.

Sister said, "Very well then, we will do our best, but I am going to ask Dr Turner to come." Then to me: "Would you go and ring him, nurse?"

In spite of his comparative affluence, Dave did not have a telephone. There would have been no point, because none of his friends or relatives had a phone, so no one would ever have rung them. The public phone box was sufficient for their needs. As I went downstairs, a stream of shouting children in paper hats, faces alight with excitement rushed past me. A voice from downstairs called out:

"Everyone hide. I'll count twenty, then I'm coming to find you. One, two, three, four …"

The children rushed higher in the house, screaming and pushing, hiding in cupboards, behind curtains, anywhere. By the time I got to the front door, all was quiet except: "Seventeen, eighteen, nineteen – cummin'."

I went out into the cold of the deserted street to find the telephone box. Dr Turner was a general practitioner who not only had a surgery in the East End, but also lived there with his wife and children. He was utterly dedicated to his work and his practice, and it seemed to me that he was always on call. Like most GPs of his generation he was a first-class midwife, with a knowledge and skill gained from the experience of his wide ranging practice.

He was expecting my call. I told him the facts.

He said, "Thank you, nurse. I will come directly." I imagined his wife sighing, "even on Christmas Day you have to go out."

Back in the house, hide and seek was still going on. The noise was terrific as children were found. As I entered the door, a cheery faced man passed me carrying a crate of empty beer bottles.

"How about joining me for one, then, nurse?" he said. "You and Sister and all. Oops, does she drink, do you think?"

I assured him that the Sisters did drink, but not on duty, and that for the same reason, I would not do so either. A paper streamer shot past my ear, blown by an invisible figure behind a door.

"Oh, sorry, nurse. I thought it was our Pol."

I unravelled the pink and orange thing from my uniform, and went upstairs.

Betty's room was wonderfully quiet and peaceful. The thick old walls and heavy wooden door insulated the sounds and Betty looked calm and content. Sister Bernadette was writing up her notes, and Betty's mother, Ivy, was sitting in a corner knitting. The click of the knitting needles, and the crackle of the fire were all that could be heard.

Sister explained to me that she would not give Betty a sedative, because it might affect the baby. She said it was difficult to tell how long the first stage of labour would last, and at present the foetal heart beat was quite normal.

Dr Turner arrived, looking as though there was nothing in the world he would rather do on Christmas Day than attend a breech delivery. He and Sister conferred, and he examined Betty thoroughly. I expected him to do another vaginal examination, but he did not: he accepted Sister's diagnosis without question. He told Betty that she and her baby seemed very well, and that he would come back at 5 p.m. unless we called him earlier.

We sat down to wait.

Much of a midwife's work involves intense, often dramatic activity, but this is balanced by long periods of waiting quietly. Sister sat down and took out her breviary in order to say the office of the day. The nuns lived by the monastic rules of the six offices of the day: lauds; tierce; sext; none; vespers; compline and Holy Communion each morning. In a contemplative community, the offices together occupy about five hours of prayer time. For a working community this is impracticable, so, in the early days of their vocation, the Midwives of St Raymund Nonnatus had had a shortened version devised for them. Thus they were able to maintain their professed religious life, and work full-time as nurses and midwives.

The sight of this fair young face in the firelight, reading the ancient prayers, turning the pages quietly and reverently, her lips moving as she read, was deeply affecting. I sat watching her and marvelled at the depth of a vocation that could make such a pretty young woman renounce life, with all its fun and opportunities, for a religious life bound by the vows of poverty, chastity, and obedience. I could understand the vocation to nursing and midwifery, which to me were fascinating both as a study and a practice, but the calling to a religious life was quite beyond my comprehension.

Betty groaned as a contraction came on. Sister smiled, got up and went over to her. She returned to her breviary, and all that could be heard in the room was the tick of a big clock and the click of Ivy's knitting needles. Beyond the door the sounds of the party continued, but within the room all was calm and prayerful.

I sat in the firelight, and allowed my mind to wander backwards. I had spent many Christmases in hospitals. Contrary to what one might think, it was a happy time. Fifty years ago, hospitals were very much more personal than they are today. The nursing hierarchy was formidable but at least everyone knew or was acquainted with everyone else. Patients stayed in hospital for much longer and, as nurses worked sixty hours per week, we really got to know our patients as people. At Christmas, everyone let their hair down, and even the most draconian old Ward Sister, after a few sherries, would be giggling with the student nurses. It was all rather like schoolgirl fun, but it was good humoured, and the aim was to give a happy time to the patients, many of whom had horrible diseases.

My most abiding Christmas memory was the carol singing on Christmas Eve. Led by Matron, all the nursing staff would go through the wards by candlelight, singing. For someone in a hospital bed it must have been a lovely sight. There may have been over one hundred nurses, twenty or more doctors, and fifty or more ancillary staff. The nurses wore full uniform, and we turned our cloaks inside out showing the scarlet lining. We all carried candles. We walked through each darkened ward, usually containing thirty beds, singing the age-old story of Christmas. All this has long since gone from hospitals, and the memory of it is all that remains, but it was very beautiful, and I know that many patients shed tears of emotion.

Overleaf. One of the author's abiding memories was of the nursing staff carol singing to the patients in hospitals that she had worked in. "For someone in a hospital bed it must have been a lovely sight."

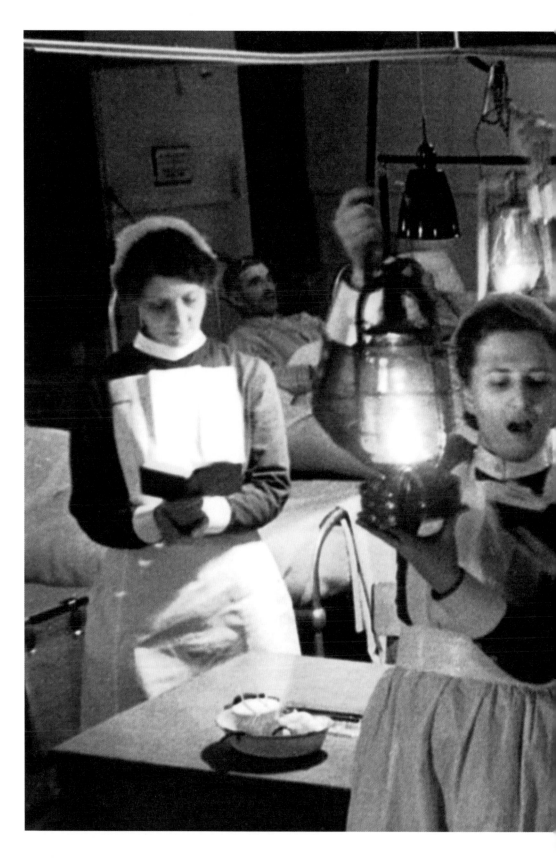

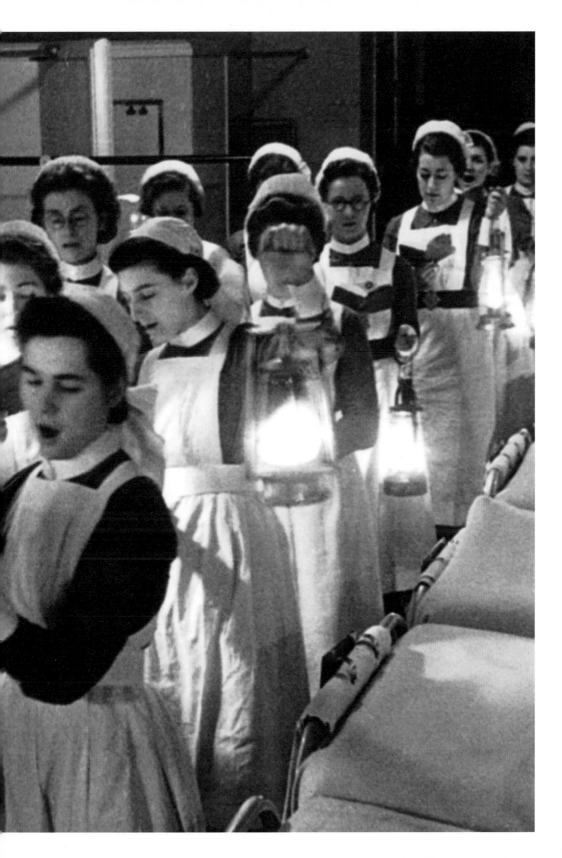

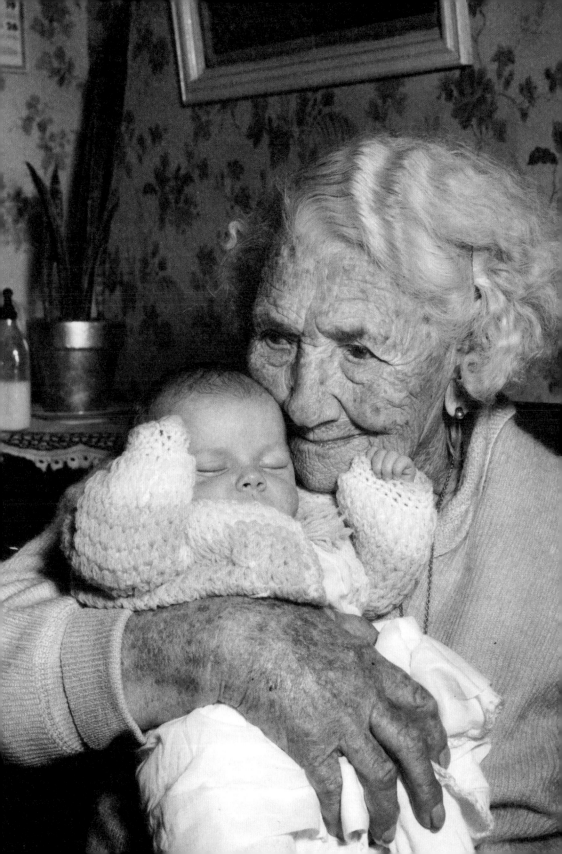

A BREECH DELIVERY

The time ticked quietly by. The sounds of "Aye, aye, aye, conga" came from below. They went round and round the sitting room, then the noise got louder and louder as the snake of people started coming up the stairs. They were all shouting at the tops of their voices, and stamping in unison. Sister thought the noise might bother Betty, but she said, "No, no, Sister. I likes to hear it. I wouldn't want this house to be quiet, not on Christmas day, like."

Sister smiled. The last few contractions had seemed stronger and were closer together. She got up, and examined Betty, and said to me, "I think you had better go and call Dr Turner if you please, nurse."

It was four o'clock when I rang him, and Dr Turner arrived within a quarter of an hour. I was excited. This was my first breech delivery. Betty was beginning to feel the urge to push.

Sister Bernadette said to her, "You must try very hard not to push at first, dear. Breathe deeply, and try to relax, but not to push."

We gowned, masked and scrubbed up again. Doctor looked at Sister Bernadette, and said, "You take this delivery, Sister. I'll be here if you need me."

He obviously had complete confidence in her.

She nodded, and told Betty that she wanted her to remain on her back,

Opposite: In the East End, families tended to be close and it was not unusual for parents to reside not just with their children but their children's children as well.

with her buttocks over the end of the bed, and she asked me and Ivy to hold a leg each. I was learning, and so Sister explained everything that she did clearly and carefully.

I could see something coming, as the perineum expanded, but it did not look like a baby's buttocks. It looked a purplish colour. Sister saw my questioning expression, and told me, "That is the prolapsed cord. It occurs quite commonly in a breech delivery, because the breech is an incomplete sphere, and the cord can easily slip down between the baby's legs. As long as it is pulsating normally, there is nothing to worry about."

The perineum continued to distend, and now I saw the baby's buttocks quite clearly. Sister was kneeling on the floor between Betty's legs because the bed was too low for her to stand.

She was explaining everything in a low voice to me, "This is a left sacro-anterior position, which means the left buttock will be born first, from under the pubic bone.

"Now don't push, Betty," she continued, "I want this baby to come slowly. The slower the better.

"The baby's legs will be curled up. I will want to rotate the baby to ensure the best position for delivery, but also the pull of gravity as the baby's body hangs from the vulva will help to maintain flexion of the head. This will be important."

The buttocks were born, and with infinite care Sister inserted a hand and hooked her fingers over the flexed legs.

"Don't push, Betty, whatever you do," said Sister Bernadette.

The legs slid out easily. It was a little girl. A long section of cord also slid out. It was pulsating quite vigorously – one could see it, there was no need to feel it.

"The baby is still fully attached to the placenta," Sister said, "and its life blood is coming through the cord. Even though the body is half born, until the head is born, or, at any rate, until the nose and mouth are clear to breathe, the baby depends upon the placenta and this cord for life."

I found it spooky that this tortuous, pulsating thing was absolutely essential to life, and said, "Shouldn't we push it back?"

"Not necessary. Some midwives do, but I really think there is no advantage to be gained."

Another contraction came, and with it the baby's body slid out as far as the shoulders.

Towels had been placed over the screen by the fire to warm. Sister asked for one and wrapped it firmly around the baby's body, saying as she did so, "The purpose of this is twofold: firstly the baby must not be allowed to get cold. Most of her body is now exposed, and if the shock of cold air makes her gasp, she will inhale amniotic fluid, which could be fatal. Secondly, the towel gives me something to grip hold of. The baby is slippery, and I have to turn her another one quarter circle so that the occiput will be under the pubic bone. I will do this as I deliver the shoulders."

With the next contraction, the left anterior shoulder impinged upon the pelvic floor, and Sister delivered it by hooking a finger under the arm, and at the same time rotating the body a little clockwise. The right shoulder was delivered in the same manner, and both baby's arms were out. Only the head remained inside the mother.

"You have a little girl," Sister said to Betty, "but from the size of her limbs I don't think she is six weeks premature. I think you got your dates wrong. I want you, Betty, to push now with all your strength and really use every contraction for delivery of the baby's head. Doctor may have to exert some supra-pubic pressure, but I would prefer it if you could push the head out by yourself."

There had been no contractions for a full three minutes, and I was beginning to feel tense and anxious, but Sister was relaxed. The baby was supported by her hands, and then she let go completely, so that it was hanging quite unsupported. I gasped in horror.

"This is the correct thing to do," Sister explained. "The weight of the baby's body will gently pull the head down a little, and will increase the flexion of the head, which is what I want. About thirty seconds like this will be enough. It will not hurt the baby."

Then she took hold of the baby again. I must say I felt relieved. A contraction came on.

"Now push, Betty, as hard as possible."

Betty did, but the head did not descend any more. Sister and Dr Turner agreed that with the next contraction he would exert supra-pubic pressure, and if that did not prove effective, a low forceps delivery of the head would be necessary. Sister explained to me, "That is because the cord will be compressed between the head and the sacral bones. The baby is all right at the moment, but if it goes on for too long, that is more than a few minutes, there is a definite risk of asphyxia."

I clenched my fingers with shock and anxiety, but Sister remained completely calm. Another contraction came, and the doctor placed his hands on Betty's abdomen just above the pubic bone and pressed down firmly. Betty groaned with pain, but there was a definite movement of the head.

"I am going to use the Mauriceau-Smellie-Veit method of extraction of the head," Sister explained to me. She was allowing the baby to hang unsupported again, and my heart was in my mouth.

"With the next contraction, all being well, we will have the airways clear, and the baby will be able to breathe. I will want my Sim's vaginal speculum, so be ready to pass it when I need it."

I looked to see where the Sim's was on her delivery tray. My hands were trembling so much that for a ghastly moment I imagined I would knock the whole tray over, or pick up the Sim's only to drop it on the floor.

Another contraction came on, and the doctor exerted the same pressure on Betty's abdomen. Sister placed her right hand over the shoulders of the baby and the fingers of her left hand into the vagina. I could see her gently moving her fingers and feeling for something. The baby was resting on her forearm.

"I am trying to hook my index finger into the mouth of the baby, in order to maintain flexion of the head, so that the mouth and nose will be the first part of the head to encounter the air. It is *not* to exert pressure by pulling. If you ever use this method of delivery, nurse, remember that. If you try pulling, you risk dislocating the jaw."

I felt sick with fear, and just hoped to God that I would never have to deliver a breech. I could see that she was manipulating the back of the skull with her right hand. She explained, "I am simply pushing upwards on the occipital protuberance of the skull to increase flexion. A little more pressure, please doctor, if you can, and I think I shall have the airways clear. That's it. The Sim's now, nurse, please."

I had to grip my wrist with my other hand to stop it trembling. All I could think was, I mustn't drop it, I mustn't drop it. My relief when I handed it over was so great that I almost laughed.

But there was more to see.

The chin of the baby was now on the perineum and Sister carefully inserted the speculum into the vagina, pushing the posterior wall backwards, rather like using a shoe-horn, so that the baby's nose and mouth were exposed. She asked for a swab, which I handed to her, and she wiped the baby's nose and mouth free of mucus.

"Now she will be able to breath, and will no longer be dependent upon the placental blood supply."

It was astonishing to hear a gasp, followed by a tiny cry. The baby's face could not be seen, yet her voice could be heard.

"That's what I like to hear," said Sister. "Did you hear that, Betty?"

"Not 'alf. Is she all right, poor little thing? I reckons as how she's goin' through it as much as what I am."

"Yes. Your baby's quite safe now, and with the next contraction she will be born, I assure you. I think you have a torn perineum, but I can't see it because it's behind the speculum, nor can I do anything about it, because if I remove the speculum your baby will not be able to breathe."

Another contraction was coming. "This is it," I thought with some relief. Delivery of the head had so far taken only twelve minutes, but it had seemed like an eternity to me.

The contraction was strong, and doctor was exerting considerable pressure. Sister drew the baby's body downwards until the nose was level with the perineum, and then swiftly upwards over the mother's abdomen. The movement took no more than twenty seconds, and the head was delivered. I nearly sobbed with relief.

The baby was blue.

Sister held her upside down by the ankles.

"This blue tinge is not serious," she said. "It is to be expected. I must make quite sure that the airways are clear. When she starts to breathe strongly and regularly the colour will improve. Pass me the mucus catheter, will you, please?"

I was not trembling any more, so was able to do this without fear of dropping it.

Sister inverted the baby, and held her in her left arm. She then inserted the catheter into the baby's mouth and sucked very gently at the other end to draw any fluid or mucus away. One could hear a bubbling sound as fluid entered the catheter. She then cleared each nostril in the same way. The baby gave two or three big gasps, and coughed, then cried. In fact she let out a tremendous scream. Her colour rapidly changed to pink.

"That's a lovely noise," observed Sister. "A few more screams like that will make me happy."

The baby obliged, and screamed lustily.

The cord was clamped and cut, and the baby wrapped in warm dry towels and handed to Betty.

"Oh she's lovely," exclaimed Betty, "bless 'er li'l heart. She's worth all the pain in the world."

It's a miracle, I thought. The mother literally forgets the agony she has been through the moment she holds her baby.

"It's Christmas Day," remarked Betty. "We must call her Carol."

"That's a lovely name," said Sister. "Now we must get the placenta out, and I think you had better stay where you are because there is a tear, as I thought, and it will be easier for the doctor to stitch you up in this position."

Doctor was drawing up a syringe and said to Sister: "I am going to give ergometrine now, to promote the expulsion of the placenta."

She nodded.

I did not ask why. It was not normal practice to give ergometrine in those days, unless there was undue delay of the third stage, or severe bleeding, or an incomplete placenta. As I noted earlier, oxytocic drugs may be given routinely today, immediately after delivery of the baby.

Within a couple of minutes a contraction came on, and the placenta plopped out into the kidney dish held by the Sister.

"Right, I'll hand over to you, doctor." she said. You can take my place, now."

This was easier said than done though. Sister tried to get up, but couldn't. She gave a gasp of pain.

"My legs! I can't feel them. I've got pins and needles."

Not surprising, poor thing! She had been kneeling on the floor for over half an hour, in the same position, concentrating wholly on the work she was doing.

"I can't move. You'll have to help me, my legs have completely gone to sleep."

The gallant doctor put his arms round her and pulled. She must have been a dead weight, because he made no impression. Ivy and I joined in, pushing and pulling. We were all laughing. Eventually we hoisted Sister to her feet, and got her stamping and moving her legs. Bit by bit the circulation and the nerve supply restored the function, and she was able to stand without help.

The doctor opened his suture case and scrubbed up again. He asked me to hold his torch, so that he had a direct light on to the tear. He anaesthetised the area with a local, and then examined it thoroughly.

"It's not too bad, Betty," he said. "I'll soon have you stitched up, and it will have healed within a couple of weeks. I want to examine you internally, though, to make sure that the cervix is not torn also, because this can sometimes happen in a breech delivery."

He inserted two fingers into the vagina and felt all around. He explained to me, "The breech is smaller in diameter than the head. Therefore the cervix may be sufficiently dilated to allow the passage of the breech, but not relatively open enough to allow the free passage of the head. This will obviously be one of the occasions when the cervix may tear. If that occurs, the mother will have to be transferred to hospital, because I do not have the facilities here to repair a cervix. However," he continued in a confident voice, "you are lucky, Betty, there is nothing torn inside you. I just have to put a few stitches on the outside." He selected his catgut and needle. He pulled the muscle together with forceps, and with a few circular movements of the wrist had made a neat repair. It only took a few minutes.

"There we are. That's that. Now let's get you back into bed, so you will be more comfortable."

Meantime, Sister had been examining the baby. "She weighs five and a half pounds, Betty. Your little Carol is certainly not six weeks premature. She may be two weeks premature, but you must have been a month out with your dates. You must keep a better record next time."

"Next time!" exclaimed Betty. "That's a good 'un. There won't be a next time. One breech delivery's enough for me."

The baby was out of danger, and the mother comfortable, and so Sister Bernadette and the doctor prepared to leave. I was left to clear up, bath the baby, and write up the notes. On her way downstairs, Sister had to shout through the crowd to get hold of Dave in order to tell him that he had a little daughter. Through the closed doors we in the delivery room heard the shouts of congratulations, and the strains of "For He's a Jolly Good Fellow".

"Who's a jolly good fellah?" said Betty. "Dave? Well, I like the sauce!" She cuddled her baby happily, and laughed.

Dave came up at once. He looked flushed, and only slightly the worse for wear, but he was proud and happy. He took Betty in his arms. I had found many East End men to be barely articulate, but not Dave. He was not a wharf manager for nothing.

"Yer wonderful, Betty, and I'm proud on yer." he said. "A Christmas babe's a miracle, and I reckons as how we can't forget this one's birthday. I reckons we should call her Carol."

He took the baby and then, with alarm, said: "Cor, ain't she little! I think I might break her. You'd best have her back, Betty."

Everyone laughed, as Carol had that moment given a little whimper and puckered her face.

I was aware that the sounds from downstairs had changed. The noise of the party had subsided, and we could all hear shuffling and whispers and giggles outside on the landing. Dave said to me: "They are all there, wanting to come and see the baby. When can they come, do you think?"

I could see no good reason why they should not do so; after all, this was not a hospital. So I said, "I will finish cleaning up with Ivy, and when I'm bathing the baby the children can come in. I'm sure they would like that. In the meantime I will need more hot water brought up."

Jugs of hot water arrived, and Ivy and I quickly cleaned up Betty and got her ready for visitors. Then I placed a tin bath on a chair by the fire and prepared water at the right temperature for the baby. Ivy opened the door, and said, "You can come in, now, but you've got to be quiet and good. Anyone who's naughty will be sent straight out."

Clearly grandmother's word was law with small children. I didn't count the number who entered the room, but probably about twenty little ones filed silently in, with big, round, awestruck eyes. It was a good thing the bedroom was large. They stood around me, sat on the bed, stood on chairs, on the windowsill, anywhere, in order to see. I looked around me with delight, for I like children, and this was an enchanting experience. Ivy told them that the baby's name was Carol.

The baby was lying on a towel on my knee, still wrapped in a flannel sheet. I took a damp swab and wiped her face, her ears, her eyes. She wriggled and licked her lips. A little voice said, "Oo, she's got a li'l tongue, look."

The baby's head was messy with blood and mucus, so I said, "I'm going to wash her hair, now."

A little boy on the windowsill said: "I don't like gettin' my hair washed."

"Shut up, you!" said a little girl bossily.

"Shan't. Shut up yourself, bossy-bum!"

"Oo, I ain't. You wait …"

"Now then," said Ivy with menace in her voice, "one more word from either of you and you'll both go out."

Dead silence!

I said, "Well, I'm not going to use any soap, and it's the soap in your eyes that is nasty."

I held the baby face upwards in my left hand, with her head over the rim of the bath, gently splashed the water over her head, and wiped it with a swab. The main purpose was to get the blood off, and really only to make the baby look more presentable. Most of the vernix or mucus is best left on the skin as a protective covering. I dried her with the towel, and said to the boy on the windowsill, "Now, that wasn't nasty, was it?"

He didn't speak. He just looked at me solemnly, and shook his head.

I loosened the flannel sheet, and the baby lay naked on my knee. There was a united gasp, and several voices cried, "What's that?"

"That is part of the cord," I explained. "When Carol was in her mother's tummy, she had a cord linking her to her mother. Now that she is born, we have cut it off, because she doesn't need it any more. You all used to have a cord where your tummy button is."

Several skirts were pulled up, or trousers down, and several tummy buttons were proudly shown to me.

I took the baby in my left hand, with her head resting on my forearm, and immersed her whole body in the water. She wriggled her tiny limbs, and kicked and splashed. All the children laughed, and wanted to join in.

Ivy said firmly, "Now mind what I says. No noise. You don't want to frighten the baby."

There was instant silence.

I patted the baby dry with a towel, and said, "Now we must put her clothes on."

All the little girls wanted to help, of course. It was just like dressing a doll. But Ivy restrained them, saying they could dress Carol later, when she was a bit bigger. Suddenly, at that moment, there was a piercing scream from a little girl. "It's Percy! It's Percy! He's come to see the baby. He knows, and he wants to say hello."

Overleaf: A midwife bathes a newborn baby, while the mother and elder sister look on. One of the joys of a home delivery was that siblings could welcome their new brother or sister into the family immediately.

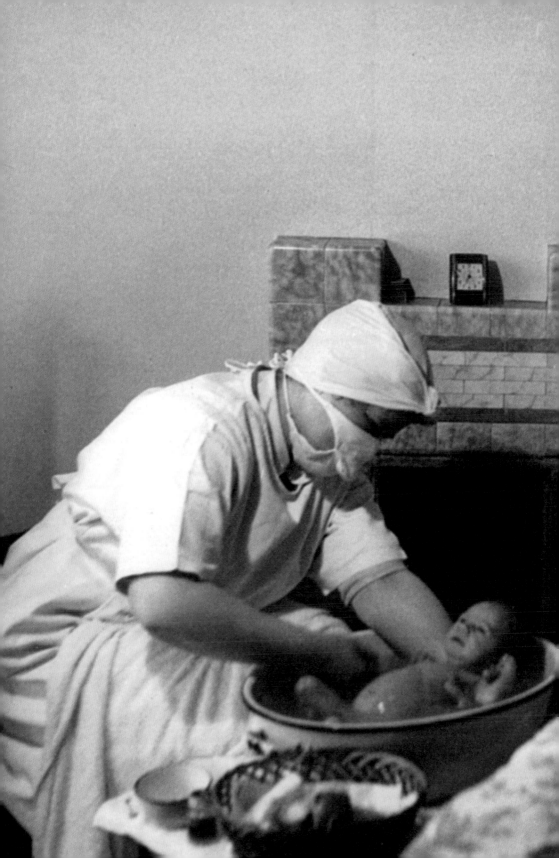

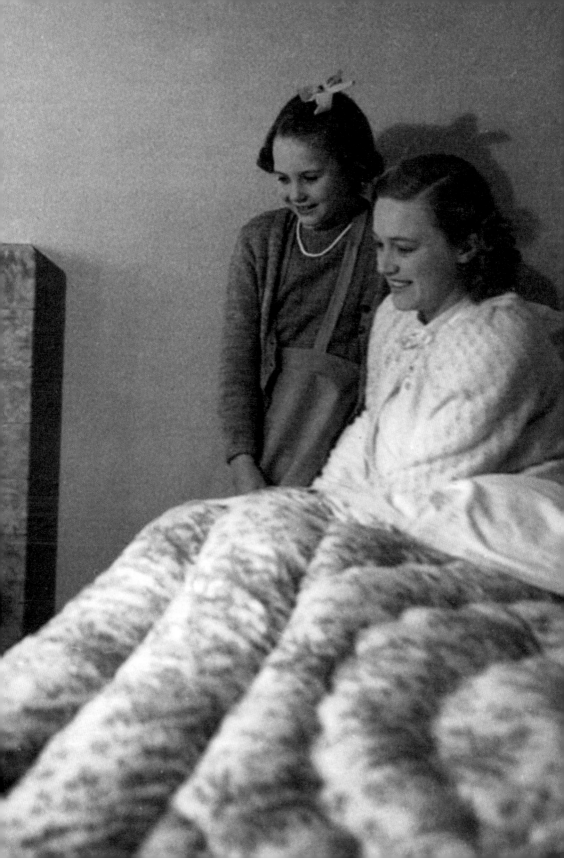

There were shrieks from the children, and Ivy's discipline ruled no more. They were all pointing in one direction, clamouring round something on the floor.

I followed their gaze and, to my astonishment saw, progressing slowly and in a stately manner from under the bed, an exceedingly large tortoise. He looked one hundred years old or more.

Dave roared with laughter. "Of course he wants to see the baby. He knows all about it. He's a clever one, our Perce." He picked the tortoise up, and the children tickled its wrinkled old skin, and felt its hard toenails.

"Perhaps he wants his Christmas dinner an' all. We'll get 'im some, shall us?" Dave said.

Most of the children were now more interested in the tortoise than in the baby, and Ivy wisely said, "Off you go, downstairs, an' see about Percy's Christmas dinner."

The children left and I was told the reason for this apparition. Percy was kept in a cardboard box under the bed to hibernate for the winter. The bedroom was usually cold. The warmth from the fire, and, perhaps, the movements for several hours, must have woken him up, and, thinking it was spring, he had made his appearance. In theatrical terms, his timing was perfect.

It was seven o' clock by the time I had packed up and was ready to leave. But Dave wouldn't let me go. "Come on, nurse. It's Christmas day. You've got to wet the baby's head."

He pulled me towards the back room where the bar was to be found.

"What's yer poison, then?"

I had to think quickly. I had had only half a Christmas lunch, and nothing to eat since then. Spirits would have knocked me out, so I accepted a Guinness and a mince pie. I didn't really want to hang around. The delivery had been a beautiful Christmas experience, but the party was really not my scene. I had loved hearing it in the background, but to be in the midst of all those buxom, hiccupping aunts with their paper hats and red-faced, sweating uncles, was more than I could take at that moment. I just wanted to be alone.

Out in the street, after the excessive warmth of the delivery room, the cold cut me like a knife. It was a cloudless night, and the stars shone brightly. There was very little street lighting in those days, so starlight was a reality. A heavy frost had descended in all its beauty, covering the black stones of the pavements, the walls, the houses, even my bicycle. I shivered, and decided I must pedal very hard to keep myself warm.

Only a mile or two away from Nonnatus House a sudden impulse made me turn right into West Ferry Road and on to the Isle of Dogs. To go all the way round the Isle before rejoining the East India Dock Road is a seven or eight mile ride, and I can't tell you what prompted me to do it.

No one was about. The docks were closed, and the ships in port were silent. The splash of the water was the only sound as I cycled over the West Ferry Bridge. On the Isle there were no lights, apart from the starlight and the Christmas tree lights in the windows of many houses. The great, majestic Thames was on my right, closely guarding all its secrets. I cycled more slowly, as though afraid to break the spell. As I turned westwards, a low moon started to rise, and a silver path shone across the river from Greenwich to my feet, or so it seemed. I had to stop my bicycle. It looked as though I could have walked on silvered feet from the north to the south bank of the Thames.

My thoughts were fleeting and flickering, like the moonlight on the water. What was happening to me? Why was the work so engrossing? Above all, why were the Sisters affecting me so deeply? I remembered my scornful reaction, only twenty-four hours earlier, to the crib in the Chapel, and then the calm beauty of Sister Bernadette's face as she said her daily office by the soft moving flames. I couldn't match the two up. I couldn't understand. All I knew was that I couldn't dismiss it.

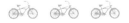

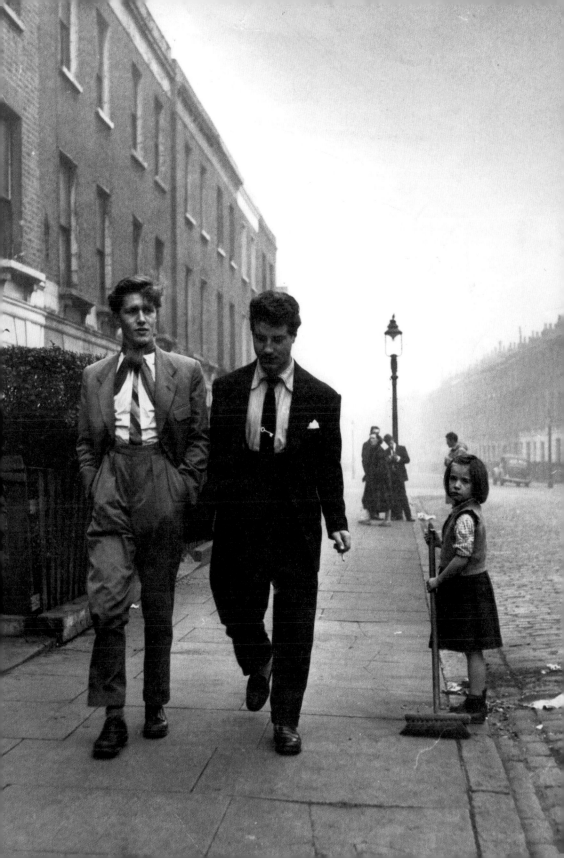

JIMMY

"Is that Jenny Lee? Where the hell have you been hiding all this time? We haven't heard from you in months. I had to get on to your mother to find out where you were. She said you are a midwife in a convent. I had to tell her, gently, that nuns don't do it, so she must be wrong, but she wouldn't listen. What? You are? You must be mad! I've always said you had a screw loose somewhere. What? You can't talk? Why not? The house phone reserved for expectant fathers! Look, that's not funny. All right, all right! I'll hang up, but not till you agree to meet us at the Plasterer's Arms on your evening off. Thursday? OK that's a date. Don't be late."

Dear Jimmy! I had known him all my life. Old friendships are always the best, and childhood friends are very special. You grow up together, and know the best and the worst of each other. We had played together for as long as I could remember, then left home and gone our separate ways, only to meet again in London. Jimmy and his friends came to all the parties and dances organised in the various nurses' homes to which I was attached, and I joined their fraternity in sundry pubs in the West End when I could. It was an excellent arrangement, because they could guarantee meeting lots of new girls, and I could enjoy their company without any commitment.

I had no boyfriends at all when I was young. This was not (I hope) because I was unattractive or boring or sexless, but because I was so in love with a

Opposite: "Dress was rather formal in the 1950s", and not just for women. Young men, like Jennifer's friend Jimmy, often wore suits out, just like the men in this photograph (1954).

man I couldn't have, and for whom my heart ached more or less all the time. For that reason no other male held the slightest romantic interest for me. I enjoyed the company and conversation of my men friends, and their lively and wide-ranging minds, but the mere idea of a physical relationship with any man other than the one I loved was abhorrent to me. In consequence I had a great many friends, and was in fact very popular with the boys. In my experience nothing arouses a young man's interest more than the challenge of a pretty girl who for some inexplicable reason does not appear to find him the sex symbol of the century!

Thursday evening came. It was nice to be stepping up west for a change. I had found life with the sisters and the work in the East End so unexpectedly absorbing that I hadn't wanted to go anywhere else. However, the chance to dress up couldn't be resisted. Dress was rather formal in the 1950s. Long full skirts that flared outwards at the hem were in vogue; the smaller the waist and the tighter the waistband the better, irrespective of comfort.

Nylon stockings were fairly new, and had seams that, *de rigueur*, had to be straight up the back of the leg. "Are my seams straight?" was a girl's constant worried whisper to her friends. Shoes were killers, with five to six inch steel-capped stiletto heels and excruciating pointed toes. It was said that Barbara Goulden, the top fashion model of the day, had had her little toes amputated in order to squeeze her feet into them. Like all the smartest girls of the day, I would totter around London in those crazy shoes, and wouldn't have been seen dead in anything else.

Careful make-up, hat, gloves, handbag, and I was ready.

There was no underground beyond Aldgate then, so I had to take a bus along the East India Dock Road and Commercial Road to pick up the tube. I have always loved the top front seat of a London bus, and to this day I maintain that no transport, however expensive or luxurious, can possibly offer half so much by way of scenery, advantaged viewing point and leisurely locomotion. There is endless time to absorb the passing scenes, perched high above everyone and everything. So my bus ambled along its route, and my mind wandered to Jimmy and his friends, and the occasion when I had very nearly got myself thrown out of nursing, had I been found out.

The hierarchy was very strict in those days, and behaviour, even off-duty, was closely monitored. Except for organised social events, boys were *never* allowed in the nurses' home. I even remember one Sunday evening, when a young man had called for his girlfriend. He rang the bell and a nurse opened the door. He gave the name of the girl he wanted, and the nurse went off to find her, leaving the front door open. It was raining quite heavily, so the young man stepped inside and stood waiting on the doormat. It so happened that the Home Sister passed at that moment. She stood stock-still, rooted to the spot, and stared at him. She drew herself up to her full 4 foot 11 inches and said, "Young man, how dare you enter the nurses' home! Kindly go outside, at once."

So intimidating were these hospital sisters of the old school, and so absolute was their authority, that the young man meekly went outside and stood in the rain, whereupon the Sister shut the door.

My behaviour over Jimmy and Mike would certainly have merited instant dismissal from the nurses' training school, and very likely the profession altogether. I was working at the City of London Maternity Hospital at the time. Early one evening, after I had come off duty, I was called to the only phone in the building.

"Is that the fascinating Jenny Lee with the fantastic legs?" a smooth voice purred.

"Come off it, Jimmy. What's up? And what do you want?"

"How could you be so cynical, my dear? You grieve me more than I can say. When have you got an evening off? Tonight! What good luck! Could we meet at the Plasterer's Arms?"

Over a convivial pint it all came out. Jimmy and Mike shared a nominal flat in Baker Street, but what with one thing and another, such as girls, beer, clothes, fags, the flicks, the occasional horse, Lady Chatterley (the communal car), and other sundry essentials, there was never quite enough money to pay the rent. The landlady who, of course, was a dragon, was lenient when the rent was two or three weeks in arrears, but when it slipped to six or eight weeks with no money forthcoming, she started breathing fire. One evening the boys returned to find all their clothes gone, and a note stating they would get them back when the arrears had been paid.

They sat down with pencil and paper, and worked out that the replacement value of their clothes would be less than the eight weeks of rent outstanding, so their course of action was obvious. At three o'clock in the morning they slipped quietly out of the house, leaving their keys on the hall table, and spent the rest of the night in Regent's Park. It was a fine September evening, and after a reasonable sleep they stepped jauntily off to work, congratulating each other on an excellent plan well executed. They reckoned they could continue such a *modus vivendi* indefinitely, and thought what fools they had been ever to have paid rent to that dragon of a landlady in the first place.

Jimmy was training to be an architect, while Mike was a structural engineer. They were both attached to the best firms in London (such training in those days was based on the old apprentice system, and students were not college based). Though they could wash and shave in the public lavatories, they could not change their clothes (they had none), and a smart London firm would not tolerate its staff turning up for work day after day covered in autumn leaves! After about a fortnight they began to think that another plan would have to be formulated. Unfortunately, both had an entire wardrobe of clothes still to purchase, so money was very tight.

A third pint was ordered as we discussed the problem. Jimmy asked, "Isn't there perhaps a boiler room or something like that in the nurses' home where we could camp out for a little while?"

Old friends are old friends. I did not even consider the risk I would be taking. I said, "Yes there is, although it's not a boiler room. It's the drying room at the top of the building. All the water tanks are in it, and it's used for drying clothes. I think there's a sink in it too."

Their eyes lit up. A sink! They could wash and shave in comfort!

"As far as I know," I continued "it's only used in the daytime – not at night. There is a fire escape that goes up the back of the building, and presumably there will be a window or door from the drying room on to the fire escape. It's probably locked from the inside, but if I opened it for you, you could get in. Let's go and have a look."

We had another pint or two before leaving for the nurses' home in City Road. The boys went round the back to the fire escape, and I entered the front door. I went straight to the drying room, and found that the slide windows opened easily from the inside. I signalled to my friends below, and each of them in turn climbed the iron ladder. It was not a staircase, just a ladder fixed to the wall, and the drying room was on the sixth floor. Normally, such a climb would be hair-raising but, fortified by several pints, it proved no trouble at all to the boys, and they entered the drying-room jubilantly. They hugged and kissed me, and called me a "brick".

I said, "I don't see why you shouldn't stay here, but don't come before about ten at night, and you must leave before six each morning so that no one sees you. You must keep quiet, too, because I will be in trouble if you are found."

No one ever found out, and they stayed in the drying-room of the nurses' home for about three months. How they managed that terrifying fire-escape in the middle of winter at six o'clock in the morning I shall never know; but when you are young and full of life and vitality, nothing is a problem.

The cry "Aldgate East – all change" broke into my reverie. I found my way to the familiar pub. It was a glorious June evening when the endless daylight lingered on and on – the kind of evening that fills you with gladness. The air was warm, the sun shone, the birds sang. It was good to be alive. By contrast the enclosed atmosphere of the pub seemed dark and gloomy. This was usually our favourite hostelry. This evening the beer was right, the time was right, the friends were right, but, somehow, the venue didn't feel quite right. We chatted a bit, drank a few glasses, but I think we were all feeling a bit restless.

Suddenly someone shouted out, "Hey! Let's all go down to Brighton for a midnight swim!"

There was a chorus of approval.

"I'll go and get Lady Chatterly."

This was the name given to the communal car. Who now remembers the furore that surrounded the proposed publication of *Lady Chatterley's Lover* by D. H. Lawrence, written in the 1920s, and the court case brought against the publishers for intending to make widely available an "obscene publication"? All that happens in the book is that the lady of the manor has an affair with the gardener, but the case went to the High Court and some pompous QC is on record as having said to a witness, "Is this the sort of book you would allow your servants to read?"

After that Lady Chatterley became synonymous with illicit pleasures and millions of copies of the book were sold, making the publishers' fortune.

Lady Chatterley was not a family car, but an obsolete 1920s London taxi. She was magnificent and huge, and on occasion actually achieved a speed of forty mph. The engine had to be coaxed into life with a starting handle, inserted beneath the elegant radiator. Considerable muscle power was needed, and the boys usually took it in turns to do the cranking. The front bonnet opened like two huge beetle wings when it was required to get at the engine and four majestic coach lamps shone on either side of the fluted radiator. There were running boards from front to back. The wheels were spoked. The capacious interior smelled of the best leather upholstery,

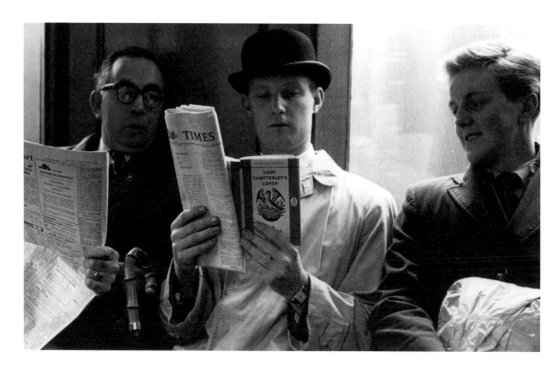

Above: Jimmy named his car after the protagonist in D. H. Lawrence's novel *Lady Chatterley's Lover.* This photograph was taken on the day the book went on general sale again after a 33-year ban (1960).

polished wood and brass. She was their pride and joy. The boys garaged her somewhere in Marylebone, and spent all their spare time coaxing her frail old engine into life, and titivating her majestic body.

But there was still more to Lady Chatterley. Chimney pots had been added and flower boxes attached. The windows were curtained, which meant that the driver couldn't see out of the rear window, but no one bothered about little things like that. The car also boasted brass door knockers and letter-boxes. Her name was painted in gold across the front, and a notice at the rear read: DON'T LAUGH, MADAM, YOUR DAUGHTER MAY BE INSIDE.

She was brought round to the pub, and everyone turned out to admire her. A few of the original enthusiasts had dropped out, but a crowd of about fifteen climbed into Lady Chatterley and she set off, amid cheers, at a steady twenty-five mph down Marylebone High Street. The evening was exquisite, warm and windless.

The declining sun looked as though it never really would decline altogether, it being already about 9 p.m. The plan included a midnight swim in Brighton, near the West Pier, then back to London with a stop at Dirty Dick's – a transport café on the A23 – for bacon and eggs.

Roads in the 1950s were not as they are today. To begin with we had to get out of central London by weaving our way through miles of suburbs – Vauxhall, Wandsworth, the Elephant, Clapham, Balham, and so on. It wasn't quite endless, but it took a couple of hours. Once through the suburbs the driver called out, "We're on the open road now. Nothing to stop us till we get to Brighton."

Nothing, that is, except the temperament of Lady Chatterley, who tended to overheat. Forty mph was her maximum, and she was being driven at that speed for too long. We had to stop at Redhill, Horley (or was it Crawley?), Cuckfield, Henfield and numerous other '-fields' so that she could rest and cool down. Tempers inside the Hackney carriage were becoming as frayed as the upholstery. The sun, which we had thought would never desert us, had relentlessly crept around to the other side of the globe, leaving us girls chilly in our flimsy summer dresses. The boys at the front called out, "Only another couple of miles. I can see the South Downs on the horizon."

Eventually, after a five-hour journey, we crawled into Brighton at about 3 a.m. The sea looked black, and very, very cold.

"Right," cried one of the boys. "Who's for a swim? Don't be chicken. It's lovely once you get in."

The girls were less optimistic. A midnight swim conceived in the warmth and security of a London pub is a very different thing from a 3 a.m. swim in the cold, black reality of the English Channel. I was the only girl who did swim that night. Having come all that way, I was not going to be beaten!

The pebbles of Brighton beach are nasty at the best of times, but if you happen to be wearing six-inch stiletto heels, they are murder. We had planned to swim in the nude, but no one had thought of what we might use for towels. It had been a cold winter and early spring, but nobody had thought about the temperature either.

About six of us stripped off, and with falsely jolly shouts to cheer each other on, we plunged into the sea. Normally, I love swimming, but the cold stabbed like a knife, taking my breath away, and brought on an asthma attack that lasted for the rest of the night. I swam a few strokes, then crawled out of the sea, gasping for breath. I sat on the wet pebbles shivering with

Overleaf. Jimmy drove Jennifer and her friends to Brighton (c. 1940/50s) in 'Lady Chatterley' for an intended midnight swim.

145

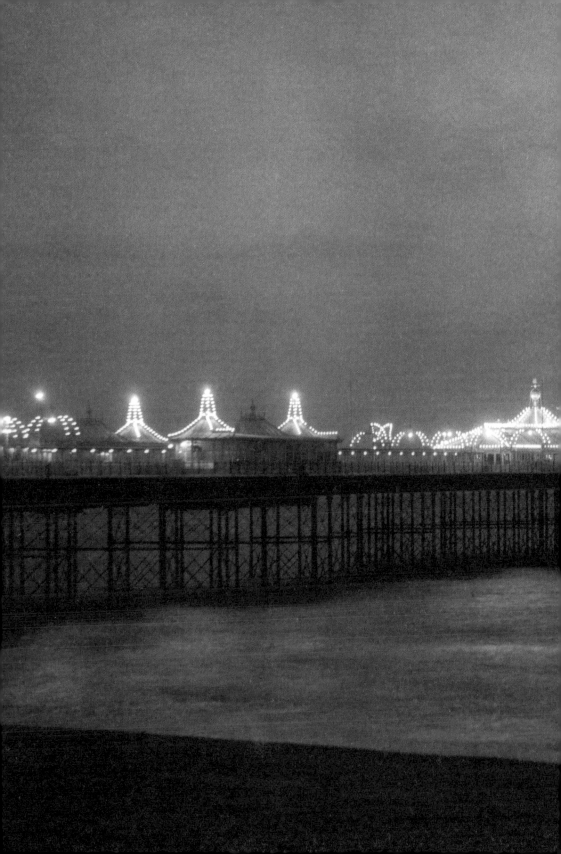

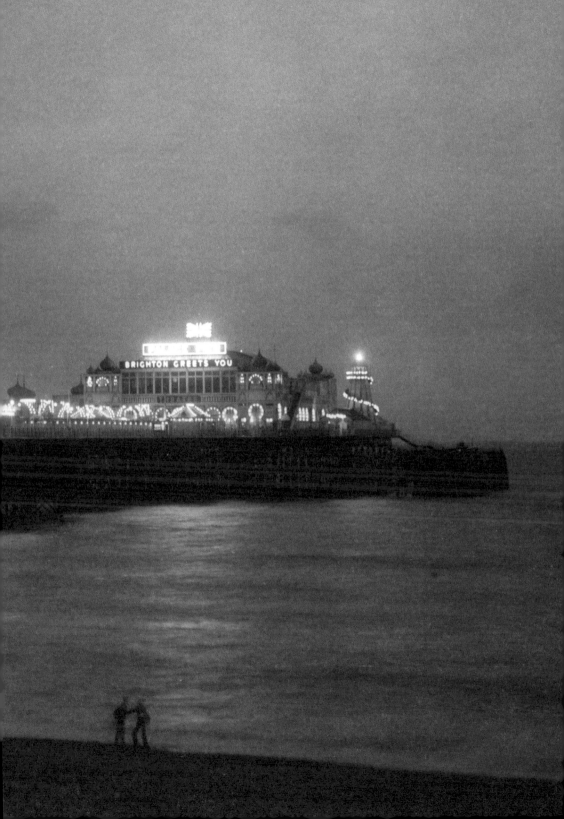

cold. I had nothing to dry myself with, nothing to wrap around me. What a fool I had been! Why did I get myself into these crazy situations? I tried to dry my shaking shoulders with a small lace handkerchief. No help. My lungs were on fire, and air just didn't seem to go into them. Some of the boys were really enjoying themselves, tumbling about with one another. I envied their vitality. I hadn't even the strength to crawl back up the beach to the car.

Jimmy came out of the water, laughing and throwing seaweed at someone. He walked towards me. We couldn't really see each other as he threw himself on the pebbles beside me, but at once he sensed that something was wrong. Perhaps he could hear me wheezing. His gaiety left him, and he became kind, concerned, thoughtful, as I had always known him when he was a little boy.

"Jenny! What's up? You're ill. You've got asthma. Oh, my dear, you are frozen. Let me dry you with my trousers."

I couldn't answer. I could only fight for breath.

He wrapped his trousers around my back and rubbed hard. He gave me his shirt with which to dry my face and wet hair, and dried my legs with his socks and underpants. He had kept his vest dry, and he put it on me, as I had none of my own. He helped me into my thin cotton dress, then put his shoes on my feet, and helped me walk up the beach to the car. His own clothes were soaking wet, but he seemed impervious to this.

Everyone was sleeping in Lady Chatterley, sprawled about all over the place, and there was nowhere for me even to sit. Jimmy soon dealt with that. He shook a boy.

"Wake up, and move over. Jenny's having an asthma attack. She needs somewhere to sit down."

Then, to another: "Wake up there, and take your jacket off. I need it for Jenny."

Within minutes he had procured a corner for me to sit comfortably and a jacket to place around my shoulders. He woke another lad, and took his jacket to put over my legs. He did it all with charm and ease, and everyone liked him so much that no one grumbled. Not for the first time I reflected on what a pity it was that I couldn't love Jimmy. I had always liked him, but no more than that. I had love for only one man, and this had eclipsed the possibility of loving anyone else.

Eventually we started back for London. The boys who had been swimming were in high spirits, invigorated by the swim and bantering with each other.

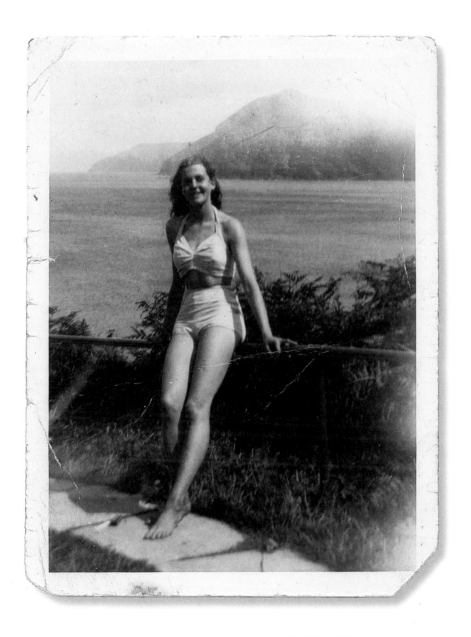

Above: Jennifer in the early 1950s. Throughout her life, she loved the sea.

All the girls were sleeping. I sat, leaning forward, elbows on my knees, by an open window, trying to get my lungs working properly again. There were no nebulisers in those days; the only treatment was the breathing exercises I was doing. An asthma attack usually passes in the end. Death from asthma is a new phenomenon related to modern living – indeed we used to say "no one dies from asthma".

A beautiful midsummer dawn was breaking as we left Brighton. We made our slow, majestic way north, several times stopping to let Lady Chatterley cool down. At the foot of the North Downs she refused to go any further.

"Everyone out. We'll have to push," cried the driver, gaily. It was all right for him. He would be sitting at the steering wheel, or so he thought.

The sun was well up, and the summer morning spread over the countryside. We all climbed out of the vehicle. Worried that the physical effort of pushing might bring on another attack of asthma, I said, "I'll take the wheel. You can push. You are stronger than me, and you don't get asthma."

I sat at the wheel of Lady Chatterley while the others pushed her up the North Downs. My heart went out to those poor girls in their stiletto heels pushing all that way, but there was nothing I could do about it, so I simply enjoyed the ride.

The rest must have done the old lady good because, over the crest, as we freewheeled down, she gave a deep cough of contentment, and the engine purred into life. We continued back to London with no further troubles. We were all working that morning, mostly starting at 9 a.m. I was supposed to be on duty at 8 a.m., miles away in the East End. I got back to Nonnatus House just after ten o'clock expecting serious trouble. But, once again, I realised how much more liberal the nuns were than the inflexible hospital hierarchy. When I told Sister Julienne about the night's adventures I thought she would never stop laughing.

"It's a good thing we are not busy," she commented. "You had better go and get a hot bath and a good breakfast. We don't want you down with a cold. You can start your morning's round at eleven o'clock, and sleep this afternoon. I like the sound of your Jimmy, by the way."

A year later Jimmy got a girl into trouble and married her. He could not support a wife and child on his apprentice pay, so he left his training in the fourth year and took a job as a draughtsman with a suburban county council.

About thirty years later, quite by accident, I bumped into Jimmy in a Tesco's car park. He was staggering under the weight of a huge box, walking beside a large, cross-looking woman carrying a potted plant. She was talking incessantly in a rasping voice that assailed my ears before I even noticed them. He had always been slight, but now he looked painfully thin. His shoulders were stooped, and a few grey hairs were brushed across his bald head.

"Jimmy!" I said as we came face to face. His pale blue eyes looked into mine, and a thousand memories of the fun of a carefree youth instantly sparked between us. His eyes lit up, and he smiled.

"Jenny Lee!" he said, "After all these years!"

The woman poked him heavily in the chest with her thumb, and said, "You come along with me, and don't hang about. You know the Turners are coming round tonight."

His pale eyes seemed to lose all their colour. He looked at me despairingly and said, "Yes, dear."

As they left, I heard her say, suspiciously: "Who is that woman, anyway?"

"Oh, just a girl I used to know in the old days. There was nothing between us, dear."

He shuffled off, the epitome of the hen-pecked husband.

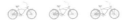

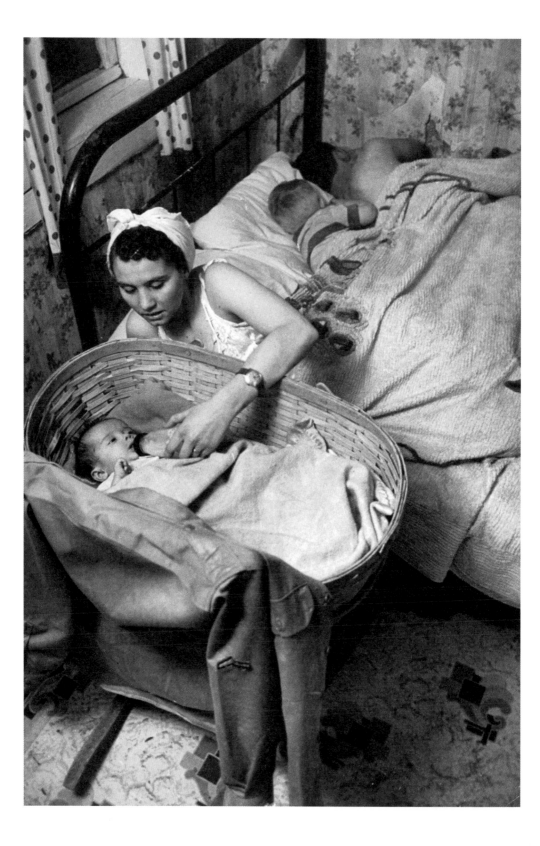

LEN AND CONCHITA WARREN

L arge families may be the norm, but this is ridiculous, I mused as I ran through my day list. The twenty-fourth baby! There must be some mistake. The first digit is wrong. Not like Sister Julienne to make a mistake. My suspicions were confirmed when I got out the surgery notes. Only forty-two years old. It was impossible. I'm glad someone else can make mistakes as well as me, I thought.

I had to make an antenatal visit to assess the mother and the viability of the house for a home delivery. I never liked doing this. It seemed such an impertinence to ask to see people's bedrooms, the lavatory, the kitchen, the arrangements for providing hot water, the cot and the linen for the baby, but it had to be done. Things could be pretty slummy, and we were used to managing in fairly primitive conditions, but if the domestic arrangements were really quite unviable, we reserved the right to refuse a home delivery, and the mother would have to go to hospital.

Mrs Conchita Warren is an unusual name, I thought as I cycled towards Limehouse. Most local women were Doris, Winnie, Ethel (pronounced Eff) or Gertie. But Conchita! The name breathed "a beaker full of the warm South … with beaded bubbles winking at the brim"*. What was

Opposite: A mother tends to her baby, while her husband and child sleep on.

---

* F rom John Keats, "Ode to a Nightingale".

a Conchita doing in the grey streets of Limehouse, with its pall of grey smoke and the grey sky beyond?

I turned off the main road into the little streets and, with the help of the indispensable map, located the house. It was one of the better, larger houses – on three floors and with a basement. That would mean two rooms on each floor, and one basement room, leading into a garden – seven rooms in all. Promising. I knocked on the door, but no one came. This was usual, but no one called out "Come in, luvvy". There seemed to be a good deal of noise inside, so I knocked again, harder. No reply. Nothing for it but to turn the handle and walk in.

The narrow hallway was almost, but not quite, impassable. Two ladders and three large coach prams lined the wall. In one, a baby of about seven or eight months slept serenely. The second was full of what looked like washing. The third contained coal. Prams were very large in those days, with huge wheels and high protective sides and I had to turn sideways to squeeze myself past. Washing flapped overhead, and I pushed it aside. The stairway to the first floor was straight ahead and was also festooned with washing. The sickly smell of soap, dank washing, baby's excreta, milk, all combined with cooking smells was nauseating to me. The sooner I get out of this place the better, I thought.

The noise was coming from the basement, yet I could see no steps down. I entered the first room off the hallway. This was obviously what my grandmother would have called "the best parlour", filled with her best furniture, knick-knacks, china, pictures, lace, and, of course, the piano. It was only used on Sundays and on special occasions.

But if *this* fine room had ever been anyone's best parlour the proud housewife would have wept to see it. About half a dozen washing-lines were attached to the picture rail just below the cornices of a beautifully plastered ceiling. Washing hung from each of them. Light filtered through a single faded curtain that appeared to be nailed across the window, screening this front room from the street. It was obviously impossible to draw this curtain back. The wooden floor was covered with what looked like junk. Broken radios, prams, furniture, toys, a pile of logs, a sack of coal, the remains of a motorcycle, and what seemed to be engineering tools, engine oil and petrol. Apart from all this, there were scores of tins of household paints on a bench, brushes, rollers, cloths, pots of spirit, bottles of thinners, rolls of wallpaper, pots of dried out glue, and another ladder. The curtain was pinned up with a safety pin by about eighteen inches at one corner, allowing sufficient light to reveal a new Singer sewing machine on a long table. Dressmaking patterns, pins, scissors, and cotton were scattered all over the table, and also, quite unbelievably, there was some very fine, expensive silk material. Next to the table stood a dressmaker's model. Also hard to believe, and the only thing that would have resembled my grandmother's front parlour, was a piano that stood against one of the walls. The lid was open, revealing filthy yellow keys, with several of the ivories broken off, but my eyes were riveted by the maker's name – Steinway. I couldn't believe it – a Steinway in a room like this, in a house like this! I wanted to rush over and try it, but I was looking for a way down to the basement, where the noise was coming from. I closed the door, and tried the second room off the hallway.

This room revealed a doorway that led down to the basement. I descended the wooden stairs, making as much clatter and noise as I could, as no one knew I was there and I didn't want to alarm anyone. I called out "Hello" loudly. No reply. "Anyone there?" I called, fatuously. There was obviously someone there. Still no reply. The door was ajar at the bottom, and there was nothing for it but to push it open and walk in.

Immediately there was a dead silence and I was conscious of about a dozen pairs of eyes looking at me. Most of them were the wide innocent eyes of children but amidst them were the coal-black eyes of a handsome woman with black hair hanging in heavy waves past her shoulders. Her skin was beautiful – pale, but slightly tawny. Her shapely arms were wet from the washing tub, and soap clung to her fingers. Although obviously engaged in the endless household chore of washing, she did not look slovenly. Her figure was large, but not over-large. Her breasts were well supported, and her hips were large, but not flabby. A flowered apron covered her plain dress, and the crimson band which held back the dark hair accentuated the exquisite contrast between skin and hair. She was tall, and the poise of her shapely head on a slender neck spoke eloquently of the proud beauty of a Spanish Contessa, with generations of aristocracy behind her.

She did not say a word. Neither did the children. I felt uncomfortable, and started babbling on about being the district midwife, and getting no reply when I knocked, and wanting to see the rooms for a home confinement. She did not reply. So I repeated myself. Still no reply. She just gazed at me with

Overleaf: A father plays with his baby and children.

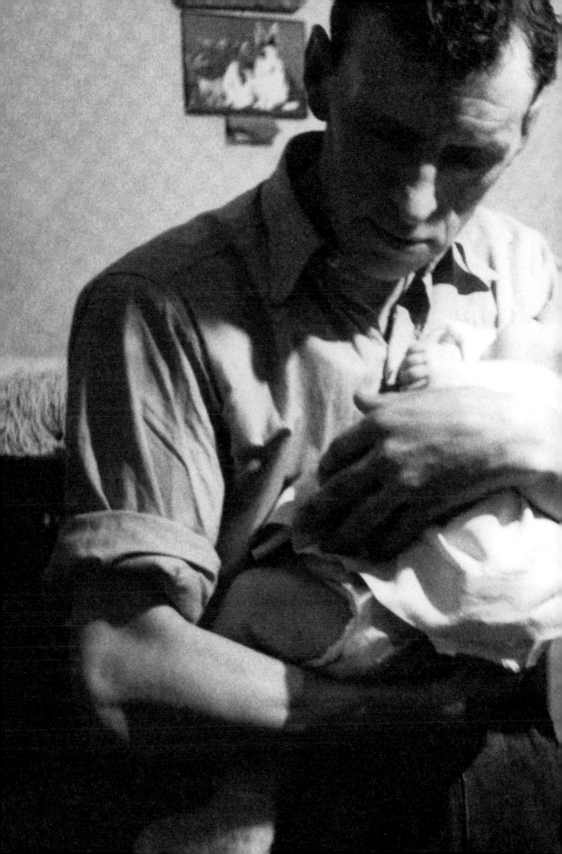

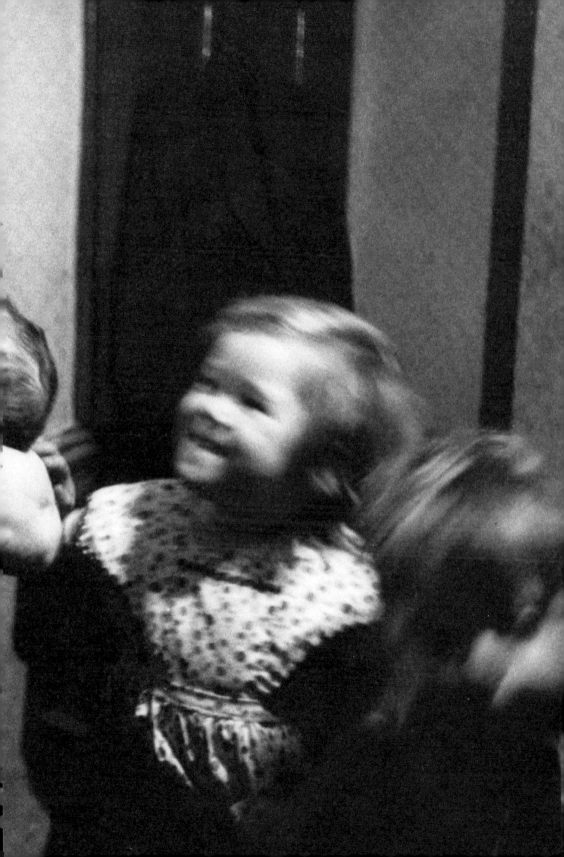

calm composure. I began to wonder if she was deaf. Then two or three of the children began talking to her, all of them at once, in rapid Spanish. An exquisite smile spread across her face. She stepped towards me and said, "*Si. Bebe.*" I asked if I might look at the bedroom. No reply. I looked towards one of the children who had spoken, a girl of about fifteen. She spoke to her mother in Spanish, who said, with gracious courtesy and a slight inclination of her sculptured head, "*Si.*"

It was clear that Mrs Conchita Warren spoke no English. In all the time that I knew her the only words that I heard her speak, apart from dialogue with the children, were "*si*" and "*bebe*".

The impression this woman made upon me was extraordinary. Even in the 1950s that basement would have been described as squalid. It contained, haphazardly, a stone sink, washing, a boiler bubbling away, a mangle, clothes and nappies hanging all over the place, a large table covered with pots and plates and bits of food, a gas stove covered with dirty saucepans and frying pans, and a mixture of unpleasant smells. Yet this proud and beautiful woman was completely in control and commanded respect.

The mother spoke to the girl, who showed me upstairs to the first floor. The front bedroom was perfectly adequate: a large double bed. I felt it – no more sagging than any other. It would do. There were three cots in the room, two wooden dropsided cots, a small crib, two very large chests of drawers and a small wardrobe. The lighting was electric. The floor covering was lino. The girl said, "Mum's got it all ready here," and pulled open a drawer full of snowy white baby clothes. I asked to see the lavatory. There was more than that. There was a bathroom – excellent! That was all I needed to see.

As we left the main bedroom I peered briefly into the room opposite, the door of which was open. Three double beds appeared to be crammed into it, but there was no other furniture at all.

We descended two flights to the kitchen, our feet clattering on the wooden stairs. I thanked Mrs Warren and said that everything was most satisfactory. She smiled. Her daughter spoke to her and she said: "*Si.*" I needed to examine the woman and take an obstetric history, but obviously I could not do that if we could not understand each other, and I did not feel that I could ask one of the children to interpret. I therefore resolved to make a repeat visit when her husband would be at home. I asked my little guide when this would be, and she told me "in the evening". I asked her to tell her mother I would come back after six o' clock, and left.

I had several other visits that morning, but my mind continually drifted back to Mrs Warren. She was so unusual. Most of our patients were Londoners who had been born in the area, as had their parents and grandparents before them. Foreigners were rare, especially women. All the local women lived a very communal life, endlessly engaged in each other's business. But if Mrs Warren spoke no English, she could not be part of that sorority.

Another thing that intrigued me was her quiet dignity. Most of the women I met in the East End were a bit raucous. Also there was her Latin beauty. Mediterranean women age early, especially after childbirth, and by custom used to wear black from head to foot. Yet this woman was wearing pretty colours, and did not look a day over forty. Perhaps it is the intense sun that makes southern skins age, and the damp northern climate had preserved her skin. I wanted to find out more about her, and intended asking some questions of the Sisters at lunch time. I also wanted to tease Sister Julienne about writing the "twenty-fourth pregnancy", when she really meant the fourteenth.

Lunch at Nonnatus House was the main meal of the day, and a communal meal for the Sisters and lay staff alike. The food was plain, but good. I always looked forward to it because I was always hungry. Twelve to fifteen of us sat down each day at the table. After grace was said I introduced the subject of Mrs Conchita Warren.

She was well known by the Sisters, although not a lot of contact had ever been made because of her lack of English. Apparently she had lived in the East End for most of her life. How was it, then, that she didn't speak the language? The Sisters did not know. It was suggested that perhaps she had no need, or no inclination to learn the language, or perhaps she just wasn't very bright. This last suggestion was a possibility, as I had noticed before that certain people can completely disguise a basic lack of intelligence simply by saying nothing. My mind flitted to the Archdeacon's daughter in Trollope, who had the whole of Barchester society and London at her feet, praising her beauty and bewitching mind, when in fact she was profoundly stupid. She achieved this enviable reputation by sitting around on gilded chairs, looking beautiful and saying not one word.

"How did she come to be in London at all?" I asked. The Sisters knew the answer to this one. Apparently Mr Warren was an East Ender, born into the life of the docks, and destined for the work of his father and uncles.

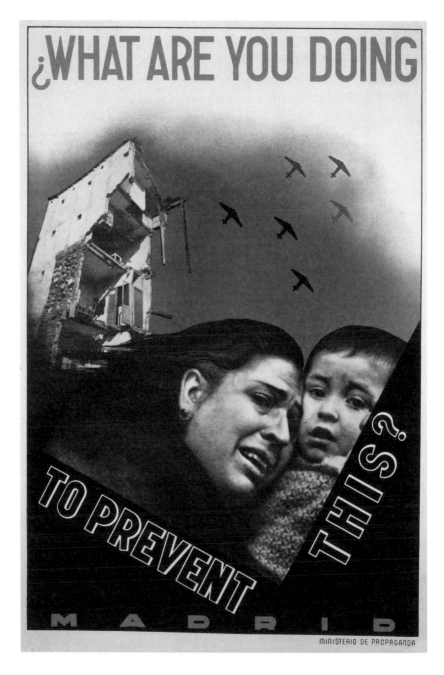

Above: A Spanish Civil War poster, issued by Ministerio de Propaganda, depicting a tearful mother and child while aircraft fly overhead, with the caption "What are you doing to prevent this?" (c.1937).

But when he was a young man, something had made him a rebel. He was not going to be cast into any mould. He cut loose, and went off to fight in the Spanish Civil War. It is doubtful if he had the faintest idea of what he was doing, as foreign affairs rarely penetrated the consciousness of working people in the 1930s. Political idealism could have played no part in it and whether he fought for the Republicans or the Royalists would have been immaterial. All he wanted was youthful adventure, and a war in a remote and romantic country was just the stuff.

He was lucky to survive. But survive he did, and came home to London with a beautiful Spanish peasant girl of about eleven or twelve. He returned to his mother's house with the girl, and they obviously lived together. What his relatives or neighbours thought of this shocking occurrence can only be conjectured, but his mother stuck by him, and he was not one to be intimidated by a pack of gossiping neighbours. Anyway, they could hardly send the girl back, because he had forgotten where she came from and she didn't seem to know. Quite apart from this, he loved her.

When it was possible, he married her. This was not easy, because she had no birth certificate and was not sure of her surname, date of birth, or parentage. However, as she had had three or four babies by then and looked about sixteen, and as she was presumably Roman Catholic, a local priest was persuaded to solemnise the already fecund relationship.

I was fascinated. This was the stuff of high romance. A peasant girl! She certainly didn't look like a peasant. She looked like a princess of the Spanish court, whom the Republicans had dispossessed. Had the brave Englishman rescued her and carried her off? What a story! Everything about it was unusual, and I looked forward to meeting Mr Warren that evening.

Then I remembered the children. I said to Sister Julienne, saucily, "I've caught you out in a mistake at last. You put in the day book the twenty-fourth pregnancy when you must have meant the fourteenth."

Sister Julienne's eyes twinkled. "Oh no," she said, "that was no mistake. Conchita Warren really has had twenty-three babies, and is expecting her twenty-fourth."

I was stunned. The whole story was so preposterous that no one could possibly have made it up.

The door was open when I returned to their home so I stepped in. The house was literally teeming with young people and children. I had seen only very young children and a girl in the morning. Now all the schoolchildren were home, as well as several older teenagers who had presumably returned from work. It seemed like a party, they all looked so happy. Older children were carrying tiny ones around, some of them were playing out in the street, some of them were doing what might have been homework. There was absolutely no discord among them and in all the contact I had with this family no fighting or nasty temper was ever in evidence.

I squeezed past the ladder and the prams in the hallway, and was directed down to the basement kitchen. Len Warren was sitting on a wooden chair by the table, comfortably smoking a roll-up. A baby was on his knee, another crawled along the table, and he had to keep pulling him back by his pants to prevent him falling off. A couple of toddlers sat on his foot and he was jigging them up and down singing, "Horsey, horsey don't you stop". They were screaming with laughter, and so was the father. Laughter lines creased his eyes and nose. He was older than his wife, about fifty-ish, not at all good-looking in the conventional sense, but so frank and open, so downright pleasant-looking, that it did your heart good to see him.

We grinned at each other, and I told him that I wanted to examine his wife and take some notes.

"That's OK. Con's doing the supper, but I spek she can leave it to Win."

Conchita was calm and radiant, standing by the boiler, which in the morning had been doing the washing and was now cooking an enormous quantity of pasta. Copper boilers were common in those days. They were tubs, large enough to contain about twenty gallons, standing on legs, with a gas jet underneath. A tap at the front was the means of emptying them. They were intended for washing, and this was the first time I had seen one used for cooking, but I surmised that this would be the only way of catering for such a huge family. It was sensible and practical, if unusual.

"Here, Win, you tek over the supper, will you, love? Nurse wants a look at yer mum. Tim, come 'ere, lad, you tek the baby, an' keep them two away from the boiler. We don't want no accidents in vis 'ouse, do we now? An' Doris, love, you lends a hand to our Win. I'll tek yer mum and the nurse upstairs."

The girls spoke rapidly to their mother in Spanish, and Conchita came towards me, smiling.

We went upstairs, Len chatting all the time to different children, "Now then Cyril, now then. Let's get that lorry off them stairs, shall we, there's a good lad. We don't want the nurse to break 'er neck, do we nah?

"Good on yer, Pete. Doin yer 'omework. He's a scholar, our Pete. He'll be a professor one of these days, you'll see.

"'allo, Sue, my love. Got a kiss for yer ol' dad, then?"

He very seldom stopped talking. In fact I would say that in all my acquaintance with Len Warren, he never stopped talking. If occasionally he ran out of something to say, he would whistle or sing – and all executed with a thin roll-up in his mouth. These days health workers would be very disapproving about smoking around babies and a pregnant woman, but in the fifties no connection had been made between smoking and ill health, and nearly everyone smoked.

We went into the bedroom.

"Connie, love, the nurse just wants to have a look at your tum."

He smoothed down the bed, and she lay down. He started to pull up her skirt, and she did the rest.

Her abdomen showed stretch marks, but nothing excessive. From appearances, this could have been her fourth pregnancy, not her twenty-fourth. I palpated the uterus – about five to six months.

"Any movements?" I enquired.

"Oh yeah, yer can feel the li'l soul kickin' an' wrigglin'. He's a right little footballer, that one, 'specially at night when we wants 'a get some sleep."

The head felt uppermost, but that was to be expected. I couldn't locate the foetal heart, but with all the kicking described, it hardly mattered.

I examined the rest of her. Her breasts were full, but firm – no lumps or abnormalities. Her ankles were not swollen. There were a few superficial varicose veins, but nothing serious. The pulse was normal, as was her blood pressure. She seemed to be in perfect condition.

I wanted to try to establish her dates. Merely going on clinical observation can be deceptive. A small baby and a large baby of the same gestation can give the appearance of about four to six weeks' difference, so you need some dates to back up observation. However, with a baby of about seven to eight months old downstairs, it seemed unlikely that Conchita had had a period at all. I was not accustomed to asking such delicate questions of a man. In the 1950s such things were never mentioned in what was called "mixed company", and I felt myself blush scarlet.

"Ah, nah, nuffink like that," he said.

"Could you ask her, please; she might not have mentioned it to you."

"Yer can tek it from me, nurse, she ain't 'ad no periods for years."

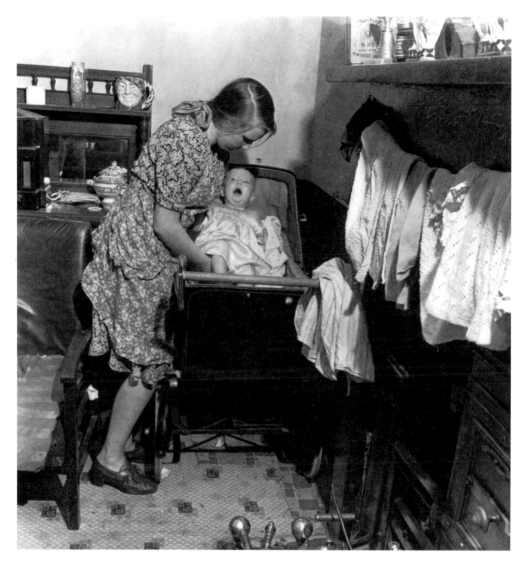

Above: Many families lived in overcrowded conditions in which space was tight and rooms often had several functions – as bedrooms, laundry areas and dining areas, among other things.

I had to leave it at that. If anyone knows, he should, I thought.

I mentioned that we had an antenatal clinic every Tuesday, and we preferred patients to come to the clinic. He looked dubious. "Well, she don't like goin' out, yer know. Not speakin' the lingo an' all, like. And I wouldn't want 'er to get lost or frightened, like. 'Sides, she's got all them babies to look after at home, yer know."

I didn't feel I could insist, so I put her down for home antenatal visits.

In all this time, Conchita hadn't said a word. She just smiled, and submitted passively to being felt and prodded all over, to hearing herself talked about in a foreign language. She got up from the bed with grace and dignity, and moved to the chest of drawers, searching for a hairbrush. Her black hair looked even more beautiful being brushed, and I observed hardly a grey hair. She adjusted the crimson band, and turned with proud confidence to her husband, who took her in his arms and murmured, "There's my Con, my gel. Oh yer looks lovely, my tresher."

She gave a contented little laugh, and nestled in his arms. He kissed her repeatedly.

Such a display of unashamed love between husband and wife was unusual in Poplar. Whatever the relationship in private, the men always kept up a show of rough indifference in front of other people. A good deal of lewd banter often went on between them, which I found very amusing, but they did not openly speak of love. I found the tender, gentle and adoring looks of Len and Conchita Warren very affecting.

I returned many times to the house over the next four months, checking Conchita's progress. I always went in the evenings, in order to speak with Len about the pregnancy. Anyway, I liked his company, liked listening to him talk, enjoyed the atmosphere of this happy family and wanted to find out more about them all. This was not difficult, due to Len's insatiable volubility.

Len was a painter and decorator. He must have been a good one because 90 per cent of his jobs were "up West". "All the nobs' houses" was how he described his work.

Three or four of his elder sons worked with their father in the business, and apparently he was never short of work. With low running costs there must have been quite a bit of money coming into the household. Len worked from home, from his shed in the backyard, where he also kept his barrow.

Workmen in those days didn't have vans or trucks to go around in. They had barrows, usually made of wood, and often home-made. Len's was made out of the chassis of an old pram, with the upholstered pram part removed, and an elongated wooden construction fitted to the highly sprung base. It was perfect. The springs made for lightness of movement, and the huge, well-oiled wheels made it easy to push. When going out to a new job, Len and his sons would load up the barrow with their equipment and push it to the address. They may have had to push for ten miles or more, but that was all part of the job. In that respect, a painter and decorator was lucky, because a job usually lasted a week or so, and they could leave their stuff at the house and go home by tube as far as Aldgate.

Plumbers, plasterers and suchlike were less fortunate. Their jobs usually lasted only a day, so they had to push the tools to the job, and then push them home in the evening. In those days you would see workmen laboriously pushing their barrows all over London. They had to walk on the road, which held up the traffic considerably. But drivers were used to it and just accepted it as part of the London scene.

I once asked Len if he had been called up in the War.

"Nah, 'cos of this Franco-job," he said, pointing to a leg wound that had rendered him unfit for military service.

"Were the family in London all through the war?" I asked.

"Not bleedin' likely, beggin' yer pardon, nurse," he said. "Wouldn' let Jerry get Con an' the kids."

He was shrewd, well informed, and above all enterprising. In 1940 Len had observed the failed strategic bombing of the air bases and ammunition fields. He had seen the Battle of Britain.

"An' I thought to meself, I though', that slippery bugger Hitler, he's not goin' to stop there, he's not. He'll go for the docks next. When the first bomb fell on Millwall in 1940, I knew as how we was in for it, an' I sez to Con, 'I'm gettin' you out of this, my girl, an' the kids an' all.'"

Len didn't wait for any evacuation scheme to come into operation. With typical energy and initiative he took a train from Baker Street out of London to the west, into Buckinghamshire. When he thought he had gone far enough, he got out at what looked to be a promising rural area. It was Amersham, which is almost a London suburb these days, on the Metropolitan Line. But in 1940 it was truly rural, and remote from London. Then he quite simply trudged around the streets, knocking at doors, telling the householders he met that he had a family he wanted to get out of London, and had they got a room they could let to him?

"I must 'ave called at 'undreds of places. I reckons as how they thought I was mad. They all sez no. Some didn't speak, jes' shut the door in my face and said nuffink. But I wasn't goin' to be put off, not by no one. I just reckons as how someone's goin' to say 'yes' some time. You jes' gotta stick with it, Len lad, I says to meself.

"It was gettin' late. I'd spent the whole day trudgin' round, 'aving doors shut in me face. I can tell you, I was feelin' down, an' all. I was goin' back to the station. I tells you, I was that depressed. I went down a road of shops with flats above 'em. I shan't never forget it. I hadn't knocked at any flats, only houses that looked like what they'd got a lo' of rooms in 'em.

"There was a lady, I shall never forget her, goin' into one o' the doors next to a shop, like, an' I just says to her 'you haven't got a room I could have, have you lady? I'm desperate.' An' I tells her, an' she says 'yes'.

"That lady was an angel," he said reflectively. "Without her, we'd be dead, I reckons."

It had been a Saturday. He had arranged with the lady that he would pack up his household on the Sunday, and move in on the Monday. This they did.

"I told Con and the kids we was goin' on 'oliday to the country."

He simply told their landlord they were moving out. They left all their furniture and only took what they could carry.

The accommodation the lady gave them was called the back kitchen. It was a fairly large stone-floored room on the ground floor leading to a small backyard with access both to the flats above, and to the shop at the side. It contained a sink, running cold water, a boiler, and a gas stove. There was a large cupboard under the stairs, but no heating, and no power point for an electric heater. There was, however, an electric light and an outdoor lavatory. There was no furniture. I don't know what Conchita thought of it all, but she was young and adaptable. She was with her man and her children and that was all that mattered to her.

They lived there for three years. Len made a few trips back to London to collect what furniture and essential bedding he could bring on his barrow. Very soon his mother came to join them.

"Well, I couldn't leave the old gel back there for Jerry to get, could I now?"

Apparently his mother passed most of the day and each night in an armchair in a corner. The older children went to school. Len took a job as a milkman. He had never handled a horse before, but it was a docile old creature that knew the round, and with native quickness Len soon learned, and whistled his way around the roads. The children came with him when they could and felt like King of the Castle sitting up behind the horse.

Conchita looked after her children, and did the lady's washing and cleaning. It was a good arrangement all round. Two more babies were born. It was when they were expecting the ninth baby that the local evacuation authorities decided Len's family needed more room, and they were allocated two rooms, a kitchen and bathroom.

It sounds pretty grim today – just two rooms for three adults and eight children, but in fact they were lucky. The times were hard, and one sees on old newsreels pathetic pictures of train loads of East End children with labels and a small bag being shunted out of London. Thanks to their father, the Warren children were not separated from their parents throughout the entire war.

Len and Conchita's children were beautiful. Many of them had raven black hair and huge black eyes like their mother. The older girls were stunners, and could easily have been models. They all talked in a curious mixture of Cockney and Spanish when together. With their mother they spoke only Spanish; with their father, or any other English person, pure Cockney. I was very impressed by this bilingual facility. I wasn't able to get to know any of them very well, principally because their father never stopped talking, and entertaining me with his chatter. The only girl I did have contact with was Lizzy, who was about twenty and a very skilled dressmaker. I have always loved clothes, and became a regular client of hers. Over several years she made me some beautiful garments.

The house was always crowded, but there was never any discord as far as I could see. If an argument arose among the younger children, the father would say good-humouredly, "Nah ven, nah ven, le's 'ave none of vis," and that would be that. I have seen internecine fighting between siblings, especially in overcrowded conditions, but not between the Warren children.

Where they all slept was a mystery to me. I had seen one bedroom with three double beds in it. Presumably the two bedrooms on the upper storey were the same, and they all slept together.

In the last month of Conchita's pregnancy I visited weekly. One evening Len suggested I had a bit of supper with them. I was delighted. It smelled good and, as usual, I was hungry. I was not at all squeamish about eating food cooked in the boiler that had been used in the morning for washing the baby's nappies, so I accepted with pleasure. Len said, "I reckons as 'ow the nurse would like a plate, like. You get 'er one, will you, Liz love?"

Liz piled some pasta on to a plate for me, and gave me a fork. It was only then that Conchita revealed her peasant origins. All the rest of the family ate from the same dish. Two large shallow bowls, the old-fashioned toilet bowls that used to be found in every bedroom, were filled with pasta and placed on the table. Each member of the family had a fork and ate from the communal bowl. I alone had a separate plate. I had seen this once before when I was living in Paris, and had spent a weekend with an Italian peasant family who had moved to the Paris area to try to find work. They all ate from a single dish in the middle of the table in just the same way.

The time came for Conchita's confinement. There were no dates to go by, and therefore no certainty when she was due, but the baby's head was well down and she looked near the end of term.

"I'll be glad when we gets this baby out. She's getting tired. I won't go to work no more, the lads can do the job. I'll stop here, and look after Con and the kids."

This he did, to my amazement. In those days no self-respecting East Ender would demean himself by doing what he would call "women's work". Most men would not lift a dirty plate or mug from the table, nor even pick their dirty socks up off the floor. But Len did everything. Conchita lay in bed late in the mornings, or sat in a comfortable chair in the kitchen. Sometimes she played with the little ones, but Len was always watching, and if they got too boisterous, he firmly took them away and amused them elsewhere. Sally, the girl of fifteen, who had left school but not yet gone out to work, was there to help him. Nonetheless, Len could do everything – change nappies, feed toddlers, clear up messes, shopping, cooking, and the endless washing and ironing. And all this was accompanied by singing or whistling and unfailing good humour. Incidentally, he was the only man I have ever met who could roll a fag with one hand and feed a baby with the other. Conchita's twenty-fourth baby was born at night. A phone call came through at about 11 p.m. that the waters had broken. As fast as I could I pedalled along to Limehouse, because I guessed it would be a quick labour. I was not wrong.

I found everything in perfect readiness. Conchita was lying on clean sheets, with the brown paper and a rubber sheet under her. The room was warm, but not too hot. The baby's crib and baby clothes were all waiting. Hot water was boiling in the kitchen. Len was sitting beside her, massaging her stomach, her thighs, her back, and her breasts. He had a cold flannel with which to wipe her face and neck, and with every contraction he took her in his arms and held her tight. He murmured encouraging noises. "That's my girl. That's my lass. Won't be long now. I've gocher. Jus' hold on to me."

I was startled to see him there. I had expected to see a neighbour, or his mother, or an elder daughter. I had never seen a man at a delivery before, apart from a doctor. But in this, as in everything else, Len was exceptional.

A glance told me Conchita was very near the second stage. I gowned up quickly, and laid out my tray. The foetal heart was steady, and the head barely palpable. It must have been already down on the pelvic floor. As the waters had broken, I did not do a vaginal examination, because any such intrusion could risk infection, and, unless absolutely essential, should be avoided. The contractions were coming about every three minutes.

Conchita was sweating, and moaning slightly, but not excessively. She smiled at her husband between each contraction, and relaxed completely in his arms. She had had no sedation.

We did not have long to wait. A change came over her facial expression, that of intense concentration. She gave a grunt of effort and with the next push, the whole baby slid out at once. It was a small baby, and delivery was so quick I had no time to do anything more than catch the child. The little thing was just lying there on the sheet with no help from me. I cleared the airway, and Len handed me the cord clamps and the scissors. He knew exactly what to do. He could have delivered the baby himself, I thought. The placenta came out fairly quickly also, and there was no excessive bleeding.

Len wrapped the baby tenderly in warm towels, and placed her in the crib. He called downstairs for hot water, and gave the message that a little girl had been born. Then he washed his wife all over, and deftly changed the sheets. He brushed her black hair, and put a white hair band on her, to match her white nightie. He called her his pet, his love, his treasure. She smiled dreamily at him.

He called downstairs for one of his children, "Here, Liz, you take these bloody sheets, and put them in the boiler, will yer, love. Then we might think about a nice cup of tea, eh?"

Then he turned back to his wife, and took the baby from the cradle, and handed it to her. She smiled contentedly, touching the baby's little head, and kissing its wee face. She didn't say anything, just chuckled with contentment.

Len was ecstatic, and started talking non-stop again. During Conchita's labour he had hardly said a thing. It was the only time I had ever known him to be silent for so long. But now nothing could stop him.

"Oh, look at her. Jes look at 'er, nurse. Isn' she beau'iful? Look at 'er li'l hands. See, she's got fingernails. Oh, she's openin' her li'l mouth. Oh, you li'l swee'heart, you. See, she's got long eyelashes, like 'er mum. She's jes perfick."

He was as excited as a young father with his first baby.

He called all the other children up, and they all sat round their mother, talking in a mixture of Spanish and English. Only the toddlers were asleep. The rest of the house was awake and excited.

I packed up my equipment and slipped silently out of the room, feeling that the unity and happiness of the family would be all the greater if I was not there. Len saw me leave and courteously came out with me. As we left, I noticed that the conversation behind us slipped into Spanish.

He thanked me for all I had done, although I had done virtually nothing. As he carried my bag downstairs, he said: "Let's have a nice cup o' tea together, shall us nurse?".

He chatted happily all the time we had our tea. I told him how much I liked and admired his family. He was a proud father. I told him how impressed I was that they all spoke Spanish so fluently.

"They're a clever lot, my kids, they are. Cleverer than their old dad. I never could pick up the lingo, meself."

Quite suddenly, with blinding insight, the secret of their blissful marriage was revealed to me. She couldn't speak a word of English, and he couldn't speak a word of Spanish.

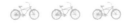

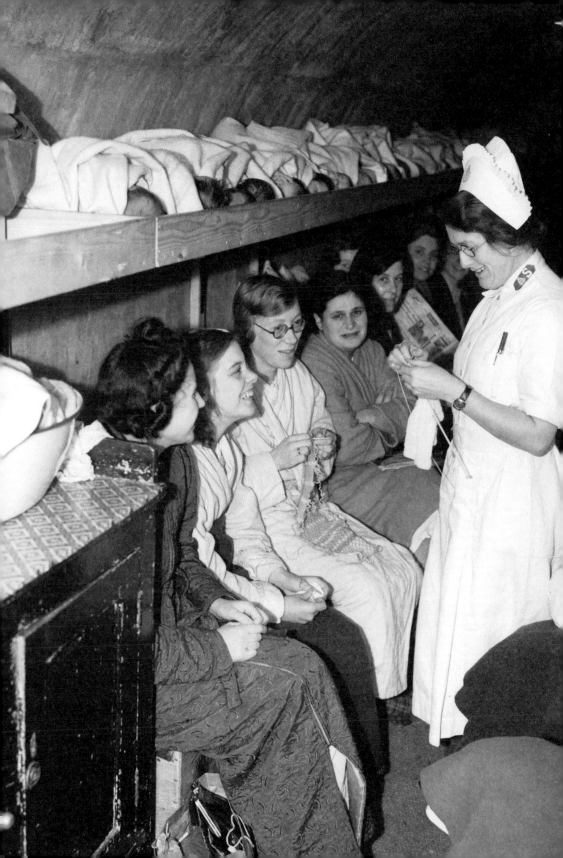

SISTER MONICA JOAN

"Light is the higher plane – life is the lower – light becomes Life. There is a fiery flash, a vision granted, a golden moment of offering."

I could listen to her all day – the beautiful modulated voice, the moving hands, the hooded eyes, the arch of her haughty eyebrows, the drape of her veil as she turned her long neck. She was over ninety, and her mind was going, but I was utterly captivated.

"Shining questions, infinite response, the astro-mental plane of man lies in the etheric. The outer darkness is a monstrous dragon, with its tail in its mouth. Did you know?"

I sat at her feet, bewitched, and shook my head, not daring to speak in case I broke the spell.

"This is the cosmic body, the critical point, the translation of parallelisms running to the neutral centre of the disappearing point. Have you seen the clouds pass and float and roll as planets do? And so we see Him come, pierced. I am the thorn that pierced His brow. Can you smell burning, my dear?"

"No. Can you?"

"I think that Mrs B.'s ahrimanic unconsciousness has prompted her to make a cake. Let us go with God in all things. I think we should investigate, don't you?"

Opposite: In the Second World War, everyone had to take cover in air-raid shelters – no matter how young they were. Here mothers, children and babies (on a shelf) gather together during the Blitz in East London (1940).

I would rather have continued listening to her talk, but I knew that once the spell had been broken, there would be no going back – for the time being – and the smell of cake for Sister Monica Joan was irresistible. She smiled appreciatively. "That smells like one of Mrs B.'s honey cakes. Come on, get a move on, don't just sit there."

She jumped up, and with quick, light steps, head held high, back straight, she sped towards the kitchen.

Mrs B. turned as she entered. "Hello, Sister Monica Joan, you're a bit early. They're not done yet. But I've kept the bowl for you to scrape, if you wants to."

Sister Monica Joan pounced on the bowl as though she had not eaten for a fortnight, scraping with the big wooden spoon, and licking both sides with murmurs of delight.

Mrs B. went over to the sink and took a wet cloth. "Nah ven, Sister, you got it all over your habit, an' a bit on your veil, an' all. Wipe your fingers, there's a good girl. You can't go to Tierce like that, can you? And the bell will go any minute."

The bell sounded. Sister Monica Joan looked round quickly, and winked.

"I must go. You can wash the bowl now. Oh the delight in Heaven as the spheres move, and the tiny grains of sand touch the stars. The Phoenix rises from the living flame, and Ceres cries ... don't forget to keep the crispy ones for me."

She tripped out of the kitchen as Mrs B. fondly opened the door for her.

"She's a caution, she is. You wouldn't fink she'd been in the Docks all through two world wars, and the Depression, would you? She's delivered thousands of our children. In the Blitz she wouldn't leave. She delivered babies in air-raid shelters and church crypts, an' once in what was left of a bombed house. Bless 'er. If she wants the crispy ones, she can 'ave 'em."

I had heard stories like that so often, from so many people – her years of selfless work, her dedication, her commitment. Sister Monica Joan was known and loved throughout Poplar. I had heard that she was the daughter of a very aristocratic English family who were scandalised when she announced in the 1890s that she was going to be a nurse. Wasn't her sister a Countess, and her mother a Lady in her own right? How could

Opposite: Sister Monica Joan qualified as a midwife in the 1900s and was one of the first in the country. Like this midwife, she probably would have reached her patients by bicycle.

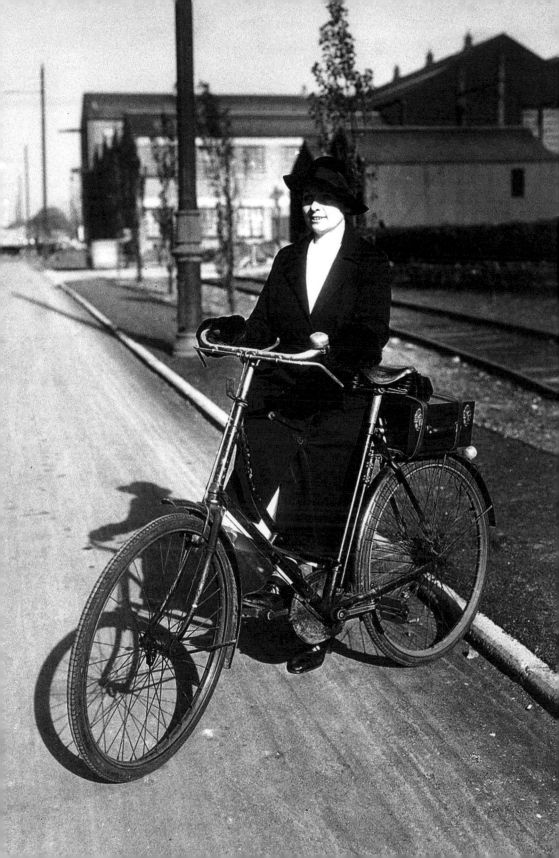

she disgrace them so? Ten years later, when she qualified as one of the first midwives in the country, they remained silent in their displeasure. But they cut her off altogether when she joined a religious order and went to work in the East End of London.

Lunch was the one occasion during the day when we all met together. Most monastic orders take their meals in silence, but talking was permitted at Nonnatus House. We stood until Sister Julienne came in and said grace, after which we all sat. Mrs B. would bring in the trolley and usually Sister Julienne would serve, with one other person carrying the plates around. Conversation that day was general: Sister Bernadette's mother's health; the two guests due to arrive at teatime.

Sister Monica Joan was peevish. She couldn't eat a chop, due to her teeth, and she didn't like the mince. Cabbage she could never abide. She would wait for the pudding.

"Do have a little mashed potato, dear, with some onion gravy. You know how you like Mrs B.'s onion gravy. You need the protein, you know."

Sister Monica Joan sighed, as though all the injustice of the world had been heaped upon her,

"'Stop and consider! Life is but a day – A fragile dew-drop on its perilous way.'"

"Yes dear, I know, but a little mashed potato wouldn't go amiss."

Sister Evangelina paused, fork in hand, and snorted, "What's that about a dew drop?"

Sister Monica Joan lost her peevishness, and said, sharply, "Keats, my dear, John Keats. Our greatest poet, though perhaps you don't know. Uh-oh, I shouldn't have said anything about dew-drops. It was a slip of the tongue."

She took out a fine lawn handkerchief, and held it delicately to her nose. Sister Evangelina was beginning to turn red around the neck.

"Your tongue slips a great deal too often, if you ask me, dear."

"No one was asking you, dear," Sister Monica Joan addressed the wall, very, very quietly.

Sister Julienne intervened. "I've put a few fresh carrots on your plate also. I know you like carrots. Did you know that the Rector has seventy-two young people from the youth club in his confirmation class this year? Just imagine! That, on top of all their other work, will keep the curates busy."

Everyone murmured interest and approval of the size of the confirmation class, and I watched Sister Monica Joan push the carrots around her plate with her forefinger. Such compelling hands, all bones and veins covered with transparent skin. Her nails were usually long, because she couldn't be bothered to cut them, and resisted anyone else doing so. The forefingers on both hands were astonishing. She could bend the first joint, keeping the rest of the finger quite straight. I sat quietly watching, and tried to do it myself, but couldn't. She got some gravy on her fingertip, and licked it off. She seemed to like it and brightened a little. She dipped her finger again. Meanwhile, conversation had turned to the forthcoming jumble sale.

Sister Monica Joan took up her fork, and ate all the potato and gravy, but not the carrots, then pushed her plate away from her with a hard-done-by sigh. She had obviously been thinking. She turned to Sister Evangelina and said loudly, but in the sweetest tone, "Keats may not be your cup of tea, but do you admire Lear, dear?"

Sister Evangelina looked at her with justifiable suspicion. Instinct told her there was a trap, but she had neither verbal skill nor wit, only a heavy, ponderous sort of honesty. She walked straight into the trap. "Who?"

It was the worst thing she could have said.

"Edward Lear, dear, one of our greatest comic poets, 'The Owl and the Pussy Cat', you know. I thought perhaps you might particularly admire 'the Dong with the Luminous Nose', dear."

There was a gasp around the table at this piece of effrontery. Sister Evangelina's face turned red all over, and the moisture began to glisten. Someone said "Pass the salt, please", and Sister Julienne asked quickly if anyone would like another chop. Sister Monica Joan looked archly at Sister Evangelina, and murmured to herself, "Oh dear, now we are back to Keats and dewdrops." She took out her handkerchief and started to sing "Ding Dong Bell, Pussy's in the Well", as though to herself.

Sister Evangelina nearly exploded with impotent rage, and scraped back her chair. "I think I can hear the telephone; I will go and answer it," she said, and left the refectory.

The atmosphere was tense. I glanced sideways at Sister Julienne, wondering what she would do. She looked exceedingly cross, but could say nothing to Sister Monica Joan in front of us all. The other Sisters looked down at their plates, discomfited. Sister Monica Joan sat erect and haughty, her hooded eyes closed. Not a muscle moved.

I had often wondered about her. Her mind was obviously going, but how much was senility, and how much downright naughtiness? This gratuitous, unprovoked attack on Sister Evangelina was a piece of premeditated malice. Why did she do it? Her history of selfless dedication in over fifty years of nursing the poorest of the poor would imply saintliness. Yet here she was, deliberately humiliating her Sister in God in front of the entire staff, including Mrs B., who had just brought in the pudding.

Sister Julienne rose, and took the tray. Serving the pudding caused the diversion she needed. Sister Monica Joan knew that disapproval was in the air. Generally she was served first with pudding, and given a choice, but on that occasion she was served last. She sat aloof, seeming not to notice. On any other occasion she would have complained bitterly, gobbled up her pudding, and asked for more. But not today. Sister Julienne took up the last bowl, placed some rice pudding in it, and quietly said, "Hand that to Sister Monica Joan, if you please." Then she said, "I will go and see Sister Evangelina, if you will all excuse me. Sister Bernadette, would you please say the closing grace?"

She rose, said a private grace, crossed herself, and left the room.

There were a few desultory remarks about the prunes being a little tough, and would it, or would it not rain for the evening visits, but we all felt a little uncomfortable, and were glad when the meal was over. Sister Monica Joan stood up with a regal toss of her head, and crossed herself elaborately as grace was said.

Poor Sister Evangelina! She was not a bad sort, and certainly did not deserve the torment she got from Sister Monica Joan. Her nose was a trifle red, admittedly, but by no stretch of the imagination could it be described as "luminous". She was heavy and plodding, both in mind and body. Her big flat feet clumped about. She banged things down on the table, rather than putting them down. She flopped down into a chair, rather than sitting down. I had seen Sister Monica Joan observing all these characteristics with pursed lips, drawing in her skirts as the heavy feet passed. She, so light, so dainty, who moved with such grace, seemed unable to tolerate the other's physical shortcomings, and called her the washerwoman, or the butcher's wife.

Nor was Sister Evangelina any match for the quicksilver mind of Sister Monica Joan. She thought slowly and pedantically, entirely concerned with practical matters. She was a careful, hardworking midwife, and an honest and devout nun; I doubt if she had ever had an original idea in her life. Sister Monica Joan's flashing wit and wisdom, her mental gymnastics, leaping from Christianity to cosmology, to astrology, to mythology, all of them thrown together in poetry and prose, and muddled in a mind on the verge of decay, was too much for Sister Evangelina. She just stood with her mouth open, looking stupid, or snorted her incomprehension and stomped off out of the room.

There was no doubt that Sister Evangelina had her cross to bear, and perched on the top was Sister Monica Joan, giggling and winking, kicking her heels in delight as she made such catty remarks as, "I think there's thunder coming – oh no, it's only you, dear. The weather is a little unsettled, isn't it, dear?"

Sister Evangelina could only grind her teeth and plod on. She never got the better of these altercations, try as she might. Had she possessed a sense of humour, she could have defused the situation with laughter – but I never saw Sister Evangelina laugh spontaneously, whatever fun was going on in the house. She would watch other people, to make sure it was funny, and then laugh when others did. Sister Monica Joan would mock this also, "The tinkling bells chime, and the stars laugh with joy. The little cherubs clap their wings and laugh with heavenly harmony. Sister Evangelina is a little cherub, and the tinkling sounds of her laughter ring the changing universe into eternal changelessness. Don't they, dear?"

Poor Sister Evangelina could only say, with solemn emphasis, "I don't know what you mean."

"Ah, so far, so far, the never star, the fruition of Joy, the husk of Despair."

Sister Julienne tried her best to keep the peace between the two Sisters, but not very successfully. How can you reprimand a nonagenarian whose mind is wandering? And would it do any good? I am sure she wondered, as I did, how much of it was due to senility, and how much was calculated mischief-making; but she could never be sure, and in any case Sister Monica Joan's wit had always flashed and gone before she could do anything about it. So Sister Evangelina's suffering continued.

The monastic vows of poverty, chastity and obedience are hard, very hard. But harder still is the task of living, day in, day out, with your Sisters in God.

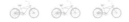

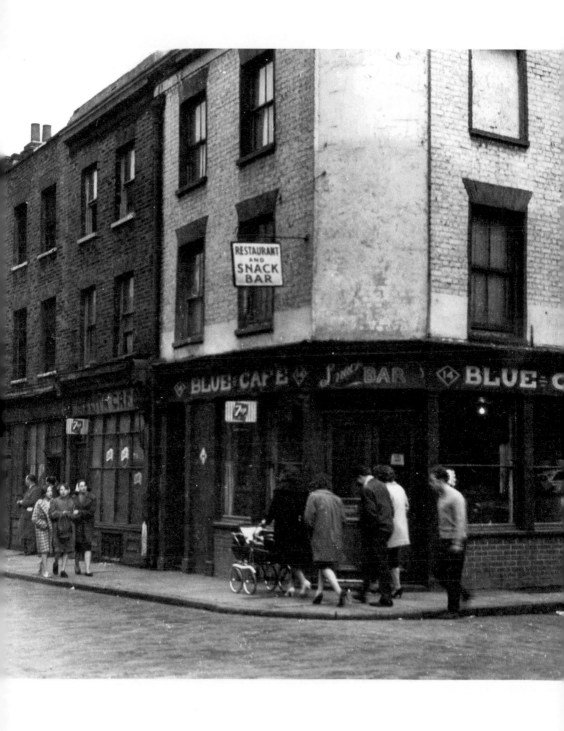

MARY

She must have planned it, and picked me out as I got off the bus at the Blackwall Tunnel. It was about 10.30 p.m. and I had been to the newly opened Festival Hall. Perhaps I looked smarter than most of the other travellers that night, which she assumed meant more affluent. She came up to me, and said quietly, in a lilting Irish voice: "Could you change a five pound note for me?"

I was staggered. Change for five pounds! I doubt if I had three shillings to last the rest of the week. It would be like someone stopping you in the street today and asking if you had change for a five hundred-pound note.

"No, I haven't," I said brusquely. My head was full of music, I was replaying the performance over and over again in my mind. I didn't want to be bothered with total strangers asking silly questions.

It was something about her despairing sigh that made me look at her again. She was very small and thin, with a perfect oval face, rather like a pre-Raphaelite painting. She could have been anywhere between fourteen and twenty years of age. She wore no coat, only a thin jacket that was quite inadequate for the cold evening. She had no stockings or gloves, and her hands trembled. She looked a very poor, ill-nourished girl – yet she obviously had five pounds.

"Why don't you go into that café and change it?"

Opposite: The corner of Cable Street and Ensign Street, Stepney in the 1950s. Prostitution was rife in the area and Cable Street was full of "notorious cafés".

She looked furtive, "I dare not. Someone would see me and tell. Then they would bash me up, or kill me."

It occurred to me that she had probably stolen the money. Stolen goods are of no value unless you can get rid of them. Sterling can usually be passed on without much trouble, but this girl was obviously too afraid to attempt it. Something made me say: "Are you hungry?"

"I haven't eaten today, nor yesterday."

No food for forty-eight hours, and five pounds in her pocket. Curiouser and curiouser, as Alice said to the caterpillar.

"Well look, let's go into that café and get you a meal. I will pay with your five pounds, and then anyone who sees will think it's mine. How's that for a scheme?"

The girl's face brightened with a joyful smile. "You had better take it now, so no one will see me giving it to you."

She looked around her, and then thrust the huge white crackling bank note into my hand. She is very trusting, I thought. She is afraid of someone, but she's not afraid that I will pocket the five pounds and run off.

In the café we ordered steak and two eggs and chips and peas for her. She took her jacket off and sat down. It was then that I saw she was pregnant. She wore no wedding ring. Pregnancy outside marriage in those days was a terrible disgrace. It was not as bad as it had been twenty or thirty years previously. Nonetheless, she would have a hard time ahead of her, I reflected.

She ate in hungry concentration, whilst I sipped a coffee, looking at her. Her name was Mary and was an Irish beauty, with tawny brown hair, delicate bone structure, and pale skin. She could have been a Celtic Princess, or the spawn of a drunken Irish navvy, it was hard to tell – perhaps there is not much difference, I thought.

The first of her hunger was assuaged, and she looked up at me with a smile.

"Where do you come from?" I asked.

"County Mayo."

"Have you ever been away from home before?"

She shook her head.

"Does your mother know you are pregnant?"

Fear, guilt and resentment came into her pretty eyes. Her lips tightened.

"Look, I'm a midwife. I notice these things. I'm trained to do so. I don't suppose anyone else has noticed yet, though."

Her face relaxed, so I said again, "Does your mother know?"

She shook her head.

"What are you going to do?" I asked.

"I don't know."

"You will have to go back home," I said. "London is a big and scary place. You can't bring up a child by yourself here. You need your mother's help. You will have to tell her. She will understand. Mothers hardly ever let their daughters down, you know."

"I can't go back home. It's impossible," she said.

She wouldn't answer any more questions on that subject, so I said, "How did you get to London, and why did you come, anyway?"

She was more relaxed now, and looked more inclined to talk. I ordered apple pie and ice cream for her. Slowly, and in bits and pieces, the story came out. I was so charmed by the lilting music of her voice, that I could have listened all night, regardless of whether she was reading a laundry list or telling me the age-old pathos of her life.

She was the eldest of five living children. Eight of her brothers and sisters had died. Her father was a farm worker and peat cutter. They lived in what she called a sheelin'. Her mother did washing for "the big house", she told me. When she was fourteen her father caught pneumonia in the west Irish winter, and died. The family was left with no protector. The sheelin' was tied to the lands worked by the father and, as none of the sons was old enough to take over the labour, the family was evicted. They moved to Dublin. The mother, a country woman who had never travelled more than walking distance from the mountains and meadows where she had been brought up, was quite unable to cope with the alien environment. They found lodgings in a tenement, and at first the mother took in washing, or tried to, but there was so much poverty and competition from other women similarly placed that she soon gave up the struggle. They couldn't pay the rent, and were again evicted. Mary took a job in a factory, working sixty hours a week for a pittance. Mick, her brother of thirteen, lied about his age and left school, taking a job in a tannery. For both of them it was child slave labour.

The combined efforts of these two might have been just enough to keep the family afloat, had it not been for their mother.

"Me poor mam! I hate her for what she did to us, yet I can't hate her really. She never could get herself away from the hills and the broad sky,

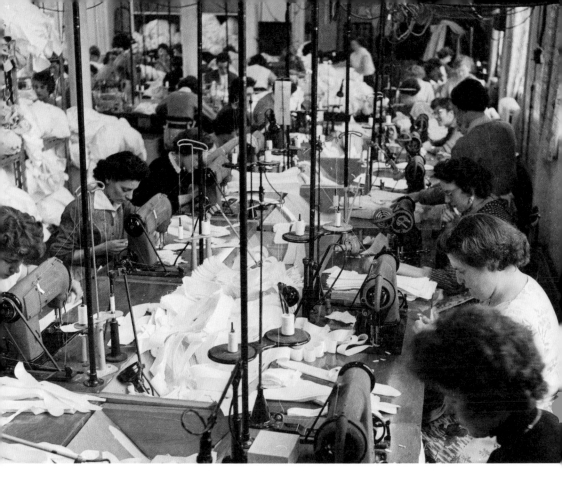

Above: Girls like Mary could work up to 60-hour weeks for a pittance in factories, such as this one in New Cross, London, but the money was often the difference between life and death for them.

from the sound of the curlew and the skylark, the sea, and the silence of the night."

Her voice was like the sad, plaintive cry of an oboe rising from an orchestra.

"At first she just drank Guinness 'because it does me good' she said. Then she took to any old sour stout that she could get. Then it was poteen, which the knife-sharpener man distilled. I don't know what she drinks now. Most likely it's meths and cold tea."

The schoolmistress reported that the three younger children were playing truant, and that when they did come to school, they were half-starving and half-naked. They were taken away from their mother, and put into an orphanage. The mother didn't seem to notice that they had gone. She had already hitched up with another man.

"It's probably a good thing that they were taken away, because I have two little sisters, and I wouldn't want what happened to me to happen to them."

I shuddered. I had heard from Child Care Officers that if a mother takes another man into the house this can frequently be the death sentence for the children.

"He was a big man. I had never seen him sober. There was nothing I could do. I never knew that anything could be so awful. He did it again and again, until I got used to it. It was when he started hitting me and my mam with anything he could get hold of that I knew I had to leave. Me mam didn't seem to notice the wallops, I think she was too drunk to feel anything. But I wasn't. I thought he would kill me."

She had slept in the streets of Dublin for a few nights, with her possessions in a string bag, but her thoughts were on London. She said, "Do you know the story of Dick Whittington and his black cat? Me mam used to tell us that story, and I always thought London must be a beautiful place."

She went to the docks, and enquired about the cost of the fare to England. It was equivalent to three weeks' wages, so she continued at the factory, and slept in a store room at night.

"I was as quiet as a mouse, and as secret as a shadow, and no one knew I was there. Even the caretaker didn't find me when he did his rounds at night, or I would have been thrown out," she said with a mischievous grin.

She spent nothing on food, scrounging what she could from other girls in the factory, and at the end of the third week, she took her wages and left, saying she wasn't coming back.

There were many cargo boats going daily from Dublin to Liverpool in those days, but nonetheless, she had to wait until the Monday before she could get a passage.

"I spent the whole of Sunday wandering around the docks. It was beautiful, with the great ships, and the water splashing, and the seagulls crying. And I was that excited about going to London, that I didn't notice I was hungry."

After another night spent in the open, she paid all her money apart from a few shillings, on a one-way ticket and boarded the vessel.

"It was the most exciting moment of my life, and as I said goodbye to Ireland, I crossed myself and prayed for the soul of me dad, and asked our Holy Mother Mary to look after me poor mam, and me brothers and sisters."

She arrived in Liverpool docks at about 7 p.m. on Monday evening. They did not seem to be quite as different as she had expected. In fact, they looked exactly like Dublin docks, only bigger. She did not know what to do. She enquired where London was, and was told three hundred miles away.

"Three hundred miles," she said. "I nearly fainted. I'd thought it was just around the corner. Can you believe I was so silly?"

She'd spent another night in the open, and found some bread that had been thrown out for the seagulls. It was stale and dirty, but satisfied the worst of her hunger. In the morning, as the sun rose, her spirits and youthful optimism rose also, and she enquired how she could get to London without any money. She was told that 95 per cent of the transport lorries leaving that day would be going to London, and all that was necessary was to ask the driver if he would take her.

"You shouldn't have any difficulties, a pretty girl like you," her informant had said.

I know this to be true from my own experience. From the age of about seventeen, I had hitch-hiked all over England and Wales, always thumbing down long distance lorries and reaching my destination safely. I was always alone. I knew it was said that lorry drivers pick up girls for one purpose only, but this had not been my experience. All the lorry drivers I met were sober, hard-working men, who knew the road, had a load to deliver, and had a schedule to fulfil. Furthermore they were in a named company lorry, and any complaint would identify them immediately, not only to the boss, but also to the wife back home!

Mary found her lorry driver, and told me, "He was such a nice man. It was a long journey and we talked all the way. I sang him songs me dad taught me when I was a child, and he said I had a pretty voice. In some ways he was like me dad. You know, he even took me into a transport café and bought me a meal, and he wouldn't take anything for it. He said 'you keep that, lassie, because I think you are going to need it.' I thought to myself, I'm going to like it in England if all the Englishmen are like this". She paused, and looked down at her plate. Her voice was barely audible when she said, "He was the last good man I have met in this country."

There was silence between us for quite some moments. I did not want to force her confidence, and in any case I am not by nature nosy about other people's affairs, so I said, "How about another ice cream? I'm sure you could manage it. And I wouldn't mind another coffee, if you think you can afford it."

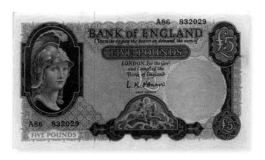

She laughed, and said, "I can afford a hundred cups of coffee."

The proprietor brought our order, and said it was 11.15 and he was closing his till, so could we pay now. But we were welcome to sit at the table until midnight.

Above: Mary asked Jennifer for change of five pounds, the author writes, the equivalent of change today for a "five hundred-pound note".

The bill was two shillings and ninepence, including coffee. That is equivalent to about twelve pence today. I drew myself to my full height, and with a grand gesture drew out the five pound note.

He jumped and spluttered, "Look 'ere, ain't you got nuffink smaller'n that? How do you expect me to change five pounds?"

I said coldly and firmly, "I'm sorry, but I have nothing smaller. If I had, I would have given it to you. My friend has no money on her at all. If you can't change the note, I am afraid we cannot pay for this meal."

I folded the note and put it back into my handbag. That did it. He said, "All right, all right, Miss Toffee-nose. You win."

He went and scratched through the till, then had to go out to the back to unlock the safe. He came back to the table, muttering and grumbling, and counted out four pounds, seventeen shillings and three pence change, whereupon I handed over the five pound note.

Mary was giggling like a schoolgirl at all this. I winked at her, and put the change into my bag. She remained just as trusting, because I could have got up and walked out with all her money.

It was getting late. Although it was my night off, I had had a very busy day, and I was on duty at 8 a.m. the next morning, with the likelihood of another busy day ahead. I was tempted to say, "Look I must get off now" but something drew me to this lonely girl, and I said, "Have you any plans for the baby?"

She shook her head.

"When is it due?"

"I don't know."

"Who are you booked with for confinement?"

She said nothing, so I repeated the question.

"I'm not booked with anyone," she said.

I was concerned. She looked about six months' pregnant, but if she had been half starved it might be a small baby, in which case she could be nearer to full term. I said: "Look Mary, you must be booked for a confinement. Who is your doctor?"

"I haven't got one."

"Where do you live?"

She didn't answer, so I asked again, still no answer. She looked angry, and a hard suspicious tone came into her voice:

"It's none of your business," she said. I think if I hadn't had her four pounds, seventeen shillings and three pence in my handbag, she would have got up and walked out.

"Mary, you might as well tell me, because you need a doctor, and antenatal care for your baby. I am a midwife and can probably arrange it for you."

She bit her lip, and picked her fingernails, then said, "I've been living at the Full Moon Café in Cable Street. But I can't go back there any more."

"Why not?" I said. "Is it because you stole five pounds from the till?"

She nodded.

"They'll kill me if they find me. And they *will* find me, somehow, I'm sure of that. Then they will kill me."

She said these last words in a flat matter of fact voice, as though she had faced and accepted the inevitable.

It was my turn to be silent. I knew that the East End was a violent place. The midwives did not see it because we were deeply respected, and on the whole only dealt with the respectable families. But this girl could easily have been in potentially violent company and if she had stolen from them that undercurrent of violence could erupt into reality. Her life might well be in danger. I had not yet heard about the notorious cafés of Cable Street.

I said, "Have you got anywhere to sleep tonight?"

She shook her head.

I sighed. The responsibility was beginning to dawn on me.

"Let's go and see if the YWCA is open. It's very late, and I am not sure what time they close, but it's worth a try."

We thanked the proprietor, and left. In the street I gave Mary her money, and we walked the mile to the YWCA. It had closed at 10 p.m.

I was weary and tired. My stiletto heels were killing me. I had another mile to walk back to Nonnatus House, and a heavy day's work to come. I cursed myself for getting involved at all. I could so easily have said at the bus stop, "No, I do not have change for five pounds", and walked away.

But I looked at Mary standing outside the closed door. She looked so small and vulnerable, and somehow utterly docile in my hands. How could I leave her in the street with, possibly, men looking for her who might kill her? Who would notice if she disappeared? I thought, There, but for the grace of God, go I, and that solemn thought was truer than you might suppose.

She shivered in the cold night air, and pulled her thin jacket around her neck. I was wearing a warm camel hair coat with a beautiful fur collar of which I was very proud. The collar was detachable, so I took it off and put it round her thin little neck. She gave a sigh of joy and snuggled into the warm fur.

"Ooh! that's lovely," she said, smiling.

"Come on," I said. "You had better come back with me."

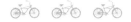

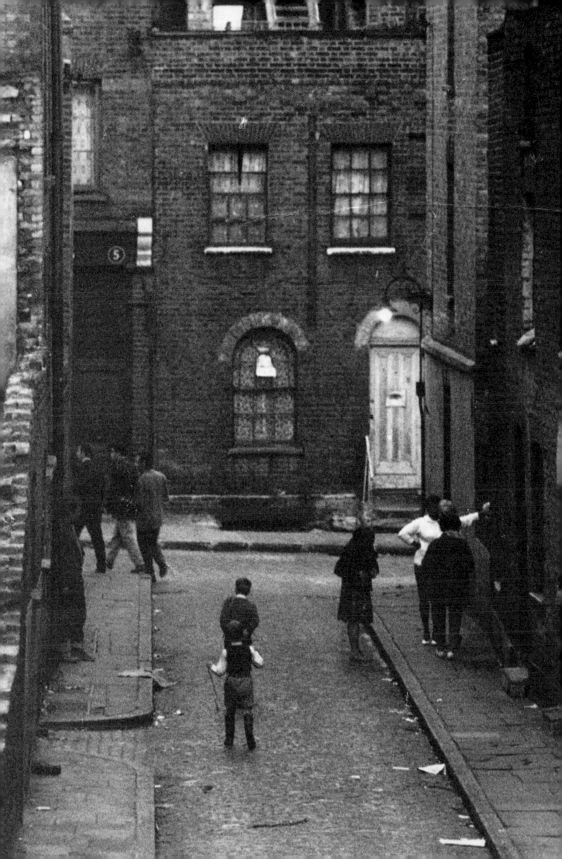

ZAKIR

The mile walk from the YWCA to Nonnatus House seemed endless. I was too tired to want to talk any more, so we walked in silence. At first all I could think about was my feet and those infernal shoes, designed for elegance, not for hiking. Suddenly the bright idea came to me to take the damned things off! So I did, and my stockings too. The cold pavement felt lovely, and cheered me up.

What was I going to do with Mary? There were only ten bedrooms at Nonnatus House, all of which were occupied. I decided to put her in the staff sitting room, and to find some blankets from the general storeroom. I knew I would have to be up before 5.30 a.m. to tell Sister Julienne as she came out of chapel. I could not risk anyone finding the girl without my first having informed the Sister-in-Charge. The nuns did not and could not take in every down-and-out who turned up at their door. If they did, they would be inundated, and the ten bedrooms would soon have ten sleeping in every bed! The nuns had a specific job to do – district nursing and midwifery – and their calling had to be directed to this end.

As I trudged along in my bare feet, I pondered Mary's words about the lorry driver, "He was the last good man I have met in this country." How tragic. There are millions of good men – the vast majority, in fact. How was it that she, a sweet and pretty girl, had never met them? How had she come to this destitute state? Was it all, perhaps, due to love? Or the absence

Opposite: Cable Street in the 1950s. Children play on the street and prostitutes deal with their customers.

of love? Would I have been in Mary's position, had it not been for love? My thoughts went, as they always did, to the man I loved. We had met when I was only fifteen. He could quite easily have used and abused me, but he didn't, he respected me. He loved me to distraction, and wanted only my ultimate good. He had educated me, protected me, guided my teenage years. Had I met the wrong man at the age of fifteen, I reflected, I would probably be in the same position as Mary now.

We trudged on in silence. I didn't know what Mary was thinking about, but my soul was longing for the sight, the sound and the touch of the man I loved so much. Poor little thing. What sort of touch had she known if the lorry driver was the only good man she had met?

We arrived at Nonnatus House. It was getting on for 2 a.m. I fixed Mary up in the sitting room with some blankets, and said, "The lavatory is down the end of this corridor, dear. Sleep well, and I will see you in the morning."

I went wearily to bed, and set my alarm for 5.15 a.m.

The Sisters were surprised to see me as they came out of chapel. It was still the time of the Greater Silence of their monastic vows, so there was no speech. I went up to Sister Julienne and told her exactly what had happened. She did not speak, but her eyes spoke their understanding. The nuns passed me in silent procession, and I went back to bed, resetting my alarm for 7.30 a.m.

At 8 a.m. I went to Sister Julienne's office.

"I have spoken to Father Joe at Church House, Wellclose Square," she said. "They can take the girl, and will look after her. I have peeped into the sitting room. She is sound asleep, and will probably sleep until midday. We will bring her some breakfast when she wakes up, and then take her along to Church House. You go and have your breakfast now, and then start your morning's work."

Her eyes smiled at me, and she added: "You could not have done otherwise my dear."

Once again, I was struck by the kindness and flexibility of the Sisters, compared with the rigid inflexibility of the hospital systems under which I had worked. Had I taken anyone into a nurses' home without permission for a night, there would have been hell to pay, simply because it was against the rules.

Mary did not wake up until four o'clock in the afternoon. It was our teatime, just before we started the evening work, so I did not have long to see her before I had to go out. Sister Julienne had taken her some tea and bread and butter, which she was eating when I went into the sitting room. Sister was explaining to Mary that she could not stay at Nonnatus House, but could go to a house where she would be welcome to stay. Antenatal care would be provided, and arrangements made for delivery. Mary looked at me with big solemn eyes, and I nodded and said that I would come to see her.

And that is how I got into the world of pimps and prostitutes, the foul brothels, masquerading as all-night café, that lined Cable Street and the surrounding area of Stepney. It is a hidden world. The same goes on in every town and city the world over, and always has done, but few people know anything about the business, nor indeed do they want to.

There are two sorts of prostitutes: the high class ones, and the rest. The French courtesans were probably the top of the market, and we read about their salons, their lavish entertainments, their artistic and political influence with amazement.

In London, the smart West End call girls today normally work within a very expensive establishmentwith a few select clients, and can command enormous fees. These are usually very intelligent women who have worked it all out, planned it, studied it, and entered prostitution with a true professionalism. One such girl said to me: "You have to go into it at the top. This is not a job where you start at the bottom and work your way up. If you start at the bottom, you just sink lower."

The vast majority of prostitutes start at the bottom, and their life is pitiable. Historically, prostitution has been the only means of earning a living for a woman who is destitute, particularly if she has children to feed. What woman worthy of the name Mother would stand on a high moral platform about selling her body if her child were dying of hunger and exposure? Not I.

Today – and indeed in the 1950s – such starvation is not seen in Western societies, but there is a different type of hunger which feeds the prostitution trade. It is starvation of love. Thousands run away from desperate circumstances, and find themselves alone and friendless in a big city. They are craving affection, and will attach themselves to anyone who appears to offer it. This is where the pimps and madams score. They offer the child food and lodgings and apparent kindness, and within days, prostitution is forced upon them. The only difference between the twenty-first century and the 1950s is that back then, the children procured for soliciting were around fourteen years of age. Today the age has dropped to as low as ten.

Mary's lorry driver was heading for the Royal Albert Docks, and so he had dropped her off in Commercial Road. She told me, "I felt so terribly alone, more alone than I had ever felt before. In Ireland, when I was making my plans to come to London, I was all excited. The journey was thrilling, because I was going to the beautiful city of London, and I didn't feel alone, because my thoughts were full of dreams. But when I got here I didn't know what I was going to do."

Who was it that said "'Tis better to travel hopefully than to arrive?" I daresay we have all experienced this in one way or another.

Mary went into a confectioner tobacconist, bought a bar of chocolate, and ate it as she wandered down the busy road. At the time, Commercial Road and East India Dock Road were said to be the busiest roads in Europe, because the Port of London was the busiest port in Europe. The continuous stream of lorries bewildered and frightened her. By contrast, Dublin had been as quiet as a country village. The shrill blast of a siren nearly gave her a heart attack, and then she saw thousands of men pouring out of the dock gates. She flattened herself against a doorway as they passed, chatting, laughing, squabbling, shouting and talking to each other. But not one of them spoke to the shy, small figure in the doorway. In fact it is doubtful if any of them even noticed her. She said, "I nearly cried with loneliness. I wanted to shout out 'I'm here, just beside you. Come and say hello to me. I've come a long way just to be here.'"

She didn't like Commercial Road much, so she turned off into a side street where she saw children playing. She was scarcely more than a child herself, but they didn't want her to join in the game. She continued on until she came to what was known as the Cuts – the canal that went under Stinkhouse Bridge on its way to the Docks. It was pleasant standing by the bridge, looking down at the moving water, and she stood there a long time watching a water rat pop in and out of his hole and seeing the shadows lengthen.

"I just didn't know what I was going to do. I wasn't cold, 'cos it was summer, and I wasn't hungry, 'cos that nice lorry driver had given me sausage and chips. But I felt so empty inside, and sick with longing for someone to talk to me."

Night came, and she had nowhere to sleep, nor the money to purchase a night's lodgings. She had already spent many nights in the open, and the prospect did not bother her. There were bomb sites all over the East End at the time, and she found one that looked as though it might do. However, it was a bad choice.

"I was woken in the night by the most terrible noise. Men screaming and fighting and cursing and swearing. In the moonlight I saw knives and flashing things. I crawled deeper into the hole I was in, and hid under some foul-smelling sacks. I just kept quite, quite still, and didn't breathe. Then I heard the police whistles and dogs barking. I was frightened the dogs would smell me, but they didn't. Perhaps the sacks I was under smelt so bad they couldn't smell anything else."

She giggled. I didn't. My heart was too full for laughter.

Apparently she had stumbled into a bomb site regularly used by the meths drinkers. After the police had cleared the place, Mary crept out, and spent the rest of the night by the Cuts.

The next day was spent in much the same way as the first, just wandering around the Stepney end of Commercial Road with nothing to do.

"There were a lot of buses around, and I wondered if I should get on one and go somewhere else, because I didn't really like it where I was. But they all said places like Wapping and Barking, Mile End, and Kings Cross, on the front, and I didn't know where these places were. I had wanted to come to London, and the lorry driver said it was London when he put me down, so I didn't get on a bus, because I wouldn't know where I was going to."

Two more days were spent like this. Completely alone, talking to no one, sleeping in the Cuts at night. On the third evening Mary spent the last of her pennies on a sausage roll.

The fourth day in London would have been without food, had she not seen an old lady in a churchyard feeding the sparrows with breadcrumbs.

"I waited until the old lady had gone, then I shooed the birds away, and crawled around scooping up the breadcrumbs and putting them in my skirt. The sun was shining, and the trees were nice. I saw a little squirrel. I sat on the grass and ate a whole lap full of breadcrumbs. They tasted all right. The

Overleaf: The bombsites, which littered the East End, became the playgrounds for local children and also the home of the homeless and meths drinkers.

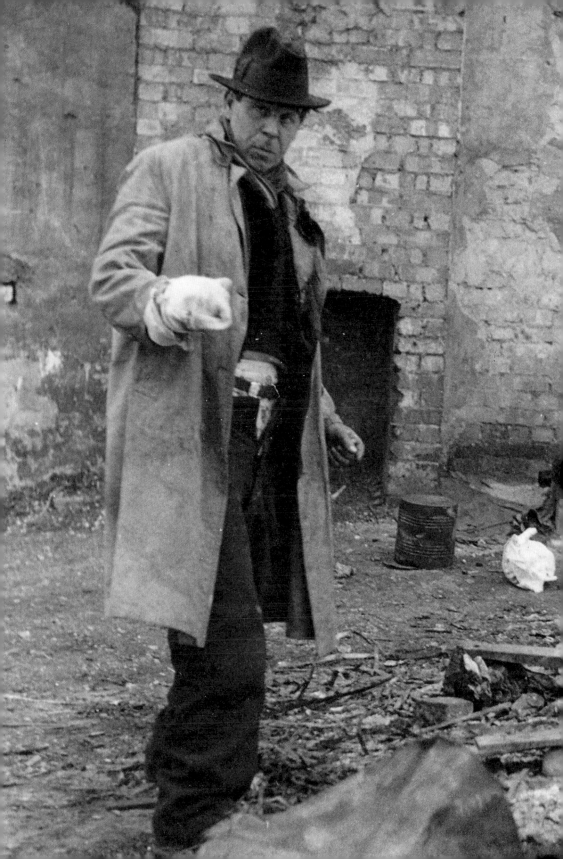

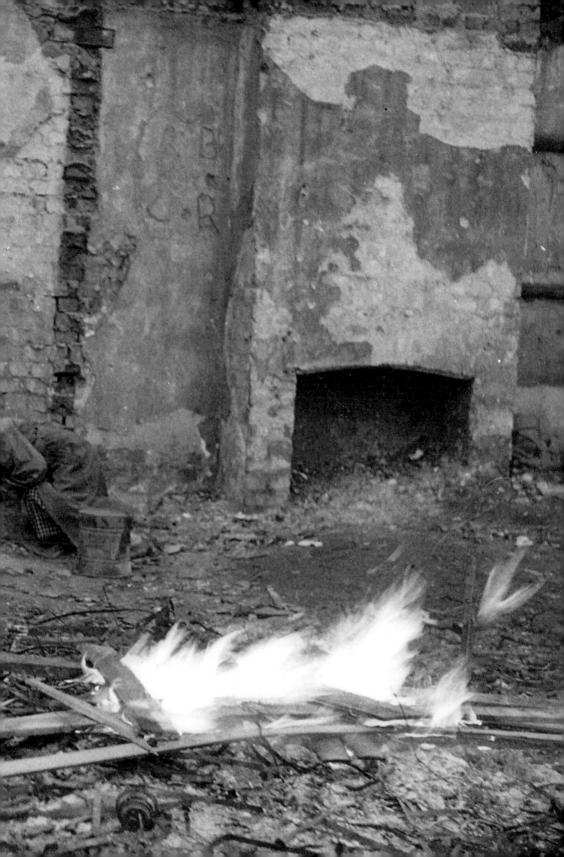

next day I went to the churchyard again, thinking that the old lady would come to feed the birds. But she didn't come. I waited the whole day but she still didn't come."

In the evening she scavenged some bits of food from a dustbin.

As she was talking, I wondered why it was that a bright young girl, who had had the initiative and enterprise to plan her journey all the way from Dublin, could not have been more resourceful and forward thinking when she arrived in London. There were places she could have gone – the police, a Catholic Church, the Salvation Army, the YWCA – where people would have helped her, sheltered her, and probably found her a job. But such a course of action did not seem to have occurred to her. Perhaps it would have done, given a little more time. But instead she met Zakir.

"I was looking in a baker's window, sniffing the bread and thinking what I wouldn't give to have some. He came and stood beside me, and said, 'Do you want a cigarette?'

"He was the first person who had spoken to me since the lorry driver. It was so nice just to hear someone say something to me, but I didn't smoke. Then he said, 'Do you want something to eat, then?' and I said: 'I'll say I do.'

"He looked down at me and smiled, such a lovely smile. His teeth were gleaming white, and his eyes were kind. He had beautiful eyes, a dark black-brown colour. I loved his eyes the moment I looked into them. He said, 'Come on, let's get some of their nice filled rolls. I'm hungry too. Then we'll go and sit by the Cuts and eat them.'

"We went into the shop, and he bought lots of rolls with different fillings, and some fruit pies, and some chocolate cake. I felt very scruffy beside him, because I hadn't washed or changed my clothes for days, and he looked so smart and well dressed, and had a gold chain on."

They sat on the grass of the towpath, leaning their backs against the wall, watching the barges go by. Mary said she was tongue tied. She felt overwhelmed by this kind, handsome youth who seemed to like her, and she couldn't think of a thing to say, even though for four or five days she had been longing for someone to talk to.

"He talked all the time, and laughed, and threw bits of bread to the sparrows and pigeons, and called them 'my friends'. I thought someone who is friends with the birds must be very nice. Sometimes I couldn't understand quite what he was saying, but the English accent is different to the Irish accent, you know. He told me he was a buyer for his uncle, who had a nice café in Cable Street and who sold the best food in London. We had such a lovely meal sitting there on the towpath in the sunshine. The rolls were delicious, the apple pies were delicious, and the chocolate cake was out of this world."

She leaned back on the stone wall, and sighed with contentment. When she woke up the sun was behind the warehouse, and his jacket was over her. She found that she was leaning on his shoulder.

"I woke up with his strong arm around me, and his beautiful brown eyes looking down at me. He stroked my cheek, and said, 'You've had a nice big sleep. Come on, it's getting late. I had better take you home. Your mother and father will wonder what has happened to you.'

"I didn't know what to say then, and he didn't talk either. After a bit, he said: 'We must get going. What will your mother think, you being out with a stranger all this time?'

"'Me mam's a long way off in Ireland.'

"'Well, your dad then.'

"'Me dad's dead.'

"'You poor little thing. I suppose you are living with an auntie in London?'

"He stroked my cheek again when he said 'you poor little thing', and I thought I would melt with happiness. So I snuggled up in his arms, and told him the whole story – but I didn't tell him about me mam's man and what he'd done to me, because I was ashamed, and didn't want him to think badly of me."

"He didn't say anything. For a long while he just stroked my cheek and my hair. Then he said: 'Poor little Mary. What are we going to do with you? I can't leave you here by the Cuts all night. I feel responsible for you now. I think you had better come back with me to my uncle's place. It's a nice café. My uncle is very kind. We can have a good meal and then we can plan your future.'"

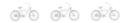

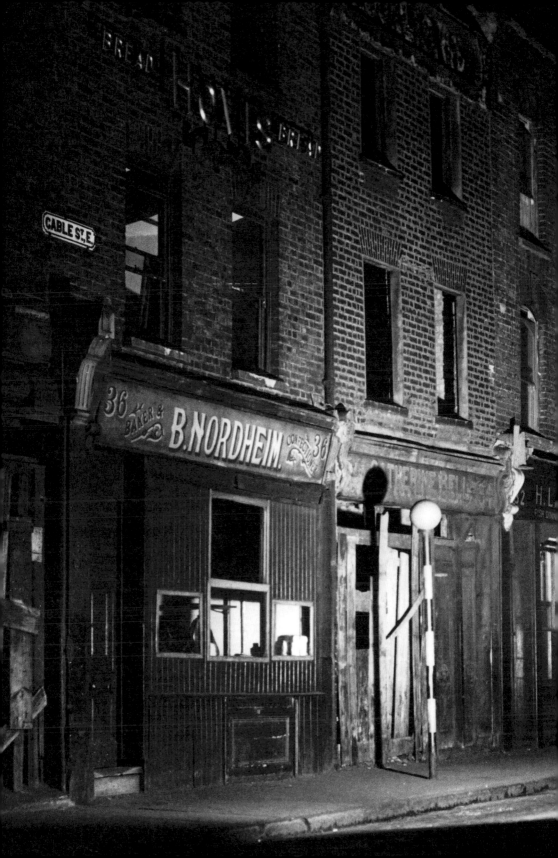

CABLE STREET

Pre-war Stepney, just east of the City, with Commercial Road to the north, the Tower and Royal Mint to the West, Wapping and the Docks to the South, and Poplar to the east, was the home of thousands of respectable, hard-working, but often poor East End families. Much of the area was filled with crowded tenements, narrow unlit alleyways and lanes and old multi-occupant houses. Often the old houses had only one tap, and one lavatory in the yard, to serve between eight and a dozen families, and sometimes a whole family of ten or more might occupy one or two rooms. The people had lived like this for generations, and were still doing so in the 1950s.

This was their inheritance and their accepted lifestyle, but after the war, things changed dramatically, for the worse. The area was scheduled for demolition, which did not actually take place for another twenty years. In the meantime, the area became a breeding ground for vice of every description. The condemned houses, which were privately owned, could not be sold on the open market to responsible landlords, so they were bought up by unscrupulous profiteers of all nationalities, who let out single, derelict, rooms for fantastically low rents. The shops were bought up in the same way and turned into all night cafés, with their "street waitresses". They were, in fact, brothels, making life hell for the decent people who had to live in the area, and bring their children up in the midst of it all.

Opposite: Cable Street in Stepney (c. 1947).

Overcrowding had always been part of the East Ender's life, but the war made it far worse. Many homes had been destroyed by the bombing and not replaced, so people lived anywhere they could find. On top of this, in the 1950s, thousands of commonwealth immigrants poured into the country with no provision made for where they were going to live. It was not uncommon to see groups of ten or more West Indians, say, going from door to door, begging for a room to let. If they did find one, in no time at all it would be filled with twenty to twenty-five people, all living together.

This sort of thing the East Enders had seen before, and could absorb. But when it came to the blatant widespread use of their streets, their alleys and closes, their shops and houses, as brothels, it was a very different matter. Life became sheer hell, and women were terrified to go out of doors, or to let their children out. The tough, resilient East Enders, who had lived through two world wars, lived through the Great Depression of the 1930s, survived the Blitz of the 1940s, and come up smiling, were to be crushed by the vice and prostitution that descended in their midst in the 1950s and '60s.

Below. 1950s' London saw increased immigration, particularly from the West Indies. As men competed for jobs, housing and, sometimes, women, racial intolerance became a problem.

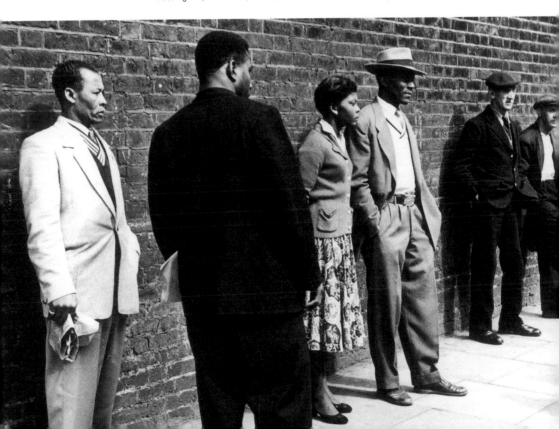

Try to imagine, if you can, living in a derelict building, renting two rooms on the second floor, with six children to bring up. And then try to imagine that there is a new landlord, and through threats, intimidation, fear, or genuine rehousing, one by one, all the families you have known since childhood have moved out. All the rooms of the house in which you live have been divided up and filled with prostitutes, as many as four or five to each room. The general store, which used to be the ground floor of the building, has been turned into an all-night café with noise and loud music, parties, swearing, fights, going on all night. The trade of prostitution goes on all night and all day, with men tramping up and down the stairs, and hanging around on the stairways or landings, waiting their turn. Imagine it, if you can, and imagine the poor woman who has to take her toddlers out shopping, or get the children off to school, or go down to the basement alone to get a couple of buckets of water with which to do her washing.

Many such families were on the council waiting list for rehousing for as much as ten years, and the biggest families had the least chance of getting other accommodation because the council (under the Housing Act) was not allowed to put a family of ten into a four-room flat, even though the two room conditions under which they were living had been condemned for human habitation.

Into this environment came Father Joe Williamson, who was appointed Vicar of St Paul's in Dock Street in the 1950s. He devoted the rest of his life, his considerable energies, his powerful mind and above all his Godliness, to cleaning up the area and helping the East End families who had to live there. Later, he began his work of helping and protecting the young prostitutes, whom he loved and pitied with all his heart. It was he who opened the doors of Church House, Wellclose Square, as a home for prostitutes, and this was the place Mary went the day after I had picked her up at the bus stop. I visited her there several times, and it was during these visits that she told me her story.

"Zakir put his coat around my shoulders, because it was getting chilly, and he carried my bag. He put his arm round me, and led me through the crowds of men leaving the docks. He escorted me over the road like a real gentleman, and I can tell you I felt like the greatest lady in London by the side of such a handsome young man."

He took her down a side street off Commercial Road, which led into other side streets, each one narrower and dirtier than the last. Many windows were boarded up, others broken, others so dirty that it would have been impossible to see through them. There were very few people around, and no children played in the streets. She looked up the height of the black buildings. Pigeons flew from ledge to ledge. A few of the windows looked as if someone had tried to clean them, and had curtains. One or two even had washing hanging out on a little balcony. It looked as though the sun never penetrated these narrow streets and alleys. Filth and litter were everywhere; in the corners, the gutters, piled up against railings, blocking doorways, half filling the little alleys. Zakir carefully led Mary through all this dirt, telling her to be careful, or to step over this or that. The few other people they met were all men, and he protectively drew her closer to him as they passed. One or two of them he obviously knew, and they spoke to each other in a foreign language.

Mary said, "I thought he must be so clever and educated to speak a foreign language. He must have been to a very expensive school to have learned it, I thought."

They came to a wider, longer street, which was Cable Street and Zakir said to her, "My uncle's café is just up there. It's the best and the busiest one in the street. We can have a meal together, just you and me. Won't that be fun? My uncle also owns the whole building and he lets out rooms, so I'm sure he would find one for you. That way you won't have to sleep by the Cuts any more. Perhaps he could find a job for you in the café, washing up, or peeling the vegetables. Or he could put you in charge of the coffee machine. Would you like to work the coffee machine?"

Mary was enchanted. Working the coffee machine in a busy London café was about the height of her dreams. She clung to Zakir in gratitude and adoration, and he squeezed her hand.

"Everything's going to be all right for you from now on," he said. "I've got that feeling."

Mary was too overcome to speak. She loved him with all her heart. They entered the café. It was dark inside because the windows were so filthy, and the net curtains that hung from halfway down were nearly black with filth. A few men sat at formica tables, smoking and drinking. One or two of them sat with a woman, and a group of women and girls sat together at a bigger

Opposite: Jennifer did not change the name of Father Joe Williamson, pictured here walking in his parish. He was Vicar of St Paul's in Dock Street in the 1950s.

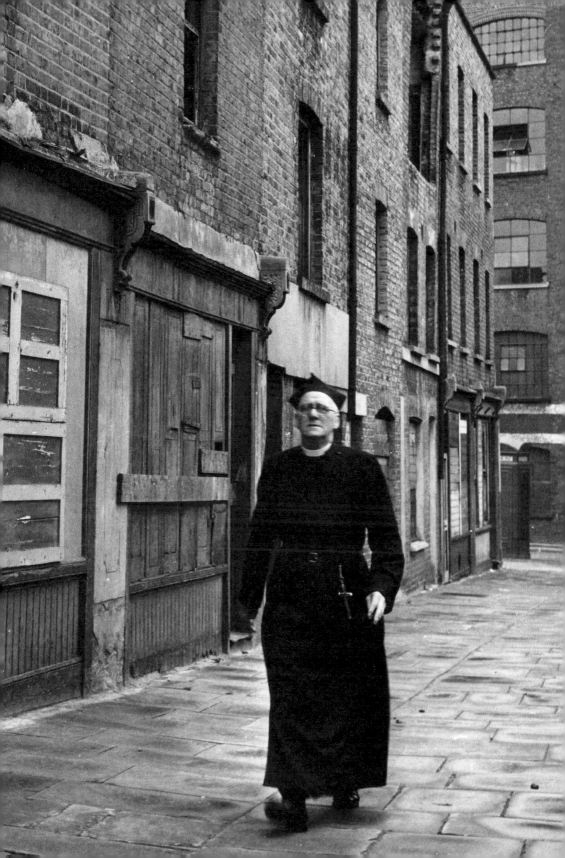

table smoking. No one spoke. The silence in the place was quite eerie, and somehow threatening. Everyone looked up as Zakir and Mary walked in, but still no one spoke. Mary must have contrasted sharply with the other girls and women in the café, who all seemed pale. Some of them looked sullen, some were scowling, and all looked haggard. By contrast, Mary's eyes were shining with expectation. Her skin was glowing with the fresh air, first from the boat trip, then from sleeping by the Cuts for four nights. Above all, the soft, sensuous glow of love filled her, irradiated her whole being.

Zakir told her to sit down while he went to speak with his uncle. He took her string bag with him. She sat at a table by the window. Several of the people in the café stared at her, but did not speak to her. She didn't mind, she smiled quietly to herself; she didn't really want to talk to anyone, now that she had Zakir. A rough-looking man came over and sat opposite her at the table, but she turned her head away haughtily. The man got up and left. She heard some sniggering from the girls in the corner, so she turned to them and smiled, but no one smiled back.

After about ten minutes Zakir came back. He said, "I have spoken to my uncle. He is a good man, and he will look after you. We will have a meal together later. It is only seven o'clock now. The fun starts at about nine o'clock. You will enjoy the evening. This café is famous for its entertainment, and for its food: my uncle employs the best chef in London. You can have whatever you want. My uncle is a very generous man, and he says you can choose whatever you fancy from the menu and the wine list. He only says this because you are a special friend of mine, and I am his favourite nephew. I am the meat buyer, and I have to travel a lot to find the best. A good café must have good meat, and I am the best meat buyer in London."

Certainly the meat in Mary's dinner was very good. She chose meat pie and beans and chips. Zakir had the same, because there was nothing else on the menu that evening. But to Mary, who had been brought up in the poverty of rural Ireland, mainly on potatoes and swede, and then the destitution of Dublin, the meat pie was the finest thing she had ever tasted, and she sighed with contentment.

They sat in the corner by the window. From his seat Zakir could see the whole of the café and his eyes roamed around it continuously, even when he was talking to Mary. From her seat, she could see about half the café, but she didn't look around, nor did she want to. She had eyes only for Zakir.

He said, "Now let us choose our wine. You must always be careful with the wine, because a good wine is essential to a good dinner. I think we will have Chateau Marseilles 1948. It is an excellent wine, full bodied, yet not too heavy, with a tantalising piquancy that lingers on the palate and suggests the warmth and brilliance of the grape. I am an expert in wines."

Mary was impressed, in fact overwhelmed by his polish and urbanity. She had never tasted wine before, and did not like it. She had expected something delicious from the dark-red liquid in her tumbler, but thought it was bitter and sour. However, as Zakir was drinking his with delight, murmuring things like "an excellent vintage, drink up, you won't find anything better than this in all of London" or "ah, what a bouquet – quite exquisite – I assure you this is a rare treat", and as she did not want to hurt his feelings by saying she didn't really like it, she swallowed the whole tumbler full in one gulp, and said, "Delicious."

He refilled her glass. All the while his eyes were roving around the café. When he spoke to Mary he smiled, but as he looked around the café neither his eyes nor his mouth smiled. Mary could not see the table where the girls and women were sitting, but they were directly opposite Zakir. Frequently he stared over towards them with cold unblinking eyes, nodded slightly, and moved his head momentarily in another direction, then back again towards the table. Each time, Mary could hear the scrape of a chair as one of the girls got up. About half a dozen times during the meal he got up and went over to the table. Mary followed him with her eyes, not because she was suspicious, but because she just couldn't take her eyes off him. She noted with satisfaction that he did not seem to like the girls very much, because he never smiled at them, but seemed to be talking with his teeth closed and his eyes fixed and hard. Once she saw him clench his fist, and push it up against a girl's face in a menacing fashion. The girl got up and went out.

Mary thought, "He likes me the best. He doesn't like those girls. They look a nasty bunch anyway. But I am his special friend," and a warm glow flooded over her.

Each time Zakir returned, he showered Mary with smiles, his beautiful white teeth flashing and his dark eyes gleaming.

"Drink up," he said. "You can't have too much of this excellent wine. Would you like some fruit or some gateau? My uncle says you can have anything you want. Soon the entertainment will begin. It is the best in

London. The night clubs of London, Paris and New York are famous all over the world, and this one is the best in London."

Mary drank up, and ate a piece of sticky, sweet cake which Zakir said was Black Forest gateau with morello cherries marinated in chartreuse. Although Mary could not find the cherries it tasted delicious, but unfortunately the wine now tasted even worse than before and the sourness made her tongue feel all furry and her lips and mouth rough.

She was vaguely aware, in a hazy sort of way, that the café was filling up. Men were coming in continuously. Zakir said, "This is our busy time. You will enjoy the entertainment, won't you?"

Mary smiled and nodded, anxious to please. In reality her eyes were hurting, because the air was getting more and more smoky, and her head was beginning to ache. She felt deeply tired after the meal, and would rather have gone to sleep, but she thought that she must stay awake to enjoy the entertainment that Zakir had so kindly brought her to see. She drank some more wine, and tried to keep her eyes open. She was not aware that shutters had been put up at the windows, the doors locked, and the lights dimmed.

Quite suddenly the most deafening noise shattered her fuddled senses. She nearly fell off her chair in fright, and had to grip the edge of the table to keep herself upright. It was louder than anything she had ever heard in her life, louder even than the dock yard siren that had frightened her in Commercial Road. And it went on and on. It was a jukebox, and the noise was rhythm music.

Zakir shouted: "The entertainment. Turn your chair and watch. It is the best in London."

All the men in the room had turned their chairs, and were silently facing a table in the centre.

A girl leapt up on to the table and started dancing. The table was only about three foot wide, so she could not really dance for fear of falling off, but she moved her body, her hips, her shoulders, her arms and neck in rhythm with the music. Her hair flew about her. The men cheered. Then she threw off a shawl that was round her shoulders. The men cheered again and scrambled to get it. Slowly, suggestively, she undid the buttons of her blouse and threw it off, revealing a crimson bra. She undid the band which kept her skirt on, and it dropped to her feet. Beneath it, she wore only a crimson string that ran round her waist and between her legs. Her bottom was enormous. She turned to face the wall, shaking her bottom and thighs then bent over with her legs apart.

Mary was stunned. All sleepiness had left her and she couldn't believe her eyes. She couldn't believe it was happening.

Zakir flashed his beautiful teeth at her and shouted: "It is good, no? I told you we have the best entertainment in London."

The girl straightened up and turned to face her audience. She stared around her in an insolent fashion, and slowly began to undo the fastenings

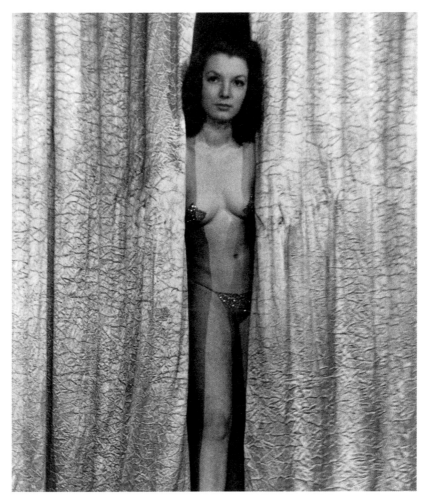

Above: A woman peeps through a curtain, wearing very little apart from nipple tassels and glittery briefs. "Exotic" dancing was one of the entertainments available to customers in special cafés.

of her bra. The men cheered and screamed and stamped as two huge breasts fell out, with crimson tassels attached to each nipple. With a skill that must have taken much practice, she began to make her breasts gyrate faster and faster, and the tassels flew round and round with ever increasing speed. Mary's eyes were hypnotised by these tassels. She was numb with amazement until gradually the gyrations slowed down, and the tassels drooped to the floor, swinging slightly. The girl undid the string around her waist, and threw it to the audience, who scrambled to get it.

Now the serious part of her dance started. She shook and moved her pelvis slowly back and forwards. Her eyes were fixed on her audience, and her tongue was hanging out. She did this for quite a long time, sometimes moving her upper body as well, sometimes swinging her breasts from side to side. The jukebox was turned down a bit, so that just the beat of the drums was heard, and all the time her pelvis moved back and forwards to the rhythm.

Mary was quite mesmerised. As suddenly as it had started, and with a scream, the girl stopped, and lay down on the table. There was not a lot of space, but she lay with her back and head on the table, and her legs high in the air, heels touching. The jukebox went up loud, louder, louder again, as she slowly opened her legs until they were almost horizontal, revealing her vast fleshy, hairy vulva. Then, with even more skill, and to the screams of delight from her audience, she started to produce ping-pong balls from her vagina, and throw them at the audience. The speed and the number were bewildering. There must be some magic in this, Mary thought, no woman can have so many ping-pong balls inside her. The balls were flying around the room, the men throwing them at each other, at the girls, at the walls, in a frenzy of excitement.

The other girls had now left their table and joined the men, some sitting on their knees and fondling them or being fondled, some going out the back in pairs, some just sitting, smoking and drinking. Two older women came up to the girl lying on the table, and each took hold of a leg. Then they beckoned to the men. There was a rush towards her, but two thickset, middle-aged men wearing knuckledusters barred the way. They snarled at the advancing men, and said something. Mary could not hear what was said because of the noise of the jukebox, but several of the men turned and went back to their seats. Some remained standing, however, and Mary saw a lot of money being handed to the knuckledusters. Then one by one, the men undid their trousers and penetrated the girl on the table. Some, whilst waiting their turn, came up the sides and rubbed her breasts with their hands. After more money was pressed into the knuckledustered hands, one went up to her head, undid his trousers, and pressed his penis into her mouth, while the girl contentedly sucked. After that, several other men did the same, one at a time.

Mary felt sick. Her experience of the Irishman had been enough to tell her what was going on, and the sight of the money passing hands told her the rest. She did not need to ask any questions. She shuddered, and crossed herself. "Holy Mary, mother of God, pray for me," she whispered.

Mary told me all this over cups of coffee and digestive biscuits as we sat in the kitchen of Church House in Wellclose Square. I visited her often. I was not a social worker, nor even a voluntary church worker. I just liked the girl, and the circumstances of our meeting gave us a bond; and she trusted me and was clearly able to talk to me. As I wanted to find out more about prostitutes and their way of life, I encouraged her to talk.

I said, "After that, why did you not just leave? You were free to do so. No one could have stopped you. Why didn't you just go?"

She was quiet, and nibbled the edge of a biscuit.

"I should have done, I know, but I couldn't leave Zakir. He took my hand and squeezed it and said, 'Is this not good entertainment? You will find nothing better in London. All the nightclubs in London are trying to get that dancer for their shows, but I found her and brought her to my uncle and he pays her well, so she will not go to another café. She performs each night for us, and makes the café famous. But my dear little Mary, you are looking tired. You need to go to bed. Come. My uncle has a room ready for you.'"

He tenderly took her hand, and led her through the crowd of men and girls, pushing them aside, putting his arm protectively around her.

She said to me, "I knew he cared for me then, because he treated me differently to all the others. He was looking after me and protecting me from all those rough men, wasn't he?"

I sighed. With the wisdom of my twenty-three years, I wondered if it was really possible that a girl of fourteen or fifteen could be so taken in by a smooth-talking scoundrel. I felt that I could not have been. But now I am not so sure.

He led her out the back to the kitchen area, and said, "This is the stairway to the upper rooms. They are very fine and beautiful. You will see. If you want the lavatory, it is over there, in the yard."

He pointed to a wood and asbestos shack.

Mary did need to go and after whispering, "Don't go away," she went over to it. It was revolting and evil smelling, but in the dark Mary could not see the magnitude of the ordure covering the wet and slippery floor.

She returned to Zakir, who led her through the kitchen and up to the first floor. He produced a key, opened a door and switched on the light.

Mary found herself in a room the like of which she had never seen, nor even imagined, in all her life. Lights shone from the walls, not the ceiling, and some even shone from the curtains. There were mirrors on the walls reflecting the lights. She gasped at the gold and silver that seemed to be everywhere although it was, in fact, just chrome. In the centre of the room stood a huge brass bed, with what looked to her like a silk covering. After the dark, dingy interior of the café below, it seemed like paradise.

She murmured, "Oh, it's beautiful Zakir, just beautiful. Is this really the room your uncle will let me have?"

He laughed, and replied, "It is the most beautiful room in London. You will not find a finer room anywhere. You are a lucky girl Mary, I hope you know that."

"Oh I do, I do, Zakir," she sighed, "and I am grateful with all my heart."

He had seduced her with practised ease. She did not want to talk about it, and I did not want to press her. I felt that the memory of that one night was sacred to her. She did, however, say, "I am sure he loved me, because no one else has ever touched me in the way that he did. All the other men were rough and horrible. But Zakir was gentle and beautiful. I thought I would die with happiness that night. It would have been best if I had died," she added quietly.

As they lay in each other's arms, watching the daylight banish the soft darkness, he whispered, "There, my little Mary, did you enjoy that? Did you think anything like that could come to you? There are many other things that I can show you also."

"Then I made a terrible mistake," she said to me. "If I had not made that mistake, he would love me still. But I thought I should tell him all the truth about myself, so that there would be no secrets between us. I told him about me mam's man in Dublin, and what he did to me."

"Zakir pushed me away from him then, and jumped up, shouting, 'Why do I waste my time with you, you little slut. I am a busy man. I have better things to do with my time. Get up, and get yourself dressed.'"

"He slapped me in the face and threw my clothes at me. I was crying, and he slapped me again, and said, 'Stop snivelling. Get your clothes on, and hurry up.'

"I got dressed as quickly as I could, and he pushed me out of the door on to the landing. Then his mood changed again, and he smiled at me. He wiped my eyes with his handkerchief and said, 'There, there, my little Mary. Don't cry. It will be all right. I am quick tempered, but it is soon over. If you are a good girl, I will always look after you.'

"He put his arm around me, and I felt happy again. I knew it had been my fault for telling him about the Irishman. You see, I had hurt his feelings. He had wanted to be the first."

Her gullibility astonished me. After all that she had been through and witnessed, did she really cling to the dream that Zakir had loved her, and prized her virginity so much that his love ceased when he knew that she had been raped by a drunken Irishman?

"He took me down to the café area, and called over to one of the women I had seen holding the leg of the girl on the table the night before. He said to her, 'This is Mary. She'll be all right. Tell Uncle when he gets up.'

"Then he said to me: 'I have to go out now. I am a busy man. You stay with Gloria and she will look after you. Do what Uncle tells you. If you do what Uncle tells you, and are a good girl, I will be pleased with you. If you do not, I will be cross with you.'"

Mary whispered: "When are you coming back?"

He said, "Don't worry, I will come back. Stay here and be a good girl, and do what Uncle tells you."

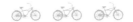

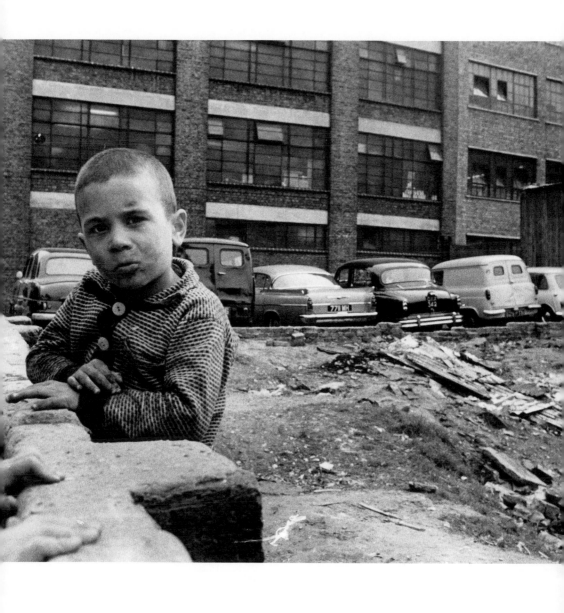

CAFÉ LIFE

During my time at Nonnatus House, I took many walks around Stepney to see what it was like. It was simply appalling. The slums were worse than I could ever have imagined. I could not believe that it was only three miles from Poplar where, although poor, badly housed and overcrowded, the people were cheerful and neighbourly. In Poplar everyone would call out to a nurse: "'allo luvvy. 'Ow's yerself? 'Ow you doin' then?" In Stepney no one spoke to me at all. I walked down Cable Street, Graces Alley, Dock Street, Sanders Street, Backhouse Lane and Leman Street, and the atmosphere was menacing. Girls hung around in doorways, and men walked up and down the streets, often in groups, or hung around the doors of cafés smoking or chewing tobacco and spitting. I always wore my full nurse's uniform, because I did not want to be propositioned. I knew that I was being watched, and that my presence was deeply resented.

The condemned buildings were still standing, nearly twenty years after they had been scheduled for demolition, and were still being lived in. A few families and old people who could not get away remained, but mostly the occupants were prostitutes, homeless immigrants, drunks or meths drinkers, and drug addicts. There were no general shops selling food and household necessities as the shops had been turned into all-night cafés, which in fact meant they were brothels. The only shops I saw were tobacconists.

Opposite: The war had left its toll on the East End and many buildings had been destroyed by bombs or were due for demolition. With little other choice, people lived, worked and played in the bombsites.

Many of the buildings apparently had no roofs. Father Joe, the vicar of St Paul's, told me he knew of a family of twelve who lived in three upper rooms, with tarpaulins to shelter them. Most of the upper storeys were quite derelict, but the lower storeys, protected by the floor above that had not yet collapsed, were teeming with humanity.

In Wellclose Square (now demolished) there was a Primary School that backed on to Cable Street. I was told that every kind of filth was thrown over the railings, so I spoke to the caretaker. He was a Stepney man born and bred, a cheerful East Ender, but he looked grim when I spoke to him. He told me that he came in early every morning to clean up before the children came to school: filthy, blood-and wine-sodden mattresses were thrown over into the school playground; sanitary towels, underwear, blood-stained sheets, condoms, bottles, syringes – just about everything. The caretaker said he burned the rubbish each morning.

Opposite the school in Graces Alley was a bomb site where the same sort of filth was thrown by the café owners every night. This was never cleaned up or burned; it just accumulated, and stank to high heaven. I could not bear to go past it – the smell from fifty yards away was enough for me – so I never did visit Graces Alley, although I was told that a few Stepney families still lived there.

The brothels, ponces and prostitutes dominated the area and the squalid derelict buildings seemed to stand gloating over the sordid trade, and evil, cruel practices. The more Cable Street became known for its cafés, the more the customers flocked there, and so the trade fed itself. The local people could do nothing. Their voice was silenced by the noise of the jukeboxes. In any case, they lived, I was told, in deadly fear of complaining and were crushed by the magnitude of the problem.

There had always been brothels in the East End. Of course there had; it was a dock land. What else would you expect? But they were always absorbed and tolerated. It was when hundreds of brothels sprang up in a small area that life became intolerable for the local inhabitants.

I could well understand the fear felt by local people, and that to complain, or in any way interfere with the profits of the café owners, would mark you out for retribution. A knifing or a beating would be all that you would get for your courage. I was glad that I walked down Sander Street in broad daylight. Through the dirty windows the haggard, painted faces of girls could be seen leaning on the windowsill, looking out, openly touting for men. As Sander Street led directly off Commercial Road, men were constantly looking into it, and going down it. These houses used to be a neat little terrace only ten or fifteen years before, a place where families lived and children played. The day I went, it looked like something from a horror film. The girls in the windows did not pester me, of course, but there were a lot of big, sinister-looking men around, who glared at me as if to say, "You get out of here." Did any Stepney family really live amid all this? Apparently yes. I saw two or three little houses with clean windows and net curtains, and a well-scrubbed doorstep. I saw one old lady shuffling along close to the wall, eyes down, till she came to her door. She looked around furtively, then opened the door with her key and shut it quickly after her. I heard two bolts slamming shut.

There is a saying amongst the masters of working dogs, be they sheep dogs, guard dogs, police dogs or huskies, 'Don't treat them with kindness, or they won't work for you.'

It is the same with pimps and prostitutes. The girls are treated like dogs, but usually far, far worse. Dogs have to be bought or bred, and in consequence are usually well looked after. They are expensive assets, and the loss of a valuable dog is a serious matter. But girls on the game are utterly expendable. They do not have to be bought, like a dog or a slave, yet they live a life of slavery, subject to the will and the whims of their masters. Most girls enter the trade voluntarily, not really aware of what they are doing, and within a very short time they find that they cannot get out of it. They are trapped.

Zakir had left Mary with the words, "Be a good girl, and do what you are told, and I will be pleased with you." Mary lived on this promise for months. Just for a smile from Zakir she would, and did, do anything.

He left her at about 8 a.m. with Gloria, a hardened old pro of about fifty who occasionally worked, but whose main job was to keep the girls up to scratch. She stared at Mary unsmiling, and said, "You 'eard what he said. You 'ave to do as you are told. You'd better get on wiv cleaning up the café and the kitchen before Uncle comes down."

Mary didn't know what to do. The whole area looked so big, and was in such a mess, that she didn't know where to begin. In the sheelin' back in Ireland, cleaning was a simple business – a bed, a table, a mat, a bench; that was all. But the café looked enormous. She stared around in bewilderment.

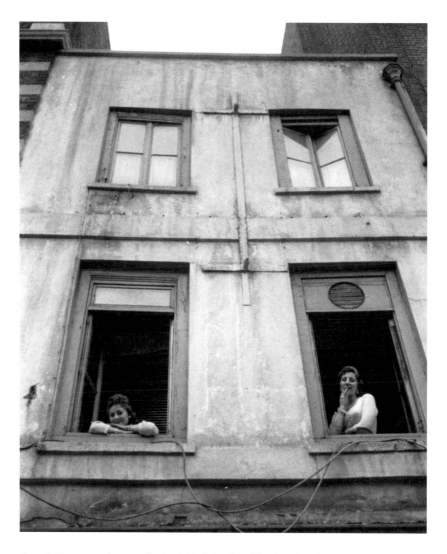

Opposite: Two women lean out of a brothel in Soho, Central London. West End prostitutes could usually charge more money to clients. In East End brothels, girls like Mary were often expected to charge as little as sixpence for sex.

A heavy foot landed in the small of her back, and she was flung forward a yard or two.

"Get on wiv it, you lazy bitch, don't just stand there starin'."

Mary jumped to it. She remembered what Zakir had said about a job in the café washing up, and she ran round collecting dirty glasses, mugs, spittoons, and a few dirty plates. She hurried with them into the kitchen, which was filthy, and over to the greasy sink. There was only cold water in the tap, but she washed everything up as best she could, and then dried the things on a filthy bit of old sheet. Gloria, in the meantime, was putting chairs up on the tables.

"Clean the floor when you've done," she called.

There wasn't a broom, but there was a wet mop, and Mary rubbed it all over the floor, in reality just pushing the dirt around.

"That's better," said Gloria. "Go and clean the kazi now."

Mary looked blank.

"The gerry, the lav, the bog, stupid."

Mary went out to the yard. It stank. The lavatory had probably been used by over a hundred men during the night, and each night before, and had not been cleaned properly for years. Most of the men peed on the ground around the shack, so the cobblestones were always wet and slippery. There was no toilet paper, only the torn up newspaper that littered the place. Some of the men had been sick, and as it was a warm summer morning, the stench was rising. This was also the only lavatory available for the girls to use, and as there was no bin, used sanitary towels lay scattered all over the yard.

Mary stared at it in horror, but fearing another kick in the back, she quickly got to work. There was a broom in the yard, so she swept up most of the more solid filth into a pile in a corner. Then she got a bucket of water, and swilled it over the yard. It seemed to be effective, so she fetched several other buckets of water, and did the same.

Gloria came out, and stared around silently. She took the fag from her mouth. "You done a good job 'ere, Mary. Zakir'll be pleased wiv you. An' Uncle an' all."

Mary glowed with pleasure. To please Zakir was her keenest desire. She said, timidly, pointing to the pile of filth in the corner:

"What shall I do with that?"

"Take it over to the bomb site in Graces Alley. I'll show you where it is."

There was no other way of picking the mess up but with her hands. Mary was not happy about it, but did so nonetheless. She had to make four trips to the bomb site to get rid of it all.

Mary felt filthy. Her last wash had been in the Cuts, and she hadn't changed her clothes for days. She went into the kitchen and washed her face and arms under the cold tap, then her feet and legs, which made her feel better. She tried to remember what had happened to the string bag, that contained her clean blouse. She remembered Zakir had carried it the night before, and she had not seen it since. She asked Gloria where he might have put it.

Gloria laughed: "You won't see that again," she said. And indeed Mary didn't.

At that moment a man entered the café. He was one of the knuckledustered pair Mary had seen the night before taking money from the men. He was thickset, with a large stomach, which hung over the belt of his trousers. Dirty slippers scraped across the floor and tattoo marks covered his arms. His face was terrifying, and robbed Mary of the power of speech. She slunk away out into the yard. The man was Uncle.

"Come back here," he shouted.

Mary was powerless to disobey. She stood before him trembling. He just stared at her with hard black eyes and sucked at his fag end. He put out a podgy hand, grabbed her shoulder, pushed her head sideways, then said, "You good girl, obey me. I look after you. You bad girl…" He didn't finish the sentence, just curled his lips and held a threatening fist up to Mary's face.

He said to Gloria, "Take her," then he walked out.

The old building consisted of the shop and back yard, two rooms in the basement, and about eight rooms on the upper storeys. All the rooms were divided into three or four small cubicles by thin boarding. In each cubicle was a narrow bed, or, in some, as many as four to six bunk beds. All the beds were filthy, grey, ex-army blankets the only cover.

Mary was taken upstairs, past the gold and silver room where she had spent the night with Zakir, to the top of the house. In the attic were about twenty girls, lying on the floor or on bunk beds. Most were asleep.

Gloria said, "You stop here. We'll want you later."

Mary sat down on the floor in a corner. She had known nothing but poverty all her life, and, since her Dublin days, had slept only in makeshift slum dwellings or outdoors, so she was not surprised or dismayed. It was hot in the attic, and she soon fell asleep.

She was woken at about 2 p.m. by movement. Most of the girls were going out. She stood up, but was told to stay where she was. She remained in the hot attic all afternoon accompanied by the heavy snores of the girl she had seen dancing on the table. She had had no food or drink, and spent the afternoon dreaming of Zakir.

In the early evening, the girl woke up. She was called Dolores, and was about twenty; a cheerful buxom wench who had been a prostitute since childhood. She knew no other life, and could not imagine any other way of earning a living. She sat up sleepily, and saw Mary, "You new?" she enquired.

Mary nodded.

"Poor little thing," she said. "Never mind, you'll get used to the game. It's all right when you get used to it. What you need is a gimmick, like me. I'm a stripper. But not one of your regular strippers. I'm an *artiste*." She said the word artiste with great pride.

"Come on, we'd better go down to the café before Gloria comes up. You need a clean blouse, here, have one of mine. And you need a bit of make up. I'll do it for you."

She chatted all the time as she dressed, doing her hair and Mary's, and making them both up. Mary liked her. Her buoyant cheerfulness was infectious.

"There now, you look lovely."

In fact, Mary looked grotesque, but she couldn't see it. The sight of her painted face in the mirror thrilled her.

"Will Zakir be there tonight?" she said.

"Yes, you'll be seeing him, don't worry."

Mary was overjoyed, and followed Dolores into the café for the evening's entertainment.

They went to the large table, where a number of girls already sat. Zakir was at the corner table, and Mary's heart leapt. She took a step towards him, but he waved her away without speaking, and she sat down sadly with the other girls. They were not talking much, and they all stared at her. One or two gave a thin smile, others openly scowled. One rough, dirty-looking girl said, "Look at her. Zakir's latest. Who does she think she is. We'll soon cut her down. You'll see, Mary, Mary, quite contrary."

Mary told me that she hadn't really liked it, and wanted to leave.

"Well, why didn't you?" I asked.

"Because Zakir was sitting in the corner, and nothing in the world could have dragged me away from him."

I supposed that was how he got and kept most of his girls.

I said, "If you had known what kind of life he was dragging you into, would you have left?"

She thought, and said: "I don't think so, at first. It was not until I saw him bring in several other young girls, and sit at the corner table with them, that I began to understand what he meant when he said he was 'the meat buyer'.

221

I wanted to run over to the girl and warn her, but I couldn't, and anyway, it would have done no good."

That night Mary had her first clients. She was auctioned as a virgin, and the highest bidder got her first, with eight others following after. The next day Zakir put his arm around her, and told her that he was very pleased with her. He flashed his smile at her and her heart melted.

She lived off this smile, and the others he condescended to give her, for months.

For the first week, the clients were arranged for her from the men who came to the café, and they paid Uncle. She hated it, and found the men revolting, but as Dolores and many of the others said, "You get used to it."

When she was pushed out on to the street, and told to find her own clients, the real horror began.

"I had to bring back one pound each day," she said. "If I didn't, Uncle would hit me in the face, or knock me down and kick me. At first I asked for two shillings [10p] but there were so many other girls on the game, asking sixpence or one shilling, that I had to cut my price too. Sometimes I would bring the men back to the café, but sometimes we just did it in alleyways or doorways, up against a wall, anywhere – even the bomb sites. I hated myself. There were dreadful fights between girls about whose pitch was whose, and fights between the men. If a girl tried to go to another protector, she might get her throat cut. You just don't know the dreadful things that go on."

"I was out all the time. I got some sleep in the mornings, but I had to go out every afternoon until about five or six the next morning. I hardly got any food, except some chips at the café , if I was lucky. I hated it, but I couldn't seem to stop. I'm filthy, I'm bad, I'm …"

I cut her short, not wanting her to dwell on self-reproval: "Well, you left in the end. What made you do that?"

"The baby," she said quietly, "and Nelly. I liked Nelly," she continued. "She was the only girl who was always kind to all the other girls. She never quarrelled and was never spiteful. She came from an orphanage in Glasgow and never knew who her father and mother were, nor if she had any brothers and sisters. She was always lonely, I think, because deep down inside, she was always looking for someone who belonged to her. She was two years older than me."

Then Mary told me the terrible truth.

* * *

Gloria found out that Nelly was expecting a baby. It had happened before, other girls had fallen pregnant, but I hadn't been involved, because I wasn't friends with them. Gloria made arrangements, and a woman came in. I don't know who she was, but the girls said she always did it. It was a morning, and I was asleep after my night out. I heard terrible screaming, and I knew at once that it was Nelly's voice. I ran downstairs and found her in a little room. She was lying on a bed screaming, and Gloria and two other girls were holding her legs open while this woman stuck what looked like steel knitting needles inside her. I rushed in and took Nelly in my arms, and told them to stop, but of course they wouldn't. I couldn't stop the pain for Nelly, either, so I just held her tight in my arms."

I asked Mary to tell me more about Nelly.

"It was dreadful. The woman went on and on poking and scraping. Then suddenly there was blood everywhere. All over the bed, and the floor, and the woman. She said, 'That's all she needs. Just keep her in bed for a few days. She'll be all right.' They cleaned up, and threw the mess into the bomb site, while I stayed with Nelly. She was dead white, and still in dreadful pain. I didn't know what to do, so I just stayed with her, and gave her water, and tried to make her comfortable. Gloria looked in sometimes, and told me to sit with her, and not to go out that night."

Mary started to cry.

"Sometimes she knew who I was, sometimes she didn't. She got terribly hot. Her skin was burning up. I wiped her with cold water, but it didn't help. All the time she was bleeding, till the mattress was soaked with blood. I sat with her all day and all night, and the pain never left her. In the early morning, she died in my arms."

She was silent – then said bitterly:

"I don't know what they did with her body. There was no funeral, and no police came. I suppose they just got rid of her, and told no one about it."

I pondered, was it really possible to dispose of a body? If the girl had no relatives or friends, who would enquire about her if she disappeared? The other girls at the café knew her, but it seemed that they all lived in so much fear of Uncle, that they would say nothing. If Gloria or the abortionist were caught, it would probably have meant a charge of murder or at the very least manslaughter, so a web of protection was woven around them. I had

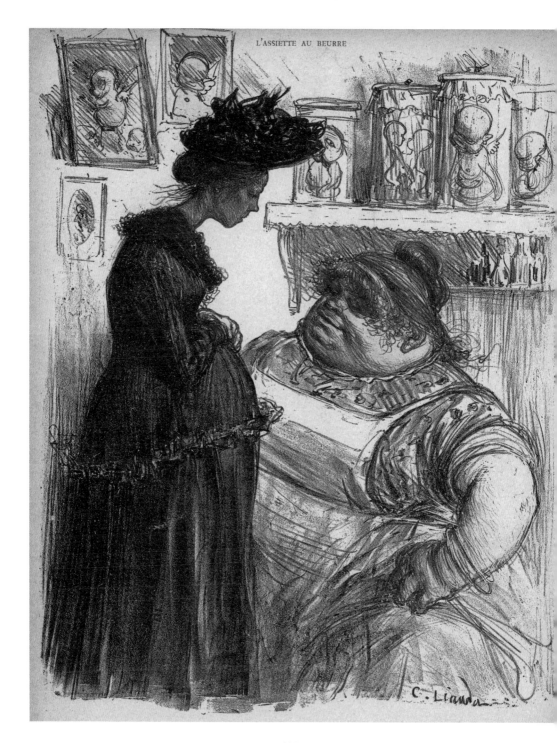

L'ASSIETTE AU BEURRE

C. Liand

little doubt that many other prostitutes had disappeared and no one ever missed them because they were usually homeless, unwanted girls.

A couple of months later, Mary realised that she, too, was pregnant but fear made her conceal the fact. She continued to go out soliciting, even though she was sick most of the time. She told me that she wanted to get away but was too afraid to try. The baby didn't mean anything to her, until she felt it moving inside her, and then a rush of maternal love swept over her. Some time later, as she was dressing in the attic one day, another girl screamed out:

"Look at Mary. There's a bun in the oven."

And then everyone knew.

Mary was frantic, and knew she had to get away. She said, "I didn't mind if they were going to kill me. But they weren't going to kill me baby."

That evening she came in with a customer, and as she went upstairs, she saw that the door of the gold and silver room was open. She told the man to undress in a cubicle, and slipped into the room. There was a lot of money on a table. She grabbed five pounds and ran like mad, out into the street and away.

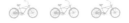

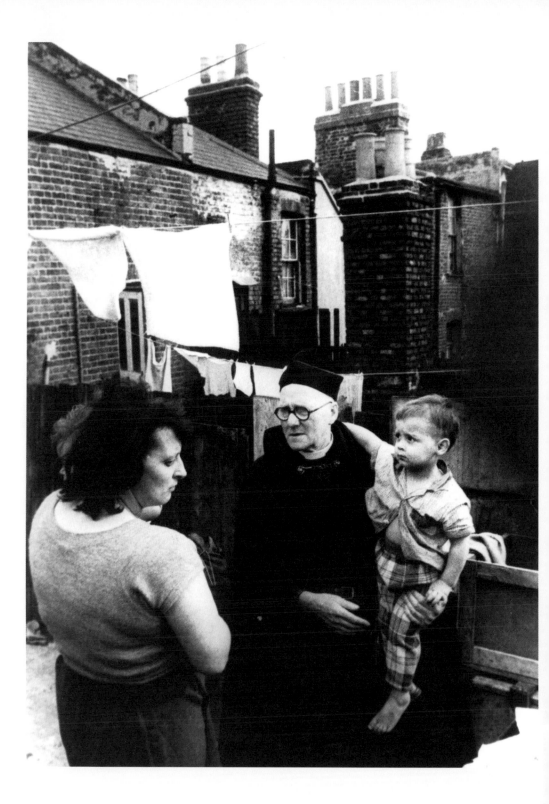

FLIGHT

Mary ran for her life, and the life of her baby. She hadn't the faintest idea of where she was going, so she just ran, driven by fear. It was night-time, and in her heightened imagination, she thought that someone was pursuing her with every step. She mainly kept to the unlit side streets, because under the lights of the main roads, she thought she would be recognised.

"I turned corner after corner, and hid in doorways, then doubled back and ran down another dark street, always avoiding the lights of the big roads. I spent nearly the whole night running."

In fact, Mary must have run round in circles, because she described the river and the docks and boats, and a church where she rested in the porch, which sounded very like the famous Bow Bells Church. She did not get very far. After her sleep in the church porch, the terrors of the night departed, and she thought she would take a bus, to get a long way away, to a place where no one would look for her. It was not until she had actually boarded the platform of a bus and saw the bus conductor clipping tickets and taking one and two penny fares, that she realised her predicament with the five pounds. She could not possibly use it. She leapt off the bus just as it started to move, and fell into the gutter. Several people came over to help her up, but she was so terrified that she brushed them aside, and ran, hiding her face in her hands.

Opposite: Father Joe Williamson speaking with some of his parishioners. "Father Joe was a saint. Saints come in all sorts of shapes and sizes – they don't have to wear halos."

Mary spent the whole day hiding. It did not seem rational. I asked her, "Why did you not go to a police station and claim protection?"

Her reply was interesting.

"I couldn't. I was a thief. They would have locked me up, or taken me back to the café, and made me give the money back to Uncle."

Her terror of Uncle was almost tangible, so she spent the whole day wandering, and hiding from people. She must have headed south again from Bow towards the river as it was in the East India Dock Road that she finally had the idea of asking someone, a lady who did not look as though she could possibly be mixed up in prostitution, to change the five pound note. As I stepped off the bus that evening she had approached me and I had taken her back to Nonnatus House where she had had the first good meal, and the first night's sleep in a secure, warm environment that she had had since leaving the sheelin' back in County Mayo.

It was Sister Julienne who made the arrangements for Mary to go to Church House in Wellclose Square. This house had been set up, and staffed by volunteers as a refuge for prostitutes by Father Joe Williamson.

Father Joe was a saint. Saints come in all sorts of shapes and sizes – they don't have to wear halos. Father Joe was born and bred in the slums of Poplar in the 1890s. Somehow he survived cold, hunger, neglect, and four years at the front during the First World War. He was a rough, tough East End street kid, crude and loud mouthed, yet when he was no more than a child, he had a vision that God was calling him to be a priest. He overcame a lack of proper education, a thick Cockney accent that no one else could understand, the inability to express himself, and class prejudice. He was ordained in the 1920s, and many years later, after serving as a parish priest in Norfolk, returned to the East End, to St Paul's parish in Stepney, right in the heart of the red-light district. He saw at first hand the appalling life these girls led. From then on, he devoted the rest of his life to helping prostitutes who wanted to escape. The Wellclose Trust still exists in the twenty-first century, and is still engaged in the same work. At Church House Mary was given a bath, clean warm clothes and good food. She was with about six other girls who, with varying degrees of success, were trying to kick the habit of prostitution. Mary was too frightened to go out, but gradually her fears about being found and murdered subsided, colour returned to her pale cheeks, and her Irish eyes began to sparkle.

I visited her several times during this period of calm, because she always seemed to want me to, and also because I wanted to learn more about prostitutes. It was during these visits that I learned the harrowing details of her life in London. I think she was relatively happy during this brief period, but it could not last. For one thing her pregnancy was advancing, and whilst she could receive antenatal care at Church House, they were not equipped to cope with a mother and baby. But more important was the fact that Church House was perilously close to Cable Street and the Full Moon Café. Whilst she did not leave the house there was no danger, but at some stage, she would want to venture out – Church House was not a prison. When she did, the chances of her being recognised, Father Joe speculated, were very real, and Mary's fears of abduction or murder were not a fantasy.

In her eighth month of pregnancy, and still only fifteen years old, she was transferred to a home for mothers and babies run by the Roman Catholic Church. It was in Kent, and I went there once, about a fortnight before the baby was born. Mary was full of excitement and happiness. She enjoyed the company and friendship of the other women and girls, who were not prostitutes, but were from the poorest and most vulnerable sections of society. Many of them had babies, and Mary was able to indulge her instincts in the gentlest and happiest of all feminine activities. The nuns held classes in baby care, and she happily bathed and dressed dolls, and listened to talks on colic, nappy rash and breastfeeding, counting the days until her baby would be born.

The staff at Church House received a postcard the same morning as one arrived for me, telling of the birth of a little girl, Kathleen. I thought one of the nuns must have written it, because I knew that Mary could read a little, but could barely write. However, her name was written in big letters across the bottom, with a row of kisses.

I was deeply touched by these straggly X's, about twenty-five of them, and I wondered who else she had communicated her wonderful news to with so many kisses. Her mother? Her brothers and sisters? Did she know where her drunken mother was, or her sisters in the orphanage in Dublin? If a postcard had been sent to the old address as she remembered it, had it been received, or had the family moved on? Did anyone else know? Did anyone else care? Tears came to my eyes as I looked at the row of X's, kisses showered with such lavish affection on someone she had merely picked up at a bus stop.

A few days later, it being my day off, I went to see Mary in Kent, feeling that someone must rejoice with her over this miraculous event. On the journey, I pondered that it might be the making of her. Motherhood brings out the best in most women, and flighty, giddy young girls often become responsible, reliable mothers, as soon as the baby is born. I had not the slightest doubt that she was a sweet and loving young girl, who was too trusting by half. I reflected that it had been her gentle, trusting nature, combined with the poverty and physical hardships of her life, that had led her to prostitution in the first place. There was no doubt that she hated it, and had been virtually a slave. Now she was liberated. The train jogged along through the countryside, and I felt a quiet wave of satisfaction and pleasure. I had not reflected upon how she was going to support herself and the baby.

I found Mary radiant with happiness. The soft glow of early motherhood emanated from her, and seemed to embrace me with its warmth as I entered the door. Two months' rest, good food and good antenatal care, had worked miracles on her. Gone was the pale, pinched look, gone the nervous hand movements; above all, the fear had disappeared from her eyes. She was completely unconscious of her beauty, which made her all the more appealing. And the baby? Well of course, every baby is the most beautiful in the world, and this little one surpassed all others without even trying! Kathleen was ten days old, and Mary told me all about her excellence: how well she slept, how well she fed, how she gurgled and laughed and kicked. She prattled on joyously, totally absorbed by her own all-consuming love. I left thinking that this was the best thing that could possibly have happened to her, and that a new life was opening up for Mary.

A fortnight or so later a postcard arrived:

ners jeny
nonatun hose
popler lundun

It is a tribute to our postal service that it arrived at all, for, apart from the address, it had no stamp. On the back was scrawled:

baby gon. cum too see mee. mary xxxxxx.

I showed the card to Sister Julienne, feeling concerned.

"Does '*gon*' mean gone? If so where? Surely it cannot mean the baby has died?" I asked.

Sister turned the card over in her hand several times, before saying: "No, I think if the baby had died, she would have written 'DED'. You had better go to see her on your day off, which is obviously what she wants."

The train journey to Kent seemed longer and more tiresome than the previous one. I had no happy thoughts to make the time fly past. My mind was puzzled, and an unpleasant feeling of foreboding would not go away The mother and baby home looked much the same as before, pleasant open grounds, prams dotted about the gardens, smiling young women, nuns going about their work. I entered, and was taken to a sitting room.

I was stunned when I saw Mary. She looked absolutely ghastly: her face was swollen, red and blotchy, with great rings under her eyes. She stared at me, unseeing. Her hair was dishevelled, her clothes were torn. I stood in the doorway looking at her, but she did not see me; instead she leapt up, rushed to the window, and began to hammer the glass with her fists, moaning all the while. Then she ran to the opposite side of the room and beat her forehead on the wall. It was hard to believe what I was seeing.

I went over to her and said "Mary" quite loudly. I repeated her name several times. She turned, eventually recognising me, and gave a cry. She grabbed me and tried to speak, but words wouldn't come.

I led her to a sofa, and sat her down.

"What is it?" I asked "What has happened?"

"They have taken my baby."

"Where?"

"I don't know. They won't tell me."

"When?"

"I don't know. But she's gone. She wasn't there in the morning."

I didn't know what to say. What can one say to such terrible news? We stared at one another in mute horror, then she winced with pain, a pain that seemed to suffuse her entire body. She threw her arms outwards and fell back against the cushions. I saw at once what the trouble was. She had been breastfeeding, and now, with no milk being drawn off, her breasts were horribly engorged. I leaned forward and opened her blouse. Both breasts were enormous, as hard as stone, and the left side was bright red and hot to touch.

"She could get a breast abscess," I thought. "In fact she probably has one already."

She moaned: "It hurts," and gritted her teeth together to stop herself from screaming.

My mind was in turmoil. What on earth had happened? I couldn't believe that Mary's baby had been taken away. When the worst spasm of pain had passed, I said, "I am going to see the Reverend Mother."

She grasped my hand. "Oh yes, I knew you would get my baby back."

She smiled, and as she did so, tears flooded her eyes, and she turned her head into the cushion, sobbing pitifully. I left, and enquired my way to the Reverend Mother's office.

The room was bare and sparsely furnished: a desk, two wooden chairs, and a cupboard. The walls were white, and only a bare crucifix broke the smooth surface. The Reverend Mother's habit was entirely black, with a white veil. She looked middle-aged, and very handsome. Her expression was serene and open. I felt at once that I could talk to her.

"Where is Mary's baby?" I demanded aggressively.

The Reverend Mother looked at me steadily, before replying, "The baby has been placed for adoption."

"Without the mother's consent?"

"Consent is not necessary. The child is only fourteen."

"Fifteen," I said.

"Fourteen or fifteen, it makes no difference. She is still legally a child, and consent is neither valid nor invalid."

"But how dare you take her baby away without her knowledge. It is killing her."

The Reverend Mother sighed. She sat perfectly straight, not resting against the back of the chair, her hands folded beneath her scapular. She looked timeless, ageless, pitiless. Only the cross on her breast moved to the rhythm of her breathing. She said evenly, "The baby is being adopted into a good Roman Catholic family who have one child. The mother, due to an illness, can have no more. Mary's baby will have a good upbringing and a good education. She will have all the advantages of a good Christian home."

"Good Christian home be bothered," I said, my anger rising. "Nothing can replace a mother's love, and Mary loves her baby. She will die, or go mad, from the grief."

The Reverend Mother sat for a moment, quietly looking at the branch of a tree that was moving just outside the window. Then she turned her head slowly, and looked straight into my eyes. This slow, deliberate movement of her head, first towards the window, and then back towards me, helped to check my anger. Her face was sad. Perhaps she is not pitiless, I thought.

"We have done all we can to trace Mary's family. We have spent three months searching parish and civil records in Ireland, with no success. Mary's mother is a drunk, and cannot be traced. There are no living uncles or aunts. The father is dead. The younger siblings are in care. If we could have found any relative or guardian who would take Mary and her baby, and pledge responsibility for them, there is no doubt at all that she would have been able to keep her baby. However, we could find no one. In the wider interests of the baby, the decision was taken for adoption."

"But it will kill Mary," I said.

The Reverend Mother did not answer this, but said: "How can a girl of fifteen, with no literacy, no home, no trade beyond that of prostitution, support and care for a growing child?"

It was my turn not to answer the question.

"She has left prostitution," I said.

The Reverend Mother sighed again, and paused for quite a long time before speaking. "You are young, my dear, and full of righteous indignation, which our Lord loves. But you must understand that it is very, very rare for a prostitute to leave the trade. It is too easy to make money. A girl is hard up, and the opportunity is always there. Why slave away all day in a factory for five shillings, when you can earn ten or fifteen shillings in half an hour? We know from experience that few things are more damaging to a growing child than to watch mother working on the streets."

"But you cannot condemn her for what she has not yet done."

"No, we do not condemn, nor blame. The Church forgives. In any case, it is quite clear that Mary was more sinned against than sinning. Our main concern is for the protection and upbringing of the baby. Mary has nowhere to go when she leaves here. Who will take her in? We endeavoured to find a residential post in service for Mary to go to, but with a baby no such post could be found."

I was silent. The Reverend Mother's logic was irrefutable. I repeated my earlier point, "But it will kill her. She already looks half mad."

The Reverend Mother sat perfectly still, the leaves fluttering outside the window. She did not speak for about half a minute. Then she said: "We are born into suffering, uncertainty, and death. My mother had fifteen children.

Overleaf: This 1930s' photograph shows National Adoption Society babies in their cots being cared for by nurses. A prospective parent studies a baby. Young girls like Mary often had their babies put up for adoption.

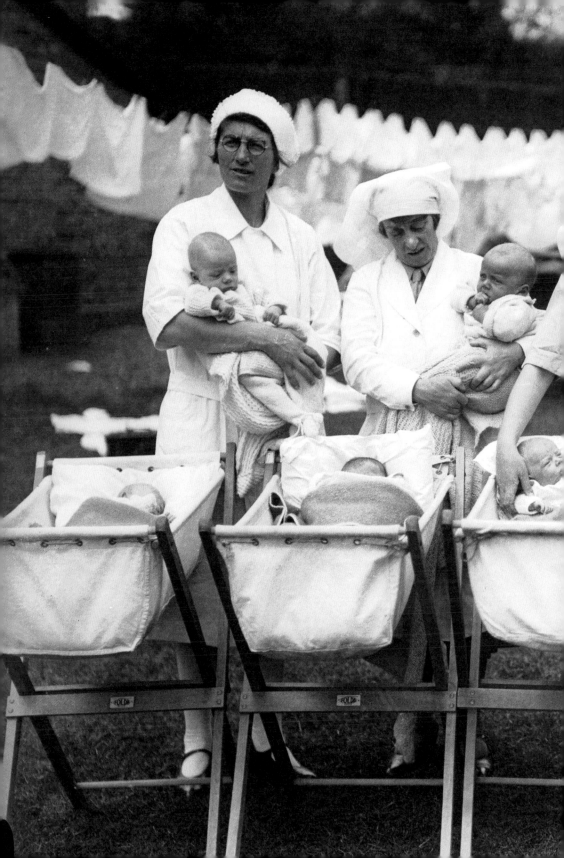

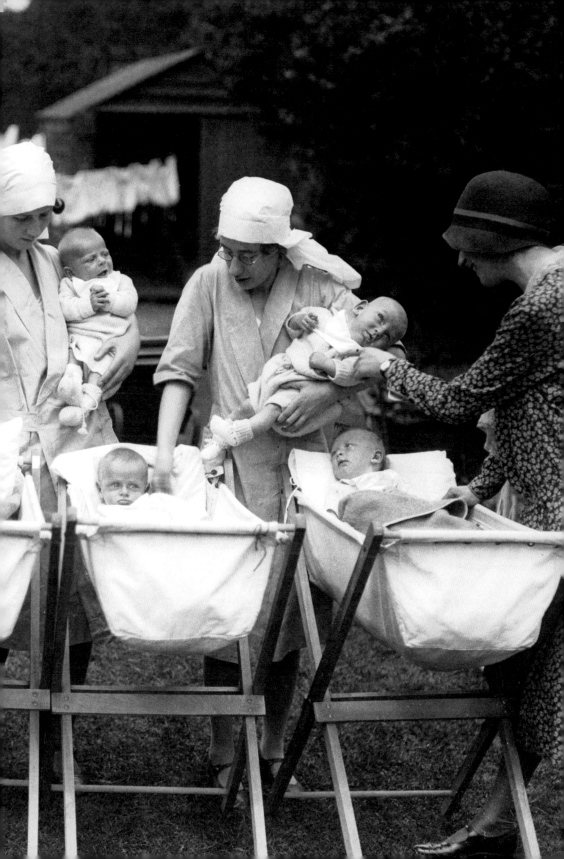

Only four survived childhood. Eleven times my mother suffered the agonies that Mary is going through. Countless millions of women throughout history have buried most of the children they have borne, and endured the sorrows of child bereavement. They have lived through it, as Mary will, and they have borne more children, as I hope Mary will."

I could say nothing. Perhaps I should have ranted and railed about the arrogance and presumption of taking the decision out of Mary's control; I could have sneered at the wealth of the Roman Catholic Church; I could have asked why could the Church not support Mary and her baby for a few years? I could, perhaps should, have said many things, but I was silenced by my own knowledge of the statistics of child mortality, by the depth of understanding in her words, and by the sadness in her eyes. I merely said, "Will Mary ever know who has adopted her baby?"

The Reverend Mother shook her head. "No. Even I do not know the actual name. None of the Sisters are ever told. The adoption is completely anonymous, but you can assure Mary that her baby has gone to a good Catholic family, and that she will have a good home."

There was nothing more to be said, and the Reverend Mother rose from her seat. This was the signal that the interview was over. She withdrew her right hand from behind her scapular and held it out to me. Long, slender, sensitive fingers. It is not often that you see such a beautiful hand, and as I took it, her grasp was firm and warm. Our eyes met, with sadness and, I think, mutual respect. I returned to the sitting room. Mary leapt from the sofa as I entered, her face alight with expectancy. But she read my features in an instant and, with a cry of despair, she fell back on to the sofa and buried her head in the cushions again. I sat beside her, trying to console her, but consolation was impossible. I told her the baby would go to a good home, where she would be well looked after. I tried to tell her how impossible it would be for her to work, and live, and support a growing child. I don't think she heard or understood anything I said. Her face remained hidden in the cushions. I told her I had to leave soon, but she did not respond at all. I tried to stroke her hair, but she pushed my hand away angrily. I crept out of the room, and shut the door quietly, too sad even to say goodbye.

I did not see Mary again. I wrote to her once, but received no reply. A month later, I wrote to Reverend Mother, enquiring, and was informed that Mary had accepted a residential post as a ward maid in a hospital in Birmingham. I wrote to her there but again, no reply. Circumstances bring people together, and take them apart. One cannot keep up with everyone in a lifetime. In any event, was there any true friendship between myself and Mary? Probably not. It was mainly a friendship of dependence on her part, with pity and (I'm almost ashamed to confess it) curiosity, on my part. I was intrigued to find out more about the hidden world of prostitution. That is no basis for a meeting of minds, and true affection, so I let the contact drop.

Some years later – by which time I was very happily married with two children – front page headlines in all the papers carried the story that a baby had been snatched from a pram in a suburb of Manchester. Desperate and tearful parents were interviewed on television, begging for the return of their baby. A nationwide police hunt was launched, and sightings of the possible kidnapper were reported from all over the country. All of them proved to be red herrings. Twelve days passed, and the story receded from public attention. On the fourteenth day, I read that a woman had been apprehended in Liverpool, boarding a boat for Ireland. She was carrying a six-week-old baby, and was being held for questioning. A few days later, a larger report carried the story that the woman questioned had been charged with the unlawful abduction of a baby two weeks earlier. The photograph was of Mary. She was held in custody for five months awaiting trial. During all that time, I wondered if I should go to see her, but did not do so. Part of my hesitation was because I wondered what on earth we would talk about, but also, with two children under three, a home to care for, and a part-time night sister's post, a trip to Liverpool and back – to what end? – was an intimidating prospect.

I followed the trial in the newspapers. Mitigating circumstances of the loss of her own baby were raised. Her counsel emphasised the fact that the baby had been well cared for, and stressed that no harm was intended. But the prosecution dwelt upon the suffering of the parents and the vagrant, unstable life that Mary had always led. Twenty-six other offences of soliciting and petty larceny were taken into consideration. The jury found Mary guilty, with a plea for mercy. Nonetheless, the judge sent her down for three years, with a recommendation that psychiatric treatment should be given whilst the prisoner was in Her Majesty's custody. Mary commenced her sentence in Manchester Prison for Women in her twenty-first year.

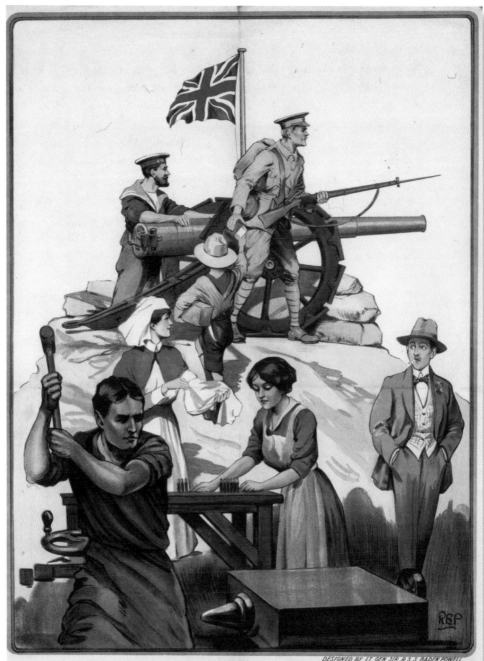

DESIGNED BY LT. GEN. SIR R.S.S. BADEN POWELL.

Are <u>YOU</u> in this?

SISTER EVANGELINA

Due to a broken shoulder I was unable to take the final midwifery exam, and had to wait several months for the next sitting. Sister Julienne suggested I might join the General District practice for added experience. Thus, I had the privilege of working with old people who had been born in the nineteenth century.

Sister Evangelina was in charge of General District nursing. Whilst I was eager to undertake the nursing, I was not at all keen to work with Sister Evangelina, whom I found ponderous and humourless. Also, she gave me to understand, subtly but unmistakably, that she did not at all approve of me. She was constantly finding fault: a door banged; a window left open; untidiness; day-dreaming ("wool-gathering" she called it); boisterousness; singing in the clinical room; forgetfulness, the list was endless. I could do nothing right for Sister Evangelina. When Sister Julienne informed her that I was to work with her, she stared at me, her heavy features set in a dour expression, then said "Humph!" and turned and stomped away. Not a word more!

We worked together for several months and, whilst I never grew close to her, I certainly grew to understand her better, and to realise that all nuns, by the very fact of their monastic profession, are exceptional people. No ordinary woman could live such a life. There must inevitably be something, or many things, that

Opposite: This British First World War poster, designed by Robert Baden-Powell, encourages everyone – from nurses and female munitions worker to boy scouts – to do their bit for the war effort.

are oustanding about a nun. To me, Sister Evangelina looked about forty-five; an unimaginable age when you are twenty-three. But nuns always look years younger than they really are, and she had, in fact, been a nurse in the First World War, so therefore must have been over sixty at the time of which I am writing.

The first morning did not start well. The clinical room boiler had gone out, and her instruments and syringes were therefore not sterile. She called loudly and crossly to Fred to come and attend to it, and grumbled about "that useless man" as he whistled his tuneless way downstairs with his shovels and rakes and pokers. She ordered me to "go to the kitchen, and boil these things up on the gas stove, whilst I sort out the dressings, and look sharp about it". On the way to the door, a glass syringe fell out of the overflowing kidney dish and broke on the stone floor. She shouted at me about carelessness and clumsiness and what she has to put up with these days. When she got to the bit about "flighty young girls" I fled, leaving the broken glass behind me. In the kitchen, Mrs B. was at the gas stove with half a dozen saucepans boiling away merrily, and she did not receive me amicably. Consequently it took quite a long time to sterilise the things, and I could hear Sister Evangelina shouting before I had even left the kitchen. She took the equipment from me to pack the bags, commenting on my "dawdling around, and wool-gathering, as usual, and didn't I realise we had twenty-three insulin injections, and four sterile dressings, and two leg ulcers, and three post-operative hernias, as well as two catheterisations, two bed-baths and three enemas to get through before lunch?".

All the midwives had gone, and we were the last to leave that morning. The bicycle shed was nearly empty. Sister Evangelina's favourite bicycle had been taken, inadvertently, by someone else. Her nose grew red, her eyes bulged, and she muttered under her breath about how she "didn't like this one, and that old Triumph was too small, and the Sunbeam was too high", and she supposed she would have to make do with the Raleigh, but it wasn't the one she liked.

Respectfully, I pulled the Raleigh out for her, fixed the black bag on the back, and watched the tyres sag as her large, heavy body clambered onto it. I think I realised then that she was not in her forties. Her square, bulky frame had no agility, and it was only by sheer determination and will power that she got herself pedalling at all.

Once out on the road her mood seemed to lighten, and she turned to me with something that resembled a smile. Along the streets numerous voices called out "Mornin', Sister Evie." She smiled brightly – I hadn't seen her smile like that before – and called gaily back. Once she tried a wave, but the bike wobbled perilously, so she didn't try again. I began to think that she was popular and well known in the area.

In the houses she was bluff and gruff, and not at all polite (I thought), but nonetheless everyone seemed to take it in good part.

"Now then, Mr Thomas, have you got your sample ready? Don't keep me waiting; I've got to test it, and I haven't all day to hang around waiting for you. Right, hold still for the injection. Hold still, I said. Now, I'm off. If you start eating sweets, they'll kill you. Not that I would care, and I dare say your missus would be glad to see the back of you, but the dog would miss you."

I was shocked. This was no way to talk to patients, according to the nursing textbooks. But the old man and his missus roared with laughter, and he said: "If I goes first, I'll keep a place warm for yer, eh, Sis Evie? An' we can share the ol' toasting fork."

I thought she would be furious at such effrontery, but she stomped downstairs in good humour, with "Out of my way, boy" to a child we met in the passage.

Her good humour, and her rough badinage with all the patients, continued throughout the morning. I ceased to be startled, because I realised that this was what the patients liked about her. She approached them all without a trace of sentimentality or condescension. The older Docklanders were accustomed to meeting middle-class do-gooders, who deigned to act graciously to inferiors. The Cockneys despised these people, used them for what they could get, and made fun of them behind their backs, but Sister Evangelina had no patronising airs and graces. She would have been incapable of them. Imagination was not her strong point, and she could not have contrived nor invented anything. She was unswervingly honest, and reacted to every person and every situation without guile or affectation.

As the months passed I began to understand why Sister Evangelina was so popular. It was because she was one of them. She was not a Cockney, but had been born into a very poor working-class family from Reading. She never told me this (she hardly ever spoke to me) but, from remarks made to the patients, it became perfectly clear. For example, "These young housewives, they don't know they're born. What! A lavatory in every flat? Remember the old middens, do you, Dad, and the newspaper on the seat, and queueing up in the frost when you're bursting?" This was usually followed by laughter, and some coarse lavatorial humour, ending up with the old chestnut about the chap who fell in a midden and came up with a gold watch. Lavatory humour was not considered vulgar or in bad taste amongst the working class during the early part of the last century, because the natural bodily functions were a conspicuous event. There was no privacy. A dozen or more families shared one midden, which had only half a door, the upper and lower portions being missing. So everyone knew who was in it, could hear everything and, above all, could smell everything. "She's a stinker" was not a moral observation, but a statement of fact.

Sister Evangelina shared this robust humour. Before an enema: "Now then, Dad, we're going to put a squib up your arse, shake your insides about a bit. Got the jerry ready, Mother, and the clothes pegs to clip on our noses." Laughter would continue about how he hadn't "been" for a fortnight, and there must be a turd inside as big as an elephant's. And no one was the slightest bit embarrassed, least of all the patient.

No, indeed, Sister Evangelina was not humourless. The only trouble was that at Nonnatus House her humour was different from everyone else's. She was surrounded by middle-class values, and the safety-valve of humour, which was common to all the nuns, was perpetually closed to her. She simply couldn't understand their jokes, so she always had to watch to see when everyone else was laughing and then joined in, somewhat half-heartedly.

Equally, her own brand of humour would definitely not have been appreciated in the convent. In fact it would have been greeted with severe disapprobation. Perhaps she had tried in the past, and been required by the Reverend Mother to do penance for loose or unguarded speech, so the young novice had simply buttoned herself up, and outwardly appeared solemn and heavily serious. It was only with her patients in the docklands that she could truly be herself.

Even her speech slipped from the middle-class pronunciation that she had acquired over the years into an approximation of the Cockney dialect. She never spoke broad Cockney – that would have been an affectation of which she was incapable – but certain phrases and idioms came naturally to her. She would talk freely about "Mystic Spec", which puzzled me greatly, until I discovered it was Cockney slang for Mist. Expect., "Mist." being medical Latin, short for "mixture", and "expect.", short for "expectorant". This meant Ipecacuanha, which could be bought at any chemist's, and was the sovereign remedy for just about everything. She also talked about "pew-monica" for pneumonia, and "the screws" for rheumatism, "Uncle Dick" for a bit sick, or "a touch of the inkey blue", meaning flu. She had a variety of expressions for an intestinal disorder – the runs, the squitters, the gripes, the cramps, the needles – all of which were greeted with howls of laughter. She obviously understood a lot of Cockney rhyming slang, although she did not use it much. Having said that, I remember being flummoxed when she told me to get her "weasel", and just stared at her, not daring to ask what she meant. Someone else fetched her coat.

She shared the older people's fear of hospitals, a fear which was widely expressed through scorn and derision. Most hospitals in England, even in the 1950s, were converted workhouses, so the buildings alone had an aura of degradation and death for people who had lived all their lives with the terror of being sent to the workhouse. Sister Evangelina did nothing to dispel this fear of hospitals; in fact she actively encouraged it, an attitude that would have been heavily censored by the Royal College of Nursing, had they known about it. She would say things like, "You don't want to go into hospital to be messed about by a lot of students", or "They only make out they treat the poor for the benefit of the rich", both statements implying that the hospitals liked to experiment on their poor patients. She proclaimed, from experience, that women who went into hospital with complications after a back-street abortion were deliberately given a rough time. That Sister Evangelina was incapable of inventing, or even exaggerating, anything, spoke to the truth of her statement. Whether or not such treatment was widespread in England in the early part of this century I am unable to say. However, in the mid 1950s, I had witnessed the appalling truth of her remark in a Paris hospital, an experience I have been unable to forget to this day.

Sister Evangelina had plenty of homespun advice to offer her patients: "Where-ere you be, let your wind go free", to which the reply was always chanted: "In Church and Chapel let it rattle". Once an old man followed this by "Oops! sorry, Sister, no disrespect", and she replied, "None taken – I'm sure the Rector does it an' all." Constipation, diarrhoea, leeks and greens, gripes and pipes, flutes and fluffs provided more hilarity than any other subject, and Sister Evangelina was always in the thick of it. After recovering from my initial shock, I realised that it was not considered to be vulgar or obscene. If the Kings of France had been able to defecate daily before his entire Court, so could the Cockneys! On the other hand, sexual obscenities and blasphemy were strictly taboo in respectable Poplar families, and sexual morality was expected and enforced.

But I digress. Sister Evangelina interested me greatly because of her background: the slums of Reading in the nineteenth century, and the fact that she had raised herself from abject poverty and semi-literacy to become a trained nurse and midwife. It would have been hard enough for a young man, but for a girl to break free from ignorance and poverty and become accepted in a middle-class profession was exceptional. Only a very strong character could have achieved it.

I discovered that the First World War had been her key to freedom. She was sixteen when war broke out, and had been working in the Huntley and Palmer's Biscuit Factory in Reading since the age of eleven. In 1914, posters appeared all over the town calling on people to join the war effort. She hated Huntley and Palmer's and with youthful optimism decided that a munitions factory could only be an improvement.She had to leave home as the factory was seven miles away – too far to walk when working hours were from 6 a.m. to 8 p.m. Accommodation was provided for the girls and women in dormitories that slept sixty or seventy females on narrow iron bedsteads with horsehair mattresses. The young Evie had never slept in a bed all by herself before, and thought this really must be an example of superior living. A uniform and shoes were provided for the workers, and as she had only worn rags and no shoes before, this was also a real luxury, even though the shoes hurt her poor young feet. Food from the factory kitchens, though plain and meagre, was better than anything she had ever had, and she lost the pale, pinched, half-starved look. She became, not a beauty, but passably pretty.

At the factory bench, where she stood all day putting nuts into military machinery, a girl talked about her sister who was a nurse, and told stories about the young men who were wounded, diseased and dying. Something stirred in young Evie's soul, and she knew that she must become a nurse. She found out where the girl's sister worked, and applied to the Matron. She was only sixteen, but was accepted as a VAD, which really meant, for a girl of her class, a skivvy in the hospital wards. She didn't mind. It was the sort of menial work she had been doing all her life, with no promise of anything else. But this time the horizons were broader and clearer. She watched the trained nurses with admiration, and decided that, however long it took, she would be one of them.

Sister Evangelina and her ageing Poplar patients spoke frequently about the First World War, and shared memories and experiences. It was from these conversations overheard during a bed bath or a surgical dressing that I was able to piece together her history. Occasionally she would speak to me directly, or answer a question, but not very often. She never unbuttoned with me much.

She spoke only once about her soldier patients. She said, "They were so young, so very young. A whole generation of young men died, leaving a whole generation of young women to weep." I looked across the bed at her – she did not know I was looking – and saw tears gathering in the corners of her eyes. She sniffed loudly, and stamped her foot, then continued bandaging up the dressing somewhat roughly, with: "There you are, Dad, that's that. We'll see you in three days. Keep 'em open," and stomped off.

She was twenty when she volunteered to go behind enemy lines. She and a patient were talking about the air force of those days, the tiny bi-planes, only invented about twenty years previously. She said, "It was after the German spring offensive in 1918. Our men were wounded, stranded behind the line with no medical help. None could be sent to them by road, so an airlift was arranged. I parachuted down."

The patient said, "You've got guts, Sister. Didn't you know that 50 per cent of all those early parachutes never opened at all?"

"Of course I knew," she said, bluntly. "It was all explained to us. No one was pressed. I volunteered."

I looked at her with new eyes. To volunteer to jump from an aeroplane, knowing full well that there was a 50 per cent chance of it being your last step, would take more than guts. It would take an inner heroism of a rare quality.

One day we were returning from the Isle of Dogs to Poplar. West Ferry Road, Manchester Road, and Preston Road were, as they are today, a continuous thoroughfare following the course of the Thames. In those days, however, the road was cut by bridges in several places. This allowed the

Overleaf. A total of 1.6 million British servicemen were wounded in the First World War. In 1914, there were two uniformed nursing organisations open to British women: the First Aid Nursing Yeomanry (FANY) and the Voluntary Aid Detachments (VAD). Initially the British Army would not allow women nurses to serve at the front, but by 1915, volunteers over the age of 23 were permitted to serve at field hospitals on the Western Front as well, as in Mesopotamia and Gallipoli. In addition to the nurses serving at the front, many more worked tending the wounded brought back to hospitals in Britain.

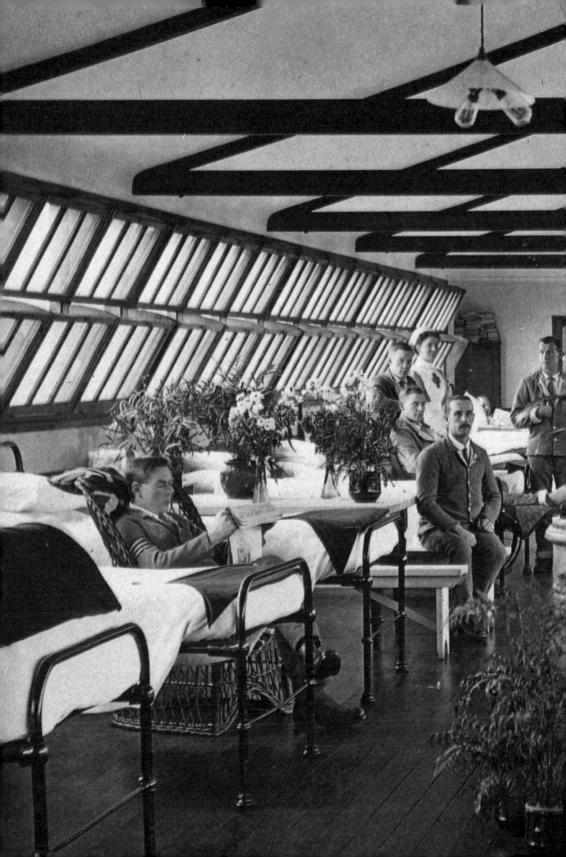

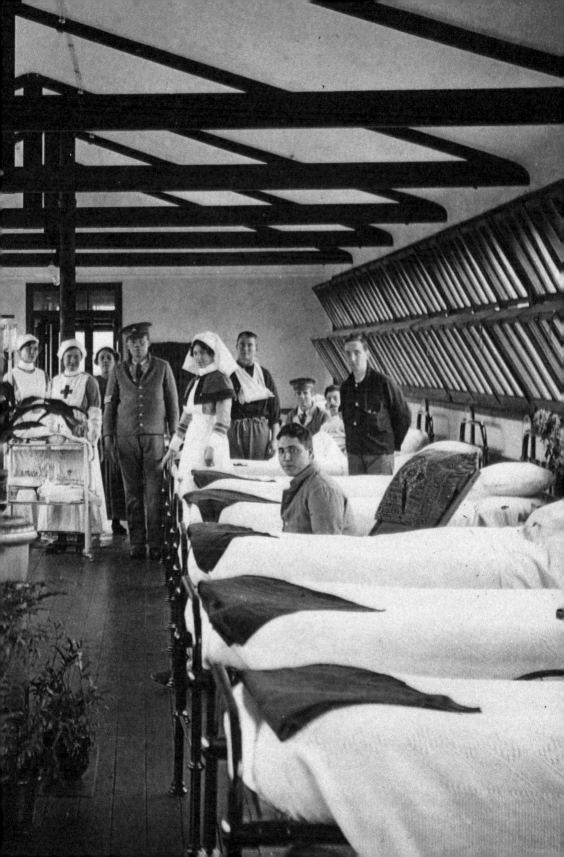

cargo boats to enter the docks, which were a mass of canals and berths and basins and jetties. Just as we approached the Preston Road Bridge, the traffic lights turned red, the gates closed, and the swing bridge rotated. This could mean as much as half an hour's closure of the road. Sister Evangelina cursed and fumed under her breath. (That was another thing, incidentally, that the Poplar people liked about her; she was not too holy to swear quietly to herself!) An alternative was open to us: we could retrace our steps, and cycle all the way round the Isle of Dogs to rejoin the West India Dock Road in the Limehouse area, a distance of about seven miles. Sister Evangelina would have none of that. Pushing her bike, she strode purposefully through the NO ENTRY, keep out gate, past DANGER signs, over the cobbles to the water's edge. Fascinated, I followed; what on earth was she up to? She stomped over towards the massed barges, calling to any dockers in sight to come and help us. Several came forward, grinning and pulling off their caps. One of them was known to her.

"Morning, Harry. How's your mother? I hope her chilblains have cleared up now the weather's better. Give her my regards. Take this bike, will you, there's a good lad, and lend us a hand."

Pulling her long skirts up and tucking them into her belt, she strode towards the nearest barge. "Give me your arm, lad," she said to a huge man of about forty. Grabbing him, she cocked up a leg, giving us a glimpse of thick black stockings and long bloomers elasticated just above the knees, and stepped on to the nearest barge. I realised what she was going to do: she was planning to cross the water as the dockers did, by jumping from barge to barge until she reached the other side.

There were eight or nine moored barges to be traversed in that way. The men, bless them, gathered round. Across the deck of the first barge there was no trouble. But then there were the two adjoining sides of the boats to be clambered over, before she could reach the second deck, and the barges were moving. It took all the strength of the big man, and two or three others besides, to get her over. I heard "gi's a leg up, there's a good lad" and "heave" and "hold me" and "push" and "good for you, Sis". I followed nimbly enough, and couldn't take my eyes off this game old nun, her veil blowing in the wind, rosary and crucifix swinging wildly from side to side, her nose growing redder with the exertion. Two men carried the bicycles, high above their heads, and she turned round and reprimanded them sharply: "Just you look after our bags. This is no laughing matter."

The second and third barges were traversed without mishap, but there was a gap of about eighteen inches before the fourth one. She looked at the water between and said "humph". She pulled her skirts even higher, rubbed a dewdrop off her nose with the flat of her hand, and said to the big man: "You go over there first and be ready to catch me." Three young men got hold of her – she was no lightweight – and she stepped up on to the side. She stood on the narrow edge of the moving barge, her two flat feet firmly planted, and looked resolutely at the big man on the other side. She was panting. She sniffed again loudly, and said: "Right, if I can put my weight on your shoulders, I'll be OK." He nodded, and raised his arms. Gingerly she leaned forward and placed her hands on his shoulders, and he caught her under the arms while the younger men steadied her from behind. My heart was in my mouth. If the barge moved at that moment, or if she slipped, there would have been nothing anyone could have done to prevent her from falling into the water. Could she swim? What if she went under the barge? It didn't bear thinking about. Slowly, carefully, she lifted one foot, brought it forward, and put it on the edge of the next barge. She waited a second, gaining her balance, and then swiftly brought the other leg over, and jumped into the arms of the big man. Cheers went up all round, and I nearly collapsed with relief. She sniffed again.

"Well, that wasn't too bad. No worse than a fart in a colander. Let's carry on." The remaining barges all adjoined each other, and she reached the other side, red faced and triumphant. She pulled her skirts down, took her bicycle, smiled at them all, and said, "Thanks, lads, you've been great. We'll be off now." And with her usual parting comment to dockers, "Keep 'em open and you won't need a doctor," she cycled out of the harbour.

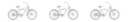

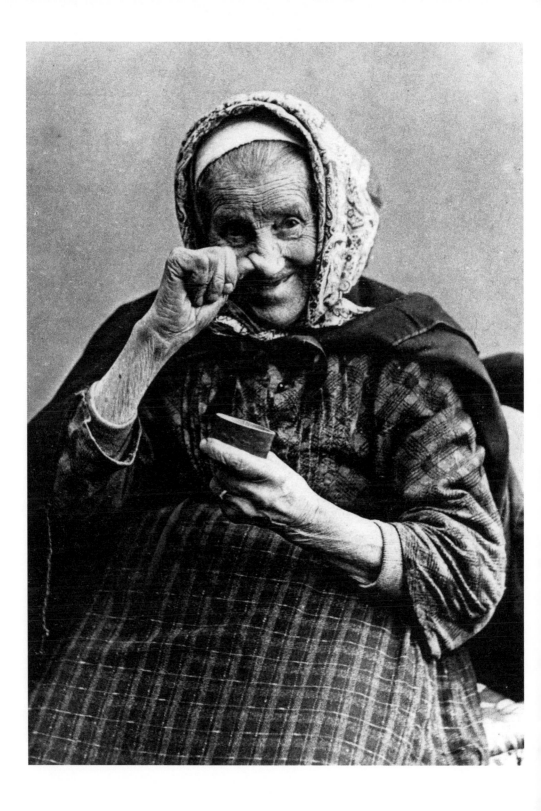

MRS JENKINS

Mrs Jenkins was an enigmatic figure. For years she had been tramping all over the Docklands, from Bow to Cubitt Town, from Stepney to Blackwall, yet no one knew anything about her. The reason for her ceaseless tramping was an obsession with babies, specifically newborn babies. She seemed to know, God knows how, just when and where a home confinement would take place, and nine times out of ten would be found hanging around in the street outside the house. She never said much, and her enquiries about "'Ow's ve baby? 'Ow's ve li'le one?" were invariably the same. On being told the baby was alive and healthy, she often seemed satisfied and shuffled away. She was always seen on a Tuesday afternoon hanging around outside the antenatal clinic, and most of the young mothers brushed past her impatiently, or pulled their young toddlers away from her, as though she were contaminated or would put an evil spell on the child. We had all heard the muttered comments, "She's an ol' witch, she is, she gives the evil eye," and no doubt some of the mothers believed it.

Mrs Jenkins was never welcome, never wanted, often feared, yet this did not deter her from going out, at any time of the day or night, often in atrocious weather, to stand in the street outside the house where a baby was born, asking "'Ow's ve baby? 'Ow's ve li'l one, ven?"

She was a tiny woman, as thin as a rake, with birdlike features, and a long pointed nose that stretched sharply between hollow sunken cheeks.

Opposite: An old woman taking snuff c. 1900. Mrs Jenkins referred to snuff as her "comfort".

Her skin was a yellowish grey, criss-crossed with a thousand wrinkles, and she appeared to have no lips because they were drawn in over her toothless gums, and she chewed and sucked them all the time. A faded black hat, greasy and shapeless, was pulled down low over her head, from which tufts of wispy grey hair escaped now and then. Summer and winter she wore the same long grey coat of indeterminate age, from beneath which protruded enormous feet. For such a tiny woman the huge feet were not only improbable, but absurd, and I am sure she received much ridicule as she shuffled her endless way around the neighbourhood.

Where she lived, no one knew. This was as much a mystery to the Sisters as it was to everyone else. The clergy had no idea. She didn't appear to go to church or belong to any parish, which was unusual among the older women. The doctors did not know, as she did not seem to be registered with any doctor. Perhaps she did not know that there was now a National Health Service and that everyone could have medical treatment free of charge. Even Mrs B., who always had her ear close to the ground as far as local gossip and information were concerned, didn't know anything about her. No one had ever seen her going into a Post Office to collect her pension.

I had always found her interesting but repugnant. My contact with her was frequent, but was always confined to her questions about the baby, and my cold reply, "Mother and baby are well", to which she invariably replied "Fank Gawd, fank Gawd fer vat." I never tried to initiate conversation, because I didn't want to get involved, but once when I was with Sister Julienne, she went straight up to the woman, took both her hands in her own and, with her all-embracing smile, said, "Hello Mrs Jenkins, how nice to see you. What a lovely day it is. How are you getting on?"

Mrs Jenkins shrank back, a half-afraid, half-suspicious look in her dull grey eyes, and pulled her hands away.

"'Ow's ve baby?" she said. Her voice was rasping.

"The baby's lovely. A beautiful little girl, strong and healthy. Do you like babies, Mrs Jenkins?"

Mrs Jenkins shrank away still further, and pulled the collar of her coat up over her chin.

"A baby girl, yer say, doin' nicely. Fank Gawd."

"Yes, thank God indeed. Would you like to see her? I'm sure I could get the mother's permission and bring the baby out for a few moments."

But Mrs Jenkins had already turned, and was hobbling away in her large, man-size boots.

An expression of infinite love and compassion spread over Sister Julienne's face. She stood quite still for several minutes, watching the bent old figure shuffling along the pavement. I watched Mrs Jenkins too, and noticed that she shuffled because she hadn't the strength to lift the boots off the ground. Then I looked again at Sister Julienne, and felt ashamed. Sister wasn't looking at the boots. She was looking, I felt, at seventy years of pain and suffering and endurance, and holding Mrs Jenkins before God in her silent prayers.

I had always been repelled by Mrs Jenkins, mainly because she was so dirty. Her hands and fingernails were filthy, and the only reason I spoke to her, reporting on the baby just born, was to avoid her grabbing my arm, which she would do with surprising strength if her questions were not answered. It was easier to answer briefly, and at a safe distance, and then to escape.

On one occasion while I was on my rounds, I saw Mrs Jenkins step off the pavement into the road. She stood with legs wide apart, and peed into the gutter like a horse. There were a lot of people around at the time, and none of them looked surprised as a torrent of urine streamed into the gutter and down the drain. Once I saw her in a little alley between two buildings. She picked up a piece of newspaper from the ground, then lifted up her coat and started rubbing the newspaper around her private parts, intent on her task, grunting all the while. Then she let the coat fall and started examining the contents of the newspaper, poking it with her fingernail, sniffing it, peering at it closely. Finally she folded it up and put it in her pocket. I shuddered with revulsion.

Another unpleasant thing about Mrs Jenkins was a brown stain on her face that extended from her nose to her upper lip, and was ingrained in the lines at the corners of her mouth. Having seen and observed her lavatorial habits, it is not hard to imagine what I assumed this brown stain to be. But I was wrong. As I got to know her better, I discovered that Mrs Jenkins took snuff (her "comfort", she called it) and the brown stain was caused by the snuff dropping out of her nose.

Not surprisingly, shopkeepers would not serve her. One greengrocer told me he would serve her outside the shop, but wouldn't allow her in.

Overleaf. A study entitled "Houseless and Hungry" (1869) by Luke Fildes, depicting homeless paupers queuing outside the casual ward of a London workhouse. A policeman stands at the left of the scene.

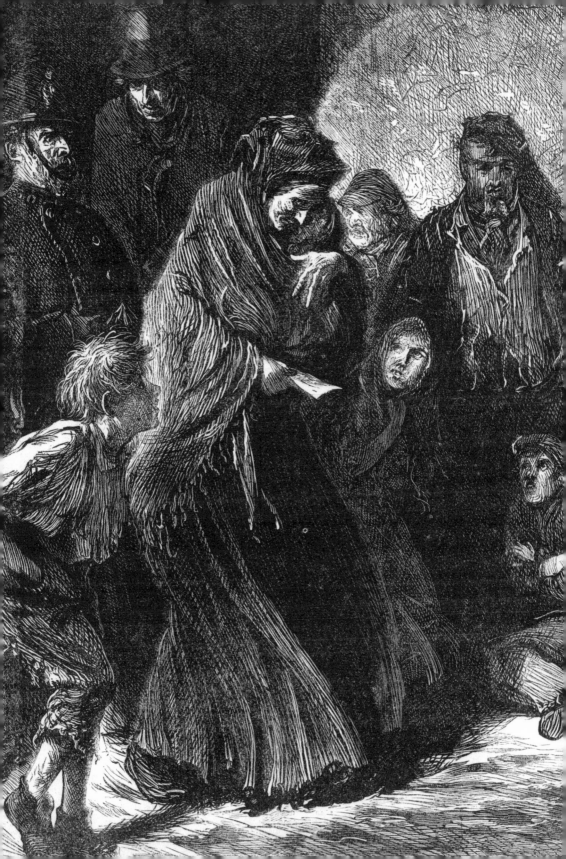

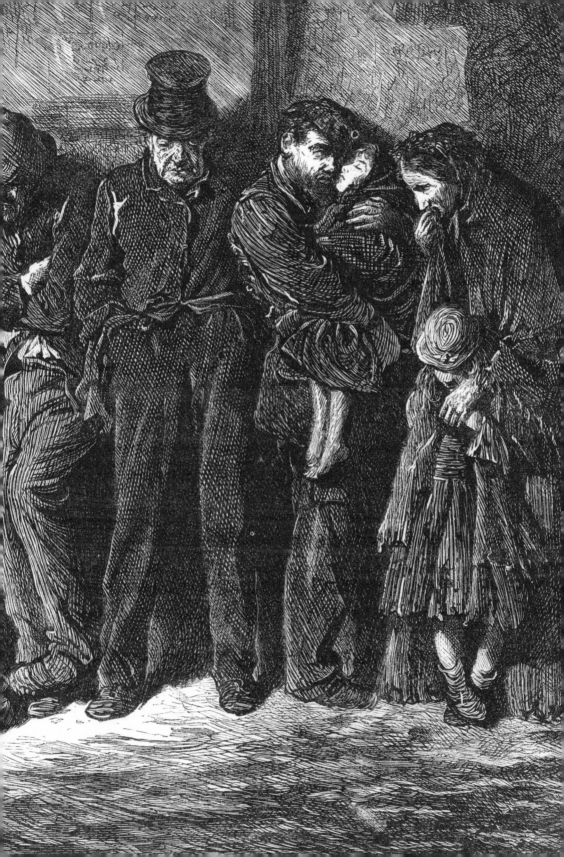

"She picks over all me fruit. She squeezes me plums an' me tomatoes, then puts 'em back. Then no one'll buy 'em. I got a business to run, I can't have 'er in 'ere."

Mrs Jenkins was a local "character", known by name only, avoided, feared, ridiculed, but a complete mystery.

The Sisters received a request from a locum doctor in Limehouse to visit a house in the Cable Street area of Stepney. This was the notorious prostitutes' area which I had explored during my brief friendship with Mary, the young Irish girl. The doctor reported that an elderly lady with mild angina was living in appalling conditions, and probably suffering from malnutrition. The patient's name was Mrs Jenkins.

I turned off Commercial Road, heading towards the river, and found the street. Only half a dozen buildings remained standing; the rest were just bomb sites with a jagged wall sticking up here and there. I found the door and knocked. Silence. I turned the door handle, expecting to find it open, but it was locked. I went round the side, which was littered with filth, but a thick layer of dirt covered the windows and I could not see through. A cat rolled sensuously on its back, whilst another sniffed at a pile of garbage. I returned to the front door, and knocked louder several times, feeling glad that it was daylight. This was not the sort of area to be alone in after dark. A window opened in a house opposite, and a female voice called out: "What you want?"

"I'm the district nurse, and I have come to see Mrs Jenkins."

"Throw a stone up a' ve second floor winder," was the advice given.

There were plenty of stones lying around, and I felt a perfect fool standing in nurse's uniform, with my black bag at my feet, throwing stones up at the second floor. "How on earth did the doctor get in?" I wondered.

Eventually, after about twenty stones, some of which missed, the window opened, and a man's voice called out in a thick foreign accent, "You see old woman? I come."

Bolts were pulled back, and the man stood well behind the door as it opened so that I could not see him. He pointed along the passage to a door at the end, saying: "She live there."

Victorian tiles flagged the passageway which passed a staircase with a fine carved oak banister. This was still in beautiful condition, although the stairs were crumbling and looked highly dangerous. I was glad that I did not have to walk up them. The house had obviously been part of a fine old Regency terrace once, but was now in the last stages of decay. It had been classed as "unfit for human habitation" twenty years previously, yet people were still living there, hidden away amongst the rats.

No sound came when I rapped on the door, so I turned the handle and walked in. The room had been the back scullery and wash house of the premises. It was a single storey extension with a stone-flagged floor. A large copper boiler was attached to an outside wall, and next to it was a coke stove with an asbestos flue running up the wall and out of the ceiling through a huge and jagged hole open to the sky. A large wood and iron framed mangle and a stone sink were the only other objects that caught my eye. The room appeared empty and abandoned and smelled powerfully of cats and urine. It was very dark, because the windows were so black with dirt that no light could penetrate. In fact, most of the light in the room came from the hole in the roof.

As my eyes became accustomed to the gloom I discerned a few other things: several saucers lying around on the floor with bits of food and milk in them; a small wooden chair and table with a tin mug and teapot on it; a chamber pot; a wooden cupboard with no door. There was no bed, no sign of a light, nor of gas or electricity.

In the corner furthest away from the hole in the ceiling was a decrepit-looking armchair in which an old woman sat, silent, watchful, her eyes filled with fear. She shrank back in the chair as far as she could go, her old coat pulled tight round her, a woollen scarf over her head and covering half her face. Only her eyes showed, and they penetrated mine as our gaze met.

"Mrs Jenkins, the doctor tells us you are not well and need home nursing. I am the district nurse. Can I have a look at you, please?"

She pulled her coat closer round her chin and stared at me silently.

"Doctor says your heart's fluttering a bit. Can I feel your pulse, please?"

I put out my hand to feel her wrist pulse, but she pulled the arm away from me with a terrified intake of breath.

I was nonplussed, and felt a bit helpless. I didn't want to frighten her, but I had a job to do. I went over to the unlit stove to read the notes by the light coming through the ceiling: there had been evidence of a mild attack of angina pectoris when the patient had fallen in the street outside the house, and an unnamed resident had carried her back to her own room. The same man had called a doctor and admitted him. The woman had obviously been in pain, but this seemed to pass fairly quickly. The doctor had been unable to examine the patient, due to her violent resistance, but as her pulse was fairly steady, and her breathing had improved rapidly, the doctor had advised a nursing visit twice a day to monitor the situation, and suggested that the Social Services department might improve the woman's living conditions. Amyl nitrite had been prescribed in the event of another attack. Rest, warmth, and good food were advised.

I tried again to feel Mrs Jenkins' pulse, with the same result. I enquired if she'd had any more pain, and got no reply. I asked if she was comfortable, and again there was no reply. I realised that I was getting nowhere, and would have to report back to Sister Evangelina, who was in charge of general district nursing.

I was not too keen on reporting my total failure to Sister Evangelina because she still seemed to think me a bit of a fool. She called me "Dolly Daydream", and spoke to me as though I needed to be directed in the most rudimentary points of nursing procedure, even though she knew I had about five years of nurse's training and experience behind me. This, of course, made me nervous, and so I dropped or spilled things, and then she called me "butter-fingers", which made it worse. We did not have to go out together very often, which was a relief, but if I reported, as I would have to, that I could not manage a patient, inevitably she would have to accompany me on the next visit.

Her reaction was predictable. She listened to my report in heavy silence, glancing up at me from time to time from under thick grey eyebrows. When I had finished, she sighed noisily, as though I were the biggest fool ever to carry the black bag.

"This evening I have twenty-one insulin injections, four penicillin, an ear to syringe, bunions to dress, piles to compress, a cannula to drain, and now I suppose I have to show you how to take a pulse?"

I was stung by the injustice. "I know perfectly well how to take a pulse, but the patient wouldn't let me, and I couldn't persuade her."

"Couldn't persuade her! Couldn't persuade her! You young girls can't do anything. Too much bookwork, that's your trouble. Sitting in classrooms all day, filling your heads with a lot of codswallop, and then you can't do a simple thing like taking a pulse."

She gave a contemptuous snort and shook her head, spraying the bead of moisture that balanced on the end of her nose all over her desk and patients' notes that she was writing up. She drew a large man's handkerchief from beneath her scapular and wiped up the fluid, which caused the ink to smudge, and so she humphed again, "There now, look what you have made me do."

The further injustice made my blood boil, and I had to bite my lips to prevent a sharp reply, which would only have made things worse.

"Well then, Miss Can't-take-a-pulse, I suppose I will have to go with you at 4 p.m. We will make it our first evening visit, after which we can both go our separate ways. We will leave here at 3.30 p.m. sharp, and don't be a minute late. I won't be kept hanging around, and I shall want my supper at seven o' clock as usual."

With that, she pushed her chair back noisily, and stomped out of the office, with another pointed "humph" as she passed me.

Half past three came round all too quickly. We pulled the bicycles out of the shed, and the nun's silence was more eloquent than her grumbling had been. We reached the house without a word, and knocked. Again no reply. I knew what to do, so told Sister about the man on the second floor.

"Well, get hold of him then, don't stand around talking, chatterbox."

I ground my teeth and started throwing stones up at the window in a fury. It was surprising I didn't break the glass.

The man shouted out, "I come", and hid behind the door again as we passed. However, he then added "I come no more. You go round back, see? I not answer no more."

In the dim light of Mrs Jenkins' room a cat came towards us, mewing. The wind made a curious sound as it hit the hole in the roof. Mrs Jenkins was huddled in her chair, just as I had left her in the morning.

Sister Evangelina called her name. No reply. I was beginning to feel justified – she would see that I had not been exaggerating. Sister walked over to the armchair. She spoke gently, "Come on, mother. This won't do. Doctor says there's something up with your ticker. Don't you believe a word of it. Your heart is as good as mine, but we've got to have a look at you. No one's going to hurt you."

The bundle of clothes in the chair didn't move. Sister leaned forward to feel her pulse. The arm was pulled away. I was delighted. "Let's see how Sister Know-all copes," I thought.

"It's cold in here. Haven't you got a fire?"

No reply.

"It's dark, too. What about a light for us?"

No reply.

"When did you first feel bad?"

No reply.

"Do you feel a bit better now?"

Again, total silence. I was feeling very smug; Sister Evangelina appeared as incapable of examining the patient as I had been. What would happen next?

What in fact did happen next was so utterly unexpected that, to this day, more than fifty years later, I blush to remember it.

Sister Evangelina muttered, "You're a tiresome old lady. We'll see what this does."

Slowly she leaned over Mrs Jenkins and as she bent down she let out the most enormous fart. It rumbled on and on and just as I thought it had stopped it started all over again, in a higher key. I had never been so shocked in all my life.

Mrs Jenkins sat upright in her chair. Sister Evangelina called out: "Which way did it go, nurse? Don't let it get out. It's over there by the door – catch it. Now it's by the window – get hold of it, quick."

A throaty chuckle came from the armchair.

"Cor, that's better," said Sister Evangelina happily; "Nothing like a good fart to clear the system. Makes you feel ten years younger, eh, Mother Jenkins?"

The bundle of clothes shook, and the throaty chuckle developed into a real belly laugh. Mrs Jenkins, who had never been heard to speak apart from obsessive questions about babies, laughed until the tears ran down her face.

"Quick! Under the chair. The cat's go' it. Ge' it off him quick, 'e'll be sick."

Sister Evangelina sat down beside her, and the two old ladies (Sister Evie was no spring chicken) rocked with laughter about farts and bums and turds and stinks and messes, swapping stories, true or false, I couldn't tell. I was deeply shocked. I knew that Sister Evie could be crude, but I had no idea that she possessed such an extensive and varied repertoire of stories.

I retreated to a corner and watched them. They looked like two old hags from a Bruegel painting, one in rags, one in a monastic habit, sharing lewd laughter with the happiness of children. I was completely out of the joke, and had time to ponder many things, not least of which was how on earth Sister Evangelina had been able to produce such a spectacular fart at that precise moment. Could she command one at will? I had heard of a performer at the Comédie-Francaise, immortalised by Toulouse-Lautrec, who would entertain the Parisian audiences of the 1880s with a rich variety of sounds emitting from his backside, but I had never heard of, still less encountered, anyone who could actually do it. Was Sister Evangelina gifted, or had she acquired the skill through hours of practice? My mind dwelled with pleasure on the possibility. Was it her party piece? I wondered how it would go down at the convent on festive occasions, such as Christmas and Easter. Would the Reverend Mother and her Sisters in Christ be amused by such a singular talent?

The two old girls were so innocently happy that my initial reaction of disapproval seemed to be churlish and mean-spirited. What was wrong with it, anyway? All children laugh endlessly about bottoms and farts. The works of Chaucer, Rabelais, Fielding, and many others are full of lavatorial humour.

There was no doubt about it. Sister Evangelina's action had been brilliant. A masterstroke. To say that a fart cleared the air may seem a contradiction in terms, but life is full of contradictions. From that moment on, Mrs Jenkins lost her fear of us. We were able to examine her, to treat her, to communicate with her. And I was able to learn her tragic history.

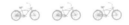

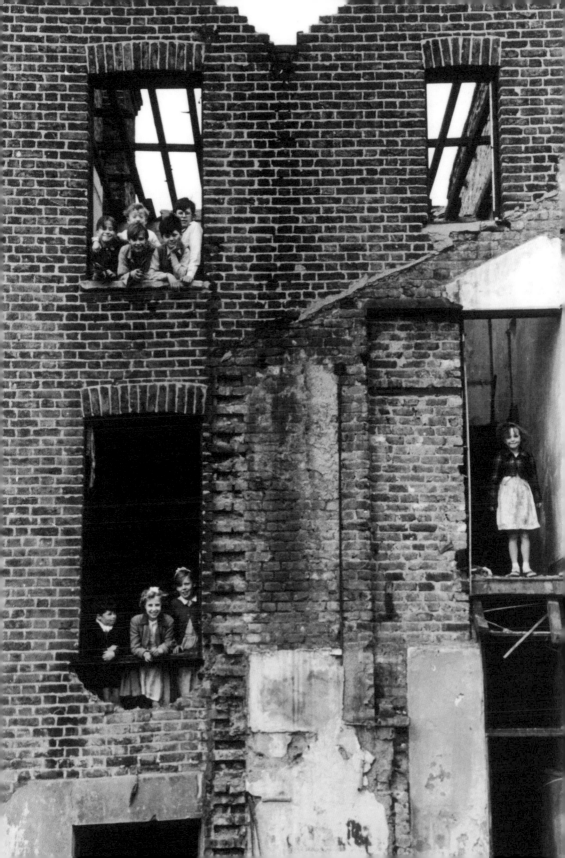

ROSIE

"Rosie? Tha' you, Rosie?"

The old lady lifted her head and called out as the front door banged. Footsteps were heard in the passage, but Rosie did not enter the room. Things were happening fast to improve Mrs Jenkins' living conditions. The Social Services had been called, and some cleaning had been carried out. The old armchair had been removed because it was full of fleas, and another donated. A bed had also been provided, but had never been slept in. Mrs Jenkins was so accustomed to sleeping in an armchair that she could not be persuaded to try the bed, so the cats slept on it. Sister Evangelina commented wryly that the new government must have more money than sense to provide Social Services for cats.

The most remarkable change was the repair of the hole in the roof which Sister Evangelina achieved through single-handed combat with the landlord. I was with her when she mounted the rickety stairs to the second floor. I would not have been surprised if they had given way under her considerable weight and warned her accordingly, but she glared at me, and strode up them to put the fear of God into the landlord.

She banged hard on the door several times. It opened a crack, and I heard, "What you want?"

She demanded that he come out and speak with her.

Opposite: Many families lived in substandard conditions, making their homes in bombed-out and often dangerous buildings due for demolition.

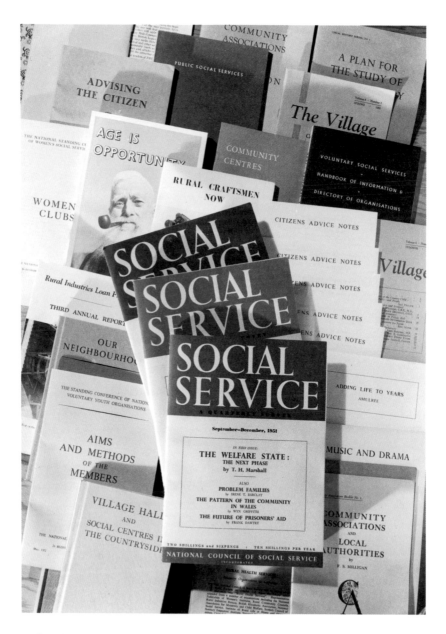

Above: Although the Social Services were set up to help those in need, the elderly – like Mrs Jenkins – often lived in fear of them, afraid that they would be put into old people's homes, away from their community.

"You go away."

"I will not. If I go away, it will be to set the police on you. Now come out and talk to me."

I heard words like "disgrace", "prosecute", "prison", and whining pleas of poverty and ignorance, but the net result was that the hole in the roof was patched up with a heavy tarpaulin, weighted down with bricks. Mrs Jenkins was delighted, and grinned and giggled with Sister Evie as they shared a cup of strong sweet tea and a piece of Mrs B.'s homemade cake that Sister Evie invariably brought with her when she visited Mrs Jenkins.

A tarpaulin to mend a hole in the roof may seem inadequate, but there was no chance of getting anything better or more durable. The building was condemned for demolition, and the fact that it was still lived in at all was due to the acute housing shortage caused by the bombing of London in the war. People were glad to live anywhere they could find.

The coke stove was usable, but furred up, and Fred, boilerman extraordinaire of Nonnatus House, cleaned and serviced it. Sister Evangelina was determined that Mrs Jenkins should stay in her own home.

"If the Social Services had their way they would put her in an old people's home tomorrow. I'm not having that. It would kill her."

When we first examined Mrs Jenkins we had found her heart to be quite fair. Angina is common amongst the elderly, and with a quiet life, warmth, and rest, it can be kept under control. Her main problems were chronic malnutrition and her mental state. She was clearly a very strange old lady, but was she mad? Would she do any harm to herself or others? We wondered if she needed to see a psychiatrist but we could not tell without assessing her over a period of weeks.

The other problems were dirt, fleas and lice. It was my job to clean her up.

A tin bath was brought from Nonnatus House, and I boiled up water on the coke stove. Mrs Jenkins was dubious about all this, but I only had to mention that Sister Evangelina wanted her to have a bath, and she relaxed and chuckled, champing her jaws.

"She's a good 'un, she is. I tells my Rosie an' all. We 'as a good laugh, we 'as. Rose an' me."

I had quite a job persuading her to undress, and she was very apprehensive. Under the old coat she wore a rough wool skirt and jumper, but no vest or knickers. Her frail little body was pathetic to behold. There was no flesh on her, and all her bones stuck out at sharp angles. Her skin hung loose, and

I could count every rib. The revulsion she had hitherto inspired in me turned to pity when I beheld her frail, skeletal body.

Pity is one thing, shock another. Shock was waiting for me when I took her boots off. I had noticed her huge man-sized boots before, and wondered why she wore them. With difficulty I untied the greasy knots and undid the laces. She wore no socks or stockings, and the boot would not budge. It seemed stuck to her skin. I eased a finger down the side, and she winced. "Leave it be. Leave it."

"I've got to get them off to put you in the bath."

"Leave it," she whimpered; "my Rosie'll do it by an' by."

"But Rosie's not here to help. If you will let me, I can get them off. Sister Evangelina says your boots have got to come off before you have your bath."

It would be a long job, so I wrapped a blanket over her and knelt down on the floor. Some of the skin was indeed stuck to the leather, and tore as I eased the boot back and forth. God knows when they had last come off. Eventually I eased the boot over her heel and pulled. To my horror there was a sort of scratching, metallic sound. What was it? What had I done? As the boot came off, an extraordinary sight met my eyes. Her toenails were about eight to twelve inches long, and up to one inch thick. They were twisted and bent, curling over and under each other, and many of the toes were bleeding and suppurating at the nail-bed. The smell was horrible. Her feet were in a terrible condition. How had she managed to tramp all over Poplar for so many years with feet like that?

She didn't even murmur as I was taking the boots off, though it must have hurt, and she looked down at her bare feet with no surprise – perhaps she thought everyone's toenails were like that. I helped her over to the bath, and it was surprisingly difficult because, without her boots, she had lost her balance and the toenails kept getting in the way, nearly tripping her up.

She stepped over the edge of the big tin bath and sat down in the water with delight, splashing and giggling like a little girl. She picked up the flannel and sucked the water noisily, looking up at me with smiling eyes. The room was warm because I had stoked up the fire, and a cat strolled up and looked curiously over the edge of the bath. She splashed him in the face with a giggle, and he retreated, offended. The front door banged, and she looked up sharply. "Rosie, that you? Come 'ere, girl, an' look a' yer ol' mum. It's a rare sight."

But the footsteps went upstairs, and Rosie didn't come.

I washed Mrs Jenkins all over, and wrapped her in the big towels provided by the Sisters. I had washed her hair and wrapped it in a turban. I had not seen too many fleas, but I applied a sassafras compress to kill any nits. The only thing I could not cope with were her toenails – a good chiropodist would have to be called in for such monsters. (I am reliably informed, incidentally, that Mrs Jenkins' toenails are to this day displayed in a glass case in the main hall of the British Chiropody Association.)

The nuns always kept a store of second-hand clothes, rescued from many jumble sales, and Sister Evangelina and I had sorted out some garments which I had brought with me. Mrs Jenkins looked at the vest and knickers and stroked the soft material with wonder.

"Is this for me? Oh, it's too good. You keep 'em fer yourself, duckie, they're too good for the likes o' me."

I had difficulty in persuading her to put them on, and when she did, she rubbed her hands up and down her thin body with amazement, as though she couldn't get over her new underwear. I dressed her in the jumble-sale clothes, which were all too big, and quietly put her old clothes out the back door.

She settled comfortably in the armchair, stroking her new clothes. A cat jumped on to her knee, and she tickled him gently.

"What'll Rosie say when she sees all this finery, eh, puss? She won' know 'er ol' mum, she won', dressed up like a queen."

I left her with the happy feeling that we were doing a great deal to improve her intolerable conditions. Outside, I put her flea-ridden clothes into a bag, and looked for a dustbin. There were none to be seen. There was no provision for waste disposal in the area because no one was supposed to be living in the condemned buildings, so no public services were provided. The fact that people *were* living there and everyone, including the Council, knew about it, made no difference to official policy. I left the bag of clothes in the street amongst the piles of rubbish already lying around.

A feeling of decay and menace hovered over the whole area like an evil vapour. The craters left by the bombs were filled with rubbish and smelled horrible. Jagged bits of wall, rose starkly towards the sky. No one was around: mornings in a red-light district are generally slow for business. The quietness had an oppressive quality about it, and I would be glad to get away.

I had barely turned the corner of the house when the sound started. I froze to the spot, the hair prickling on the back of my neck as a sort of terror gripped me. It was like the howl of a wolf, or an animal in dreadful pain. The sound seemed to come from everywhere, echoing off the few buildings, and filling the bombsites with an unearthly pain. The noise stopped, but I literally couldn't move. Then it started again, and the window in the house opposite opened. The woman who had told me to throw stones to attract the landlord leaned out, shouting, "It's that mad old hag. Yer lookin' after 'er. Tell 'er to shu' up, or I'll come and kill 'er, I will. You tell 'er from me."

The window banged shut. My mind raced.

Mad old hag? Mrs Jenkins? It couldn't be! She couldn't be making that anguished noise. I'd left her contented and happy only a few minutes ago.

The noise stopped and, trembling, I went back into the house, down the passage to her door and turned the handle.

"Rosie? That you, Rosie?"

I opened the door. Mrs Jenkins was sitting just as I had left her, with a cat on her knee and another preening itself beside her chair. She looked up brightly.

"If you see Rosie, tell 'er I'm coming. Tell 'er not to lose 'eart. Tell 'er I'm comin', an' the li'l ones, an' all. I'll scrub an' scrub all day, an' they'll let me come this time, they will. You tell my Rosie."

I was bewildered. She couldn't have made that howling noise; it was impossible. I took her pulse, which was normal, and enquired if she felt all right, to which she did not reply but smacked her lips together and looked steadily at me.

There seemed no point in my staying, but I left with misgivings that morning.

Sister Evangelina took the morning report, and I told her that Mrs Jenkins seemed to enjoy her bath. I reported on the toenails and the fleas. I reported that her mental condition seemed fairly stable – she loved her new clothes, was chatting companionably to the cats, and was not at all withdrawn and defensive. I hesitated to report the unearthly noise I had heard in the street; after all it might not have come from Mrs Jenkins. It was only the woman opposite who had suggested it had.

Sister Evangelina looked up at me, her heavy features expressionless.

"And?" she said.

"And what?" I faltered.

"And what else? What have you not reported?"

Was she a mind reader? There was clearly no way out. I told her of the ghastly cry I had heard from the street, adding that I couldn't be sure it was Mrs Jenkins.

"No, but you cannot be sure that it was *not* Mrs Jenkins, can you? Describe the cry."

Again I hesitated, as it was so difficult to describe, but I ended by likening it to the howl of a wolf.

Sister looked down at her notes, not moving, and when she spoke her voice was different, subdued and low. "Those who have heard that sound can never forget it. It makes your blood run cold. I think the cry you heard probably did come from Mrs Jenkins, and it was what used to be called 'the workhouse howl'."

"What is that?" I enquired.

She did not reply straight away, but sat tapping her pen with impatience. Then, "Humph. You young girls know nothing of recent history. You've had it too easy, that's your trouble. I will come with you on your next visit, and I will also see if we can get hold of any medical or parish records about Mrs Jenkins. Proceed with your report."

I completed the report and had time to wash and change before lunch. At table, it was hard to join in the general conversation. I was hearing in my mind that horrible wolf-howl, thinking of Sister Evangelina's explanation, and remembering. Her words brought to mind something my grandfather had told me years before, about a man he knew well who had fallen on hard times. The man had applied to the Board of Guardians for temporary relief, and had been told that he could not have it, but would be sent to the workhouse. The man replied, "I would rather die" and went away and hanged himself.

When I was a child the local workhouse had been pointed out to me with hushed and terrified whispers. Even the empty building seemed to evoke fear and loathing. People would not go down the road in which it stood, or would pass on the other side with faces averted. The dread even affected me, a little child who knew nothing about the history of the workhouses. All my life I have looked on those buildings with a shudder.

Sister Evangelina frequently accompanied me on my visits to Mrs Jenkins, and I had marvelled at the way in which she got the old lady talking. Reminiscing was obviously good therapy for her, as she relived the pain of the past with a loving and sympathetic person.

The Council supplied Sister with the old records of the Board of Guardians of Poplar Workhouse. Mrs Jenkins had been a pauper inmate from 1916 to

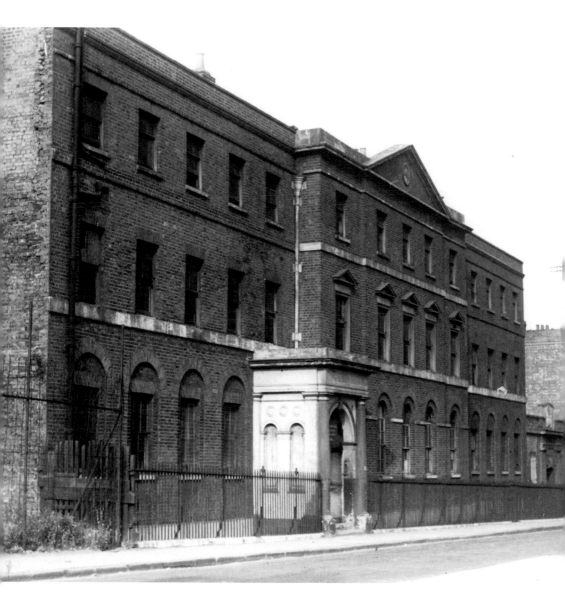

Above: Poplar Workhouse (c. 1945) was located on the high street. It opened in 1812 and was demolished in 1960.

1935. "Enough to drive anyone mad," Sister Evie commented wryly. She had been admitted as a widow with five children, unable to support herself. She was described as an "able-bodied adult". The records stated that Mrs Jenkins was discharged in 1935, with the gift of a sewing machine, the use of which would enable her to support herself, and twenty-four pounds, which was her accumulated earnings after nineteen years in the workhouse. No further mention was made of the children.

The records were dry and scant. Mrs Jenkins herself filled in the missing details in her conversations with Sister Evie. Little bits of the story came out here and there, relived with a complete lack of emotion or melodrama as though her story were nothing unusual. I felt that she had seen and experienced so much suffering for so long that she had accepted it as inevitable. A happy life seemed unthinkable to her.

She had been born in Millwall, and like most girls had gone to work in a factory at the age of thirteen, and then married a local boy when she was eighteen. They rented two rooms over a tailor's shop in Commercial Road, and six children were born to them over the next ten years. Then her young husband developed a cough that did not get better. Six months later he was spitting blood. "He jus' wasted away," she said in a matter-of-fact tone. Three months later he was dead.

Mrs Jenkins was strong and less than thirty years of age at the time. She left the two rooms and took a small back room for herself and her children. She returned to work in the shirt-making factory, working from 8 a.m. to 6 p.m. Her baby was only three months old, but Rosie – her eldest daughter – was already ten and left school in order to look after the younger children. Extra hand-sewing was taken in, and she often sat half the night sewing by candlelight. Rosie learned to sew too and became a good needlewoman, often sitting up with her mother into the night hours. These silent hours of female labour brought in a little extra money – enough to feed the family – after the rent was paid.

Then catastrophe struck. The machinery of the factory was completely unguarded, and the sleeve of Mrs Jenkins' dress caught in a wheel, dragging her right arm towards the cutting blades. Her arm was badly injured, she lost a lot of blood, and tendons were severed before the machine was stopped. She was lucky not to lose her arm. She showed us the six inch scar. The lacerations were never stitched because she could not afford to pay a doctor, and the scar, though healed, was wide, deep red, and irregular. Her

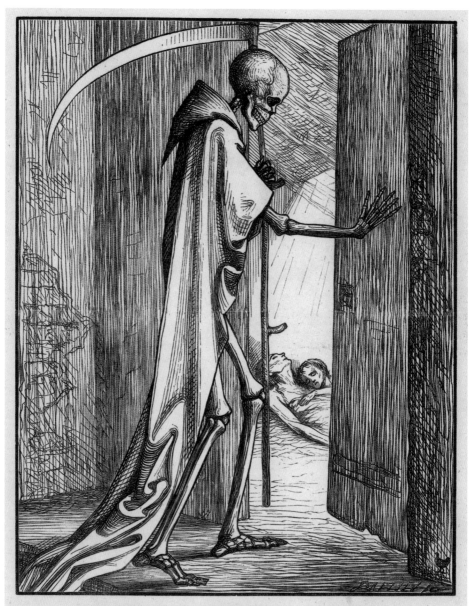

THE TRUE RELIEVING OFFICER!

DEDICATED WITHOUT PERMISSION TO THE POOR LAW BOARD.

Above: A woodcut depicting Death, "the True Relieving Officer" (1868).

arm was slightly withered because the tendons had not been sutured. It was surprising that she could use her hand at all.

She looked at the scar without emotion. "This is wha' done fer us," she said.

The family moved out of the back room, and found shelter in a basement with no window. It was close to the river's edge, and at high tide, when the water level rose, moisture seeped through the brickwork and ran down the walls. For this hovel, the landlord demanded one shilling a week, but with the mother not earning, how was this to be found?

She went out begging, but was driven off the streets by the police who saw her as an undesirable vagrant. She pawned her coat, and with the money bought matches, then went out into the streets as a match seller. The profits from her sales brought in a little money, but not enough to pay the rent as well as feed the children.

Bit by bit she pawned everything they had – the furniture, pots, saucepans, the plates and mugs, clothes, linen. Last to go was the bed in which they all slept. She constructed a platform out of orange boxes to raise them off the damp floor, and on this the family slept. Finally the blankets had to go in to be pawned, and mother and children clung to each other for warmth at night.

She asked the Board of Guardians for outdoor relief, but the chairman said she was obviously lazy and workshy, and when she told them of the accident in the factory, and showed them her right arm, she was told not to be impertinent, or it would count against her. The gentlemen debated amongst themselves, and offered to take two of her children off her hands. She refused, and returned to the basement with six hungry mouths to feed.

With no light, no heat, constant damp and mildew, and virtually no food, the children became sickly. The family struggled on for six months like this, and still the mother could not work. She sold her hair; she sold her teeth, but it was never enough. The baby became lethargic and ceased to thrive. She called it "wasting fever".

When the baby died no money could be spared for burial, so she sealed him in an orange box weighed down with stones, and slipped him into the river.

That furtive journey in the middle of the night with her dead baby was the moment when she finally accepted defeat, and knew that the inevitable had come. She and the children would have to go to the workhouse.

The New Poor Law

with a description of the new Workhouses

Look at the Picture—See

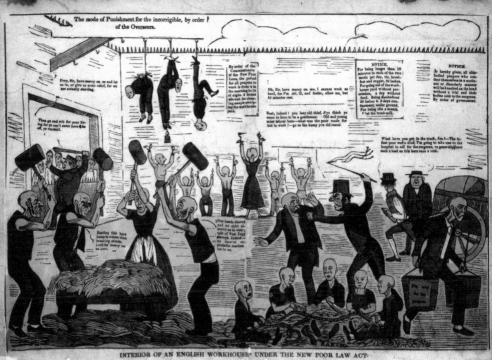

INTERIOR OF AN ENGLISH WORKHOUSE UNDER THE NEW POOR LAW ACT.

THE WORKHOUSE

The Poor Law Act of 1834 started the workhouse system. The Act was repealed in 1929, but the system lingered on for several decades because there was nowhere else for the inmates to go, and long-term residents had lost the capacity to make any decisions or look after themselves in the outside world.

It was intended as a humane and charitable Act, because hitherto the poor or destitute could be hounded from place to place, never finding shelter, and could lawfully be beaten to death by their pursuers. To the chronically poor of the 1830s the workhouse system must have seemed like heaven: a shelter each night; a bed or communal bed to sleep in; clothing; food – not lavish, but enough, and, in return, work to pay for your keep. The system must have seemed like an act of pure Christian goodness and charity. But, like so many good intentions, it quickly turned sour.

Mrs Jenkins and her children left the basement with three weeks' rent owing. The landlord had threatened to put the whip to her back if she did not pay the following day, so they had left during the night. The family had nothing to take with them; neither she nor the children wore any shoes, their clothes were just rags thrown over their thin bodies. Dirty, hungry, and shivering they stood in the unlit street, ringing the great bell outside the workhouse.

Opposite: A nineteenth-century Anti-Poor Law poster showing the interior of an English workhouse under the new Poor Laws (c. 1834).

The children, were not particularly unhappy as yet; in fact, it seemed something of an adventure to them, creeping out in the dead of night and making their way along dark roads. Only their mother was crying, because only she knew the dreadful truth: that the family would be separated once they entered the workhouse gates. She could not bring herself to tell the children, and hesitated before ringing that fateful bell. But her youngest child, a boy of nearly three, started coughing, so she pulled the handle resolutely.

The sound echoed through the stone building, and the door was opened by a thin, grey man who demanded, "What do you want?"

"Shelter, and food for the little ones."

"You'll have to come to the Reception Room. You can sleep there till morning, unless, of course, you're 'casuals' and go to the Casual Centre. There's no food until morning."

"No, we are not casuals," she said wearily.

They were the only people in the reception room that night. The sleeping platform, a raised wooden construction, was covered with fresh straw and looked inviting. They cuddled up together in the sweet-smelling hay, and the children fell asleep at once. Only the mother lay awake, her arms around her children, until dawn. Her heart was breaking. She knew it would be the last time she would be allowed to sleep with her children.

Morning sounds, keys clanking, and doors opening, were heard long before anyone unlocked the door of the reception room. Finally, the Mistress entered. She was a resolute looking woman, not unkind, but one who had seen too many paupers to be swayed by emotion. She took their names, and briefly told them to follow her to the washhouse, where they were stripped, and made to wash all over with cold water in shallow stone troughs. Their clothes, such as they were, were removed, and workhouse uniforms provided. These were of coarse grey serge, cut to fit almost any size of person. There were a variety of odd shoes. No undergarments were provided, but that did not matter, because none of them were accustomed to vests or pants, even in the coldest weather. Then their heads were shaved. The boys thought this was great fun, and giggled and pointed at the girls, cramming their fists into their mouths to stop themselves from laughing aloud. Mrs Jenkins did not have to be shaved because she had no hair, having sold it some weeks previously; she was given a bonnet to cover her bare head. She timidly asked if there would be any food for the little ones, and was told that it was too late for breakfast, but that lunch would be served at 12 noon.

They were taken to the Master's office for segregation. Everyone dreaded this moment, including the Master and Mistress, and four strong pauper inmates were brought in to take the children away. Mrs Jenkins had persuaded herself that it would not be too bad for the younger ones, because they would all be with Rosie, who had looked after them while she was at work. But this was not to be.

The Master looked at the little ones. "Ages?" he demanded.

"Two, four, and five," she whispered.

"Take them to the children's ward. And the older boy? What age is he?"

"Nine."

"He'll go to the boys' ward. The girl?" he demanded, pointing at Rosie.

"Ten."

"Take her to the girls' ward," he ordered.

Rough hands were laid on the children. The Master turned and walked out. He was not going to stay to watch the scene. As he left, he barked to the helpers, "Mind you do as you are bidden. You know the rules."

Mrs Jenkins could not give Sister Evangelina or me the details of the parting. It was too terrible to talk about. The children were dragged away screaming, and she was pushed into the women's quarters. Great doors were shut behind her, and keys were turned. She heard the sounds of screaming children and doors banging. Then she heard no more. She was told much later by a friendly woman who worked in the kitchens that there was a little boy who cried all the time, and whose eyes never left the great door of the children's quarters, watching every person who came in. He never said a single word except "mummy" from the day he entered to the day he died. Was it her little boy? She never knew, but it might have been.

I asked Sister Evangelina about this segregation, which seemed so utterly inhuman that it could not be true, but she assured me that it was. Segregation was the first rule of all workhouses throughout the country, and the one most rigorously applied. Husbands and wives were separated, parents and children, brothers and sisters. Usually, they never saw each other again.

If Mrs Jenkins was odd, it was not surprising.

Overleaf: Four interior shots of Poplar Workhouse, c. 1908.

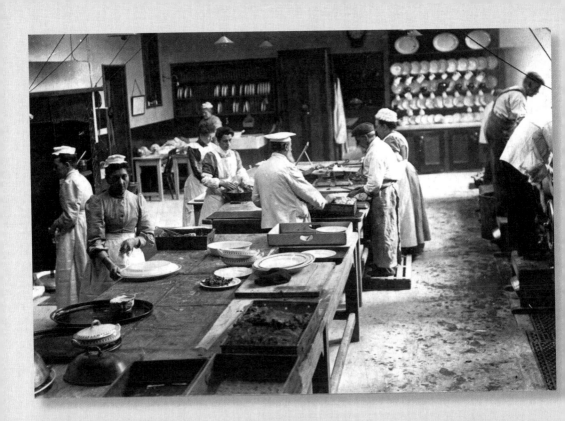

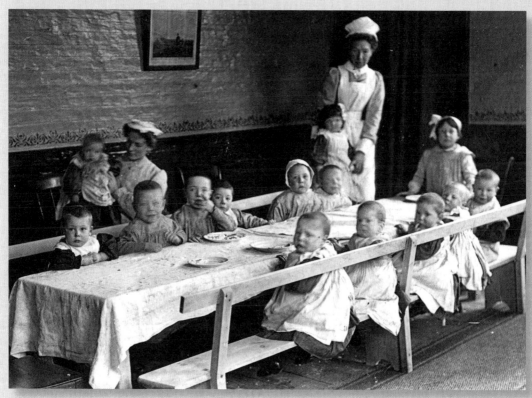

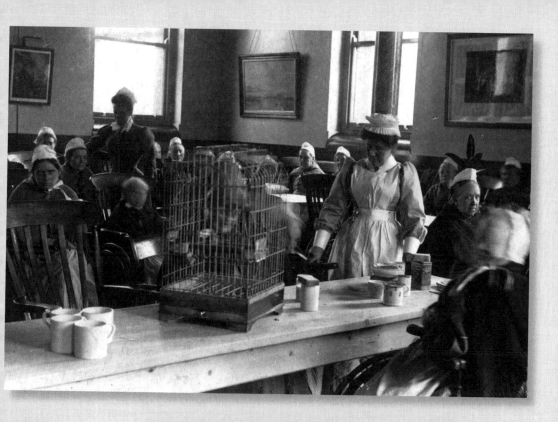

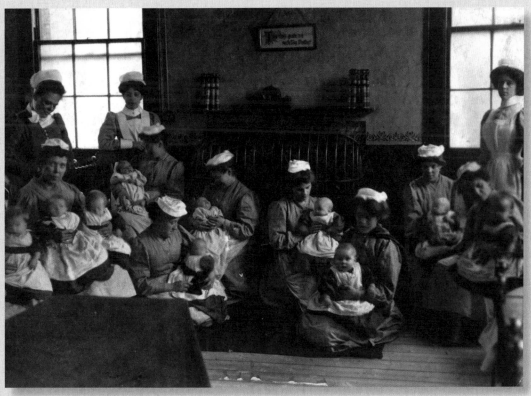

One evening I visited her quite late. It was dark and, down the side passage leading to her back door, I heard a strange, subdued human voice that was chanting in a rhythmic way. I peered through the window and saw Mrs Jenkins on her hands and knees on the floor, scrubbing. An oil-lamp stood beside her, throwing a huge and ghostly shadow of her small figure on to the wall. She had a pail of water beside her, and a scrubbing brush, and she was scrubbing the same square of floor obsessively. All the while she seemed to be repeating a rythmic pattern of words that I could not distinguish but she did not change her position.

I rapped on the door and entered. She lifted her head, but did not turn round.

"Rosie? Come 'ere, Rosie. Look a' this, girl. Look 'ow clean it is. Master'll be pleased when 'e sees how clean I scrubbed it."

She looked up at the great shadow of herself on the wall.

"Come an' see here, Master. It's so clean, an' I done it all. It's clean, an' I done it to please you, Master. They says I can see my li'l ones if I please you, Master. Can I? Can I? Oh, let me, just once."

Her cry lifted, and her tiny body fell forwards. Her head hit the bucket, and she gave a whimper of pain. I went over to her.

"It's me, the nurse. I'm just doing my evening visit. Are you all right, Mrs Jenkins?"

She looked up at me, but didn't say a word. She sucked her lips, and gazed at me steadily as I helped her to her feet and led her to the armchair.

On the bare table was a cooked lunch, left for her by the Meals on Wheels ladies. It was untouched, and quite cold.

I moved the plate, and said, "Didn't you fancy your lunch, then?"

She grabbed my wrist with unexpected strength and pushed my arm away. "For Rosie," she said in a hoarse whisper.

I checked her physical condition, and asked a few questions, none of which she replied to. She just gazed at me unblinkingly, and continued sucking her lips.

On another occasion when I called, she was chuckling to herself as she played with a piece of elastic. She was stretching and releasing it and twisting it round her fingers. She said to me, as I entered, "My Rosie brought me a bit of elastic las' night. Look 'ow it stretches. It's good an' strong. She's a clever girl, my Rose. She can always get hold of a bi' of elastic for you, if you wants it."

I was beginning to get irritated with Rosie. She wasn't much help to her old mother. A bit of elastic, indeed! Was that the best she could do?

But then I saw the tenderness and happiness on the old face, and the warmth and love in her voice as she fiddled with the elastic. "My Rosie give it me, she did. She go' it fer me, she did. She's a dear girl, my Rose."

My heart softened. Perhaps Rosie was as simple as her mother, her mind also unhinged by her early life in the workhouse. I wondered how long she had spent there, and what had happened to her brothers and sisters.

Life in the workhouse was terrible. All inmates were locked into their quarters, which consisted of a day room, a sleeping room and an airing yard. They were confined to the dormitory from 8 p.m. to 6 a.m., and there was a drain or channel running down the centre, into which they relieved themselves at night. The day room was their dining room, where they sat at long benches to eat. All windows were above eye level so that no one could see out of them, and the window sills sloped downwards, so that no one could climb up and sit on them. The airing yard was an enclosed gravel square, from which no door or gate issued. It was, effectively, a prison.

Misery and monotony blurred days into weeks, and weeks into months. The women worked all day, mostly rough work: in the laundry, washing for the entire workhouse; scrubbing – the Master was fanatical about scrubbing; cooking poor quality food for all the inmates; heavy sewing, such as sacks, sails, matting; and, strangest of all, picking oakum. This was old rope, usually tarred, which had to be untwisted and unpicked into strands, which were then used for caulking the seams of wooden ships. This sounds easy; but it was not. The rope, especially if caked in oil or tar or salt, could be as hard as steel, and unpicking it tore the hands and left the fingers raw and bleeding.

Yet the working hours were less terrible than the hours of rest. Mrs Jenkins found herself among about one hundred other women of all ages, including the sick and infirm. Many of them appeared to be mad or demented. Tired from their physical work, there was nowhere to sit down, except on benches in the middle of the day room or the airing yard. In order to rest themselves, the women sat back to back on a bench, each supporting the other. There was nothing to do, nothing to look at or listen to, no books, nothing with which to exercise the mind. Many of the women just walked up and down, or round and round in circles. Most of them talked to themselves, or rocked backwards and forwards continuously. Some moaned aloud, or howled into the night air.

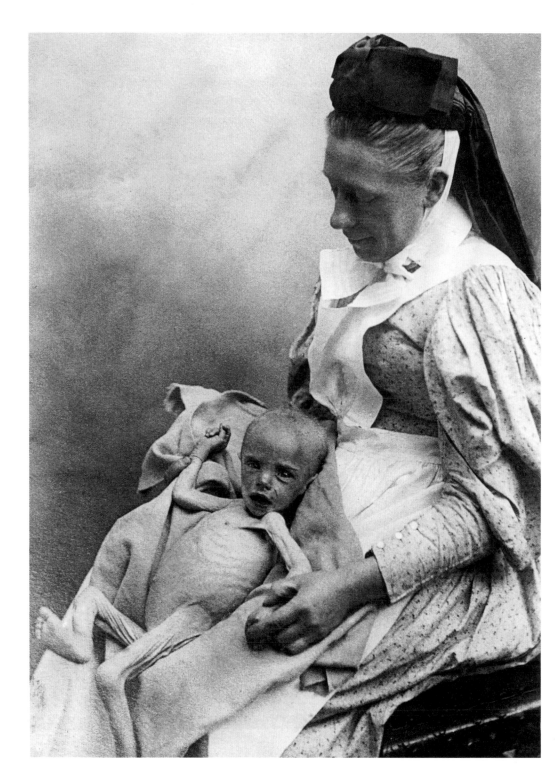

"I will ge' like tha' meself," thought Mrs Jenkins.

They were ushered into the airing yard twice a day for half an hour of exercise. From the yard, Mrs Jenkins could hear the sounds of children's voices, but the walls were fifteen feet high, and she could not see over them. She tried calling the names of her children, but was ordered to stop, or she wouldn't be allowed out into the yard again. So she just stood by the wall where she thought the sounds came from, whispering their names, and straining her ears to catch the sound of a voice she would know to be her child's own.

"I didn' know wha' I done wrong to be in there. I jus' cried all the time. An' I didn' know wha' they done wiv the li'l ones."

When the spring came, and the days grew warmer and longer, and new life was surging all around in the world that she could not see beyond the workhouse walls, Mrs Jenkins was informed that her youngest child, a boy aged three, had died. She asked why, and was told that he had always been sickly, and that no one had expected him to live. She asked if she might attend the funeral, and was told that he had already been buried.

The little boy was the first to go. Mrs Jenkins never saw any of her children again. Over the next four years, one by one, they all died. The mother was merely informed of each death, she was given no cause. She did not attend any of the funerals. The last to die was a girl of fourteen. Her name was Rosie.

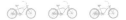

Opposite: A workhouse nurse holds an emaciated baby (c. 1880). Many children died in the workhouse, and while the mothers might be informed of their children's deaths, they were not usually given a cause of death.

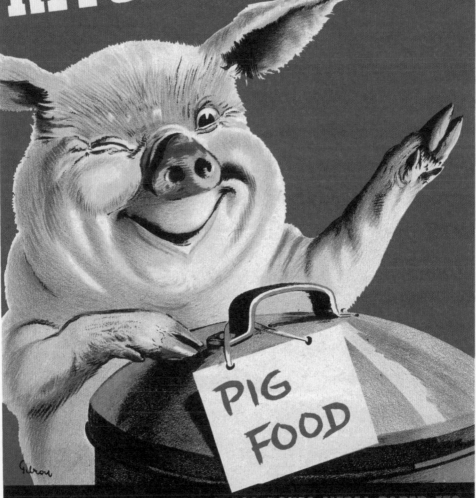

THE BOTTOM DROPPED OUT OF PIGS

Always expect the unexpected, and you will never go wrong. Fred had suffered a severe setback from the enforced closure of his quail and toffee-apple empire, and was looking round for something new. The unexpected came from a chance remark from Mrs B. as she came bustling into the kitchen muttering, "I don' know what fings is comin' to. The price o' bacon these days! I've never seen nuffink like it."

Fred slapped his shovel down on the floor, raising a cloud of ash, and shouted: "Pigs! That's the answer. Pigs. They was doin' it in the war, an' it can be done again."

Mrs B. rushed over to him, broom in hand. "You messy bugger, messin' up my kitchen."

She held the broom aggressively, ready to strike. But Fred neither heard nor saw. He grabbed her round the waist, and twirled her round and round in a frenzied dance.

"You got it, old girl, you 'as. Why didn't I think on it. Pigs."

He made snorting, honking noises, supposed to represent a pig, which did not improve his looks at all. Mrs B. extricated herself from his embrace, and poked him in the chest with the broom handle.

"You crazy …" she started shouting, and he yelled back. When two Cockneys are engaged in a shouting match it is impossible to understand the lingo.

Opposite: This poster from the Second World War asks people to keep their kitchen waste for pig food.

Breakfast was over, and we heard the Sisters' footsteps. They appeared in the doorway, and the slanging match stopped.

In high excitement, Fred explained that he had just had a brilliant idea. He would keep a pig. It could live in the chicken run, which he could easily convert into a pigsty, and in no time at all the pig would be ready for the bacon factory, and his fortune would be made.

Sister Julienne was enchanted. She loved pigs. She had been brought up on a farm, and knew a lot about them. She said that Fred could have all the peelings and waste from Nonnatus House, and advised him to go round the local cafés begging similar favours. Shyly she asked if she might come to see the pig when it was installed in the hen/pig house.

Fred wasn't one to hang around. Within a matter of days the pigsty was complete. He and Dolly pooled their resources and a pink, squealing little creature was soon purchased. Sister Julienne was profuse in her praise.

"You've got a fine pig, there, Fred. A real beauty. You can tell by the width of the shoulders. You've made a good choice."

She gave him one of her sparkling smiles and Fred turned as pink as the pig.

Fred yielded to Sister Julienne for advice about bran mash and nut mix, as well as supplies of food waste from local cafés and greengrocers. They were frequently seen in deep and earnest conversation, Fred sucking his tooth and whistling inwardly as he concentrated on the detail. Sister also advised him on hay and water and mucking out, and she impressed us all with her knowledge in the art of pig rearing.

It was a busy and happy time for Fred. Each day at breakfast we heard details of the pig's progress, her lusty appetite and rapid growth. As the weeks passed, mucking out consumed more of Fred's time and labour. However, this proved to be a money-maker. Most small houses had tiny back gardens, no more than a yard in most cases, but quite sufficient to grow a few things. Tomatoes were popular, and so, surprisingly, were grapevines, which grew exceedingly well in Poplar and produced succulent fruit. Word soon got round, and Fred's pigshit was in great demand. He concluded that there was no losing with pigs. The more he fed her, the more thick, black stuff she excreted, and the more money he made. Within a few weeks the sale of manure had covered the initial cost of the piglet.

The whole of Nonnatus House, Sisters and lay staff alike, took a deep interest in the pig and Fred's financial aspirations. We read in the papers that the price of meat was rising, and concluded that Fred had been very shrewd.

However, the vagaries and vicissitudes of the market are notorious. Demand fell. The bottom dropped out of pigs.

The blow was heavy. Fred was glum. All that feeding and mucking and raking. All the plans and hopes. And now the pig was hardly worth the cost of slaughter. No wonder the bounce had gone out of Fred's bent little legs. No wonder his North-East eye drooped.

Sunday was a day of rest in Nonnatus House. After church we were all gathered in the kitchen, having coffee and cakes left by Mrs B. from her Saturday bake. Fred was packing up to leave, but Sister Julienne invited him to join us at the big table. Conversation turned to the pig; his fag drooped.

"What'm I goin' to do wiv 'er? She's costin' me money to feed 'er an' I can't ge' nuffink for 'er."

Everyone sympathised and muttered "hard luck" and "shame", but Sister Julienne was silent. She stared at him intently, and then said, clearly and positively, "Breed from her, Fred. You could keep her as a breeding sow. There will always be a market for good healthy piglets, and when prices pick up, as they will, you could get a good price for them. And don't forget, a sow always delivers between twelve and eighteen piglets."

Such advice – so obvious, so simple, yet so unexpected! Fred's mouth fell open, and his fag dropped on to the table. Picking it up with an apology, he stubbed it out in the ashtray. Unfortunately it was not an ashtray; it was Sister Evangelina's meringue, which she had been on the point of eating. She remonstrated with characteristic vigour.

Fred was abashed and apologetic. He picked up the meringue, brushed off the ash, picked the fag end out of the cream, and handed it back to Sister Evangelina. "Piglets. Tha's the answer. I'll be a pig breeder. I'll be the best pig breeder on the Isle."

Sister Evangelina snorted, and pushed the meringue away from her with disgust. But Fred noticed none of this. He was in a trance, muttering, "Piglets, piglets, I'll breed pigs, that's what I'll do, I will."

Sister Julienne, practical and tactful, handed another meringue to Sister Evangelina, and said, "You will have to take the *Pig Breeders' Guide*, Fred, and find a good stud boar. I can help you, if you need help in the first instance. My brother is a farmer so I can ask him to send a copy."

And that was how it all started. *The Pig Breeders' Guide* arrived, and Fred and Sister Julienne were soon poring over it. It was disconcerting to see Fred attempting to read, because he had to hold the page to the left of his South-West eye in order to read anything at all. Even when he could make out a sentence or two, the language of pig breeders was completely foreign to him, and he could not have managed without Sister Julienne, who translated the strange jargon into comprehensible Cockney.

A good stud boar was selected, a telephone call made, an agreement reached, and a small open truck arrived from Essex.

Sister Julienne could hardly contain her excitement. Instructing Sister Bernadette to take charge of the House in her absence, she put on her outdoor veil and cloak, pulled a bicycle out of the shed, and cycled off to Fred's house.

The Essex farmer was a rural gentleman of settled habits. He had scarcely ventured beyond the peaceful confines of Strayling Strawless to Market Sodbury. His thoughts, as he drove his open truck with his stud boar into the heart of London's Docklands, have not been revealed to us. The boar, resting his head contentedly on the side of the truck, jogged along for several miles without arousing much interest, but once in the more densely populated streets of London it was a different story. All the way through Dagenham, Barking, East Ham, West Ham, and down to Cubitt Town on the Isle of Dogs, the pig drew crowds. He was a large animal whose only exercise was that of copulation. His nature was comparatively docile, but in ten years his tusks had never been cut, and in consequence he looked more ferocious than he really was.

As the truck turned in at the end of the street Sister Julienne arrived on her bicycle and met Fred. Together they approached the farmer, who stared at them without saying a word. Sister Julienne stood on tiptoe, looking over the edge of the truck, and brushed back her veil which had been blowing towards the pig's tusks.

"Oh, he's a beautiful fellow," she whispered excitedly.

The farmer looked at her, sucked his pipe, and said, "I don't believe this."

He asked to see the sow. The entry to Fred's yard was via a side passage that ran between the houses, at the end of which was the boundary wall to the docks. The Thames ran behind it. The farmer was thus confronted with the towering sides of ocean-going cargo vessels.

"They are never going to believe this. Never," he muttered, as he stooped to pick up his pipe and the keys that had fallen from his hands.

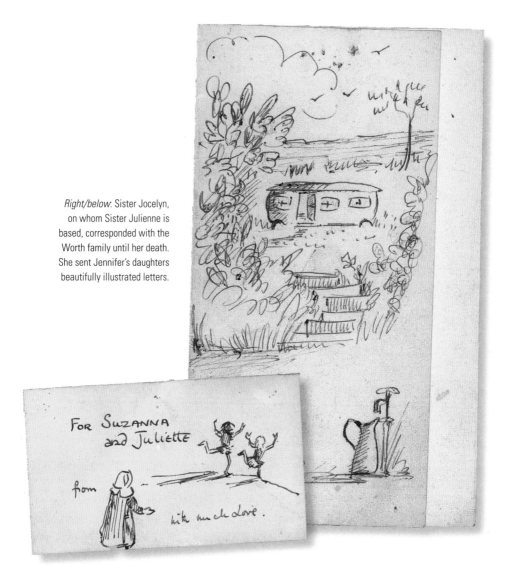

Right/below. Sister Jocelyn, on whom Sister Julienne is based, corresponded with the Worth family until her death. She sent Jennifer's daughters beautifully illustrated letters.

He was directed into Fred's yard.

"There she is, an' lookin' for a bi' of fun from that there big bugger o' your'n."

"Fun!" growled the farmer, "This bit of fun will cost you one pound, cash in hand."

Fred knew the cost, and had the money ready, but grumbled nonetheless. "Cor – pound a poke – that's more'n they gets up West, that is."

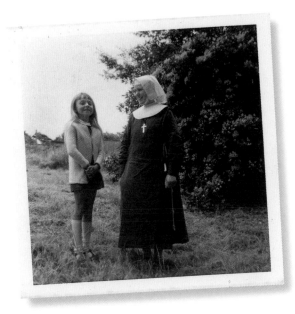

Left: Sister Jocelyn with Suzannah, Jennifer Worth's daughter, in the 1970s.

Sister Julienne remonstrated: "It's no good grumbling, Fred. A pound is the going rate, so you had better pay up."

The farmer eyed the nun strangely, but Fred handed over the money without another word.

The farmer pocketed the cash, and said, "Right! We'll bring him round."

But that was easier said than done.

A crowd had gathered, and was growing all the time – word travels fast on the Isle. The farmer backed his truck up against the passage, lowered the rear trailer board, and leaped into the truck to drive the boar down, but the boar refused to budge. A pig's eyesight is poor, and, to a creature accustomed to the open countryside of Essex, the passage must have looked like the black hole into hell.

"Get up and help me," shouted the farmer to Fred.

Together they pushed and walloped and shouted at the boar, which got nasty, and looked as if looked as if it might be tempted to use its tusks after all. The crowd in the street gasped, and mothers pulled their children back as the boar slowly and tentatively, descended the ramp on its tiny trotters and entered the passage. Even then it was not plain sailing. The alley was narrow, and the bear very nearly got stuck. The two men pushed from behind. Sister Julienne ran through the house, through the pig yard and the outside gate, and into the passage with turnip tops in her hand, which she said would entice the pig forward. She held them under its nose, but still it would not move.

Fred had an idea, "Wha' we needs is a red hot poker to stick up his arse, like wha' they do with camels in the desert when they wants 'em to go over a bridge. Camels won' go over water, you know."

"You stick a red hot poker up his arse, and I'll stick one up yours, mate," the farmer threatened, and continued pushing.

Eventually the boar was coaxed down the passage into Fred's yard. A crowd of children followed, and more went into neighbouring gardens and hung over the fence.

The farmer got cross. He spoke with slow emphasis.

"You'll have to clear this crowd away. Pigs are shy animals, they won't do anything in front of an audience."

Again, Sister Julienne took charge. She spoke with quiet authority to the children, and they crept away. She, Fred, and the farmer went into the house and shut the door. But Sister could not resist the temptation to peep out through the curtains to see how the sow took to her "husband", as she insisted on calling the boar.

"Oh Fred, I don't think she likes him – look, she's pushing him away. He's definitely interested, do you see?"

Fred stood by the window, sucking his tooth.

"No, no, not like that!" cried Sister Julienne, wringing her hands in anguish. "You mustn't bite him. That's not the way. Now she's running. Fred, I'm afraid she might not accept him. What do you think?"

Fred didn't know what to think.

"That's better. There's a good girl. She's getting more interested, do you see, Fred? Isn't it wonderful?"

Fred grew alarmed. "He'll kill 'er, he will. Look at 'im, the big bugger. He's biting her. Look 'ere, I'm not standin' fer this, not no 'ow. He'll kill 'er, he will, or break 'er legs or somefink. I'm gonna put a stop to this, I am. It's barbaric, I tells yer."

Sister had to restrain him.

"It's all perfectly natural. That's the way they do it, Fred."

Fred was not easily pacified. Sister and the farmer had to hold him back until it was all over.

* * *

The Nuns were assembled in the Chapel, kneeling in private prayer. The bell for Vespers sounded just as Sister Julienne entered Nonnatus House. Flushed and excited, she raced along the corridor, leaving behind footsteps of a sticky and highly pungent substance on the tiled floor. In haste, she composed herself, took her place at the lectern, and read:

> *"Sisters, be sober, be vigilant, for your adversary*
> *the Devil roareth around like a raging lion, seeking*
> *whom he may devour."*

One or two of the Sisters looked up from their prayers and glanced sideways at her. A few sniffed suspiciously.
  She continued:

> *"Thine adversary roareth in the midst of thy congregation.*
> *Thine enemy hath defiled thy holy place."*

The sniffs got louder, and the Sisters glanced at each other.

> *"But as for me, I walk with the godly."*

The sacristan filled the censer with an unusually large quantity of incense and swung it vigorously.

> *"In my prosperity I said I shall never be cast down."*

Smoke filled the air.

> *"But thou, oh Lord, hath seen my pride*
> *and sent my misfortune to humble me."*

There was unrest amongst the Sisters. Those kneeling closest to Sister Julienne shuffled a little distance from her. It cannot be easy to shuffle sideways whilst on your knees and wearing monastic habit, but in extremis it can be managed.

> *"But thou dost turn thy face from me,*
> *and I was troubled, and I gat me to my*
> *Lord, right humbly."*

The incense swung furiously, smoke billowing out.

> *"And I will say unto my Lord, I am*
> *unclean. I am unfit to dwell in Thy Holy Place."*

Coughing broke out.

> *"And I cried aloud What profit is there in me?*
> *I am undone. I shall go down into the Pit.*
> *Oh Lord, hear my prayer. Let my cry*
> *come unto Thee."*

Eventually, and not before time, Vespers concluded. The Sisters, red-eyed, choking and spluttering, filed out of the chapel.

It took a long time for Sister Julienne to live down the opprobrium of having filled the chapel with the odour of pigshit, and I am sure that God forgave her long before her Sisters did.

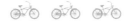

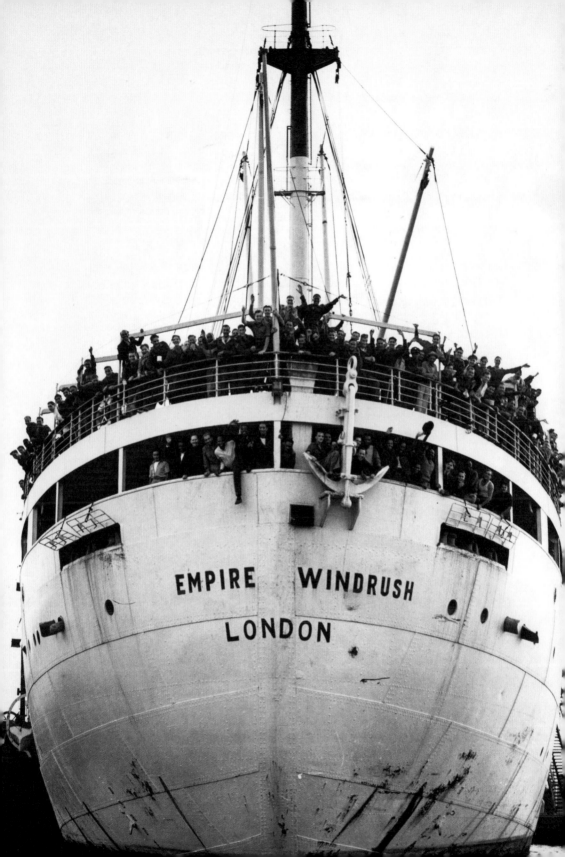

OF MIXED DESCENT I

In the 1950s the African and West Indian population in London was very small. The ports of London, like those of any nation, had always been a melting pot for immigrants. Different nationalities, languages, and cultures were flung together and intermingled, usually bound to each other by poverty. The East End was no exception, and over the centuries just about every race had been absorbed and propagated. Tolerant warm-heartedness has always been a hallmark of the Cockney way of life, and strangers, though they may have been regarded with distrust and suspicion at first, were not resisted for long.

Most of the immigrants were young, single men. Men have always been mobile, but not so women. In those days it would have been virtually impossible for a young, poor woman to go jaunting around the world by herself. Girls had to stay at home. However bad the home, however great the hardships and poverty, however much their spirits longed for freedom, they were trapped. This indeed is still the fate of the vast majority of the women of the world today.

Men have always been luckier, and a footloose young man in a foreign place, once his stomach is full, is after one thing – girls. The East End families were very protective of their daughters and, until recently, pregnancy out of wedlock was the ultimate disgrace and a catastrophe from which the poor

Opposite: In 1948, the Empire Windrush sailed up the English Channel into London's Tilbury Docks. It carried hundreds of Jamaicans, all seeking a new life in the "Motherland".

girl never recovered. However, it did occur quite frequently. If the girl was lucky, her mother stood by her and brought up the baby. Occasionally the father of the child was forced to marry her, but this was a mixed blessing, as many a girl found to her cost. Whatever the social hardship for the girl, it did mean a continuous infusion of new blood – or new genes, as we would say today – into the community. This may, in fact, account for the distinctive energy, vitality, and boundless good humour of the Cockney.

Whilst daughters were protected, married women were in a different situation altogether. A young unmarried girl who became pregnant could not hide from anyone the fact that she was unmarried. A married woman could bear anyone's child, and no one would be any the wiser. I have often felt that the situation is loaded against men. Until recently, when genetic blood tests became possible, how could any man know that his wife was carrying his child? The poor man had no other assurance of paternity than his wife's word. Unless she is virtually locked up, he can have no control over her activities during the day while he is at work. All this does not matter very much in the broad spectrum of life, because most men are quite happy with a new baby, and if a husband happens to be fathering another man's child, he is not likely to know, and, as they say, "what the eye does not see, the heart does not grieve over". But what happens when his wife brings forth a black man's child?

The East Enders had hardly faced this before, but after the Second World War the potential was there.

Bella was a lovely young redhead of about twenty-two. She was well named. Her pale skin, slightly freckled, her cornflower blue eyes would captivate any man, and her red curls would bind him to her for ever. Tom was the happiest and proudest young husband in the East India Docks. He talked about her incessantly. She came from one of the "best" families (the East Enders could be incredibly snobbish and class-conscious in their social gradings) and they had married after four years of courtship, when Tom was finally able to support her.

They had a slap-up wedding. She was the only daughter and her family were determined to do her proud. No expense was spared: a wedding gown with a train that reached halfway down the church; six bridesmaids and four pageboys; enough flowers to give you hayfever for a week; choir; bells; a sermon – the lot! That was just to show the neighbours what could be done. The reception was designed to prove the unrivalled superiority of the family to all the friends and relations. A fleet of Rolls Royces, eighteen in all, drove the most important people from the church a hundred yards down the road to the church hall hired for the occasion. The rest had to walk – and got there first! The long trestle tables had been spread with white cloths, and nearly collapsed under the weight of hams, turkeys, pheasants, beef, fish, eels, oysters, cheeses, pickles, chutneys, pies, puddings, jellies, blancmanges, custard, cakes, fruit drinks and, of course, the wedding cake. Had he seen the wedding cake after he had constructed St Paul's Cathedral, Sir Christopher Wren would have broken down and wept! It was seven storeys high, each layer supported on Grecian columns, with towers and balustrades and flutings and minarets. It boasted a domed roof bearing a coy-looking bride and bridegroom surrounded by lovebirds.

Tom was a bit abashed by all this, and didn't quite know what to say but, as he had said the all-important words "I do", none of the family really cared whether he said anything else. Bella was quietly enjoying being the centre of attention. She was not a loud or showy girl, but her enjoyment of being the occasion for such extravagance was notable. Her mother was in her element, and bursting with pride. She was also just about bursting out of her tight-fitting purple taffeta suit. (Why is it that women always dress so outrageously for weddings? Look around you, and you will see middle-aged women in things that should have been left behind with their twenties, drawn tightly across expanding backsides, pulled in at the waist, emphasising folds of flesh that would be better covered; ridiculous hairdos; ludicrous hats; kamikaze shoes.) Bella's mother and several of her aunts had fashionable veils to their hats, which made eating rather difficult, so they pushed their veils up, and pinned them to the tops of their heads, which made the hats look even more absurd.

Bella's father held the floor for forty-five minutes whilst he gave his wedding speech. He spoke at length of Bella's babyhood, her first tooth, her first word, her first step. He went on to discuss her brilliant school career, and how she had got a school certificate which was now framed and hanging on the wall. No doubt he would have gone on to the swimming certificate and the cycling test had Bella's mother not said, "Ow gi' on wiv it, Ern."

So he turned his attention to Tom, and told him what a lucky chap he was, and how all the other chaps had been after her, but that he (Ern) had reckoned that he (Tom) was the best of the bunch, and would look after his little Bella, because he was a good hard-working lad, and would remember that success in life and marriage depends upon "early to bed and up with the cock".

The uncles guffawed and winked, and the aunts affected to look shocked and said to each other, "Ow, 'e is a one, 'e is."

Tom turned pink and smiled because everyone else was laughing. It was possible that he didn't understand. Bella kept her eyes firmly on her jelly, it being prudent that she shouldn't be seen to understand.

After the delights of the honeymoon spent in one of the best boarding houses in Clacton, they returned to a small flat, near to Bella's mum. Flo was determined that her daughter should have the best of everything, and had purchased fitted carpets in their absence. Such a luxury was virtually unknown in the East End in those days. Tom was bemused and kept rubbing his toes up and down the soft pile to see how it moved. Bella was enchanted, and it triggered an orgy of spending on household items, most of them relatively new and unheard of among her neighbours: an upholstered three-piece suite; electric wall lights; a television; a telephone; a refrigerator; a toaster; and an electric kettle. Tom found them all very novel, and was glad that his Bella was so happy playing the little housewife. He had to take on more and more overtime to keep up the payments, but he was young and strong, and didn't mind, as long as she was content.

Bella booked with the Nonnatus Midwives for her first pregnancy, because her mother advised it. She attended antenatal clinic each Tuesday afternoon, and was perfectly healthy. She was about thirty-two weeks pregnant when Flo came to see us one evening. It was outside our routine hours, but she seemed agitated. "I'm worrit about our Bell, I am. She's depressed or summat. I can see it, an' Tom can see it an' all, 'e can. She won't talk, she won't look at no one, she won't do nuffink. Tom says, 'e says, often the dishes aren't even washed up when he gits in, an' the place is a real pigsty. Somefinks up, I tells you."

We said that clinically Bella was quite healthy, and the pregnancy was normal. We also said that we would visit her at home, in addition to her Tuesday antenatal clinic.

Bella was certainly depressed. Several of us visited, and we all observed the same symptoms – lethargy, inattention, disinterest. We called in her doctor. Flo made heroic efforts to try to get her out of it, by taking her out to buy piles of baby clothes and various paraphernalia considered necessary.

Tom was very worried, and fussed and fretted over her whenever he was at home; but as he worked such long hours, even longer now in order to pay for all the baby things, most of the burden fell on Flo, who was a solicitous and devoted mother.

Bella went into labour at full term. She was neither early nor late according to her dates. Her mother called us around lunchtime to say that the pains were coming every ten minutes, and that she had had a show. I finished my lunch, and stocked up on two helpings of pudding as a precaution against missing my tea. A primigravida with contractions every ten minutes is not an emergency.

I cycled in a leisurely manner round to Bella's house. Flo was waiting on the doorstep to greet me. It was a sunny afternoon, but she looked worried. "She's like I says, no change, but I'm not 'appy. Somefink's up. She's not 'erself. It's not normal, it's not."

Like most women of her generation, Flo was an experienced amateur midwife.

Bella was in the sitting room on the new settee, digging her fingernails into the upholstery. She was pulling out bits of stuffing. She stared at me dully as I entered and ground her teeth. She continued grinding her teeth for some time after she had withdrawn her attention from me. She didn't say a word.

I said, "I must examine you, Bella, if you are going into labour. I need to know how far on you are, and what the baby's position is, and listen to its heartbeat. Could you come into the bedroom, please?"

She didn't move. More stuffing came out of the sofa. Flo tried to coax her along. "Come on, luvvy, it won't be long now. We all has to go through it, but it's over in next to no time. Yer'll see. Come on, now. Into ve bedroom."

She made to help her daughter up, but was pushed roughly away. Flo almost lost her balance and fell. I had to be firm.

"Bella, get up at once and come with me into the bedroom. I have to examine you."

She looked like a child who knows the voice of command, and came quietly.

She was two to three fingers dilated, foetal head down, a normal anterior presentation, as far as I could assess, and waters unbroken. The foetal heart was a steady 120. Bella's pulse and blood pressure were good. Everything seemed perfectly normal, except this curious mental state, which I could not understand. The tooth-grinding continued all through the examination, and was getting on my nerves.

I said, "I'm going to give you a sedative, and it would be better if you stayed in bed and slept for a few hours. Labour will continue while you are asleep, and you will be refreshed for later on."

Flo nodded wisely in approval.

I laid out my delivery things, and told Flo to ring Nonnatus House when contractions were every five minutes, or sooner if she was worried. I noted with satisfaction that there was a telephone in the flat. We might need it, I thought, in view of Bella's mental state. Post-partum delirium is a rare and frightening complication of labour, requiring swift and skilled medical attention.

The phone rang about 8 p.m., and Tom's voice asked me to come. I was there within ten minutes, and he let me in. He seemed anxious but excited.

"This is it, then, nurse. Cor, I hopes as 'ow she'll be all right, her an' the baby. I can't wait to see my li'l baby, yer know, nurse. It's somefink special, like. Bell's bin a bit down of lates, but she'll perk up when she sees the baby, won't she, now?"

I went into the bedroom just as Bella was starting a contraction. It was powerful, and she was moaning in pain. Her mother was wiping her face with a cold flannel. We waited for and timed the next contraction. Every five minutes. I thought, I doubt if it will be long now. The girl looked drowsy and lethargic between contractions, and I did not want to give more sedative or analgesic if delivery was close.

"How is she?" I said to Flo, slightly tapping my head to indicate my real meaning.

She replied: "She hasn't said a word since you lef', not a word she 'asn't. She wouldn't even look at Tom when 'e comes 'ome, nor say nothin' to 'im neither. No' a word, nuffink. Poor lad, 'e feels it, 'e do."

She patted her heart to indicate the feeling.

With the next contraction the waters broke, and Bella's breathing became more rapid. She grabbed her mother's hand.

"There, there, my pet. It won' be long."

The contraction had passed, but Bella still clung to her mother's hand with a vice-like grip. Her eyes were staring wildly.

Bella gave a low scream – "No!" then, with her voice rising with every reiteration, "No! No! No! Stop it. You gotta stop it."

Then she emitted horrible high-pitched gurgling sounds. She threw herself around the bed, making this dreadful noise, something between a scream and a laugh. It was not a cry of pain, because she was not having a contraction. It was hysteria.

I said, "I must ask Tom to ring for the doctor at once."

Bella cried out, "No! I don' want no doctor. Oh Gawd! Don' chew understand? The baby's goin' to be black. He'll kill me, Tom will, when 'e sees it."

I don't think Flo understood what she had said. So uncommon were black people in the East End at that time that her daughter's words didn't make any sense to her.

Bella was still screaming. Then she swore at her mother and yelled at her, "Can' chew understand, you silly ol' cow. Ve baby's goin' ter be black!"

This time Flo understood. She leaped away from her daughter, and stared at her in horror. "Black? Yer jokin'. Yer must be. You mean it's not Tom's baby?"

Bella nodded.

"You filthy slut, you. Is this what I brings you up for, is it? To disgrace me and yer dad!"

Her hand flew to her face, and she drew in breath with a horrified gasp.

"Oh my Gawd," she whispered to herself. "They've got a big knees-up planned for yer dad at the Club, an' they was keepin' it a surprise. He's President this year, an' the lads wanted a real old knees-up when 'is first gran'child's born. It'll be the joke of all Poplar, it will. He'll never live it down. They won't let 'im."

She wrung her hands silently, then screamed at her daughter. "Oh, I wish you'd never been born, I do. I 'opes as how you dies now, you an' that bastard inside yer an' all, I 'opes."

Another contraction came on, and Bella screamed with pain. "Stop it. Don't let it come. Stop it some'ow."

"I'll give you 'don't let it come'," screamed Flo. "I'll kill you afore it comes, yer filthy bitch, you."

They were both screaming at each other. A terrified Tom appeared in the doorway. Flo turned on him, her face red with passion. "Get out of here," she said. "Vis is no place for a man. Just get out. Go for a walk, or somefink. An don't come back 'til termorrer mornin'."

Tom withdrew with speed. Men were accustomed to being ordered about in that way when it came to childbirth.

His appearance must have made Flo think more clearly. She became practical. "We've gotta get rid of it," she said. "No one mus' know, least of all 'im. When it's born I'll take it away and put it in an institution. No one will know."

Bella grabbed her hand, her eyes alight. "Oh mum, will yer? Will yer do that fer me?"

My head was spinning. Up to that moment I had been flattened morally and emotionally, by all the noise, and the high drama going on between mother and daughter. But this was a new turn of events.

"You can't possibly do that," I said. "What are you going to tell Tom when he gets home tomorrow?"

"We'll tell 'im it's dead," said Flo confidently.

"But you can't do that in this day and age. You can't spirit away a living baby and announce that it died. You would never get away with it. Tom thinks he's the father. He would ask to see the baby. He would ask why it died."

"He can't see ve baby," said Flo with less confidence. "He's got to think it's dead and buried."

"This is ridiculous," I said. "We are not living in the 1850s. If I deliver a living baby, I have to make my report, and that has to go to the health authorities. The baby can't just die or disappear. Someone will have to account for it."

Just then another contraction came on, and the dialogue had to be suspended. My head was racing. They were mad, both of them, beyond all reason.

The contraction passed. Flo had also been thinking furiously and making her plans. "Well you go away, then. Say you 'ad to go to another patient, or summat. I can deliver the baby myself, an' I don't 'ave to make no bleedin' report to no bleedin' authority. I can just take the baby away when it's born, an' no one'll know where it's gorn to, they won't. An' Tom'll never see it."

I reeled under the impact of this suggestion. "I can't possibly do that. I'm a professional midwife, trained and registered. Bella is my patient. I can't walk out on her in the first stage of labour, and leave her in the hands of an untrained woman. I still have to make my report. What am I to tell the Sisters? How am I to account for my actions?"

Another contraction came on. Bella was screaming. "Oh, stop it. Don' let it come. Let me die. What'll 'e say? 'e'll kill me!"

Her mother, defiant, said, "Don't you fret, my luvvy. He'll never see it. Yer mum'll get rid of it for yer."

"But you can't," I shouted. I felt myself getting hysterical, too. "If a living baby is born, it can't just be 'got rid of'. If you try anything like that, you will have the police after you. You will be committing a crime, and then your situation will be worse than ever."

Flo sobered up a bit. "It'll have to be adopted, then."

"That's more like it," I said. "But even then the baby has to be registered, and adoption papers have to be drawn up and signed by both parents to give consent. Tom thinks it is his baby. You can't hide it from him and then tell him he's got to sign his baby away for adoption. He wouldn't agree to that."

Bella started screaming again. Dear God, what's her blood pressure doing, I thought. Maybe, with all this second stage trauma, the grandmother will get her way after all and the baby will die! I got out my foetal stethoscope to listen to the heartbeat. Bella must have read my thoughts. She pushed the stethoscope away.

"Leave it alone. I wants it to die, can't you see that?"

"I must ring for the doctor," I said. "Anything could happen, and I need help."

"Don't you dare," Flo snarled at me. "No one mus' know – no doctors. I've got to get rid of it somehow."

"Don't let's start on that again," I shouted. "I need a doctor, and I'm going to ring for one now."

Quick as a flash, Flo was in front of me. She grabbed my surgical scissors from the delivery tray, rushed into the other room, and cut the wire of the telephone. She glared at me in triumph.

"There now. Yer can go down ve road an' telephone ve doctor."

I didn't dare do such a thing. The second stage was imminent. The baby might be born in my absence, and I might return to find it had been "got rid of".

There was another contraction. Bella seemed to be bearing down. She was still crying hysterically, but definitely giving a push. Flo started wailing.

"Shut up," I said in a cold, hard voice. "Shut up, and get out of this room."

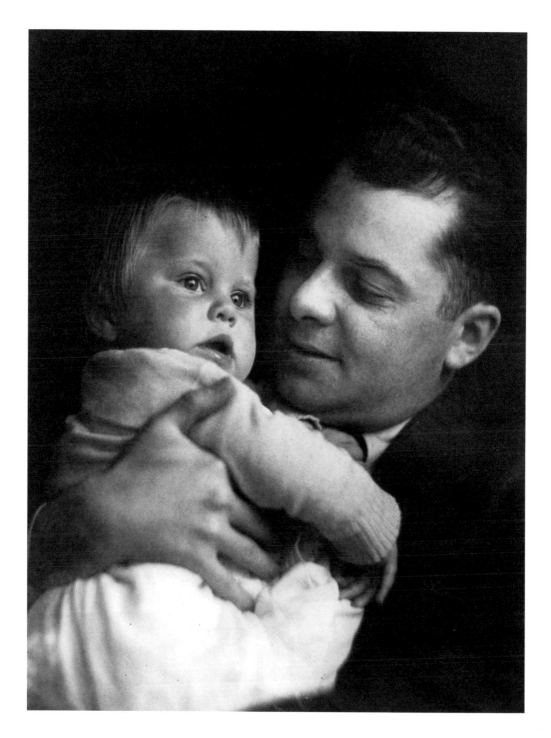

She looked startled, but stopped her noise.

"Now, leave this room at once. I have a baby to deliver, and I cannot do it with you present. Go."

She gasped, and opened her mouth to say something, but thought better of it and left, shutting the door quietly behind her.

I turned to Bella. "Now roll over on to your left side, and do exactly as I tell you. This baby will be born within the next few minutes. I don't want you to have a tear or a haemorrhage, so just do as I say."

She was quiet and cooperative. It was a perfect delivery.

The baby was pure white and looked just like Tom. She was the apple of her father's eye, and was doted upon by her proud grandfather. Her wise grandmother kept the secrets of the delivery room to herself.

I was the only person outside the family to know, and until this moment, I have never told a soul.

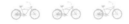

Opposite: This young baby is held lovingly in his father's arms. Some babies weren't so lucky and were put up for adoption, particularly if they were of mixed heritage.

305

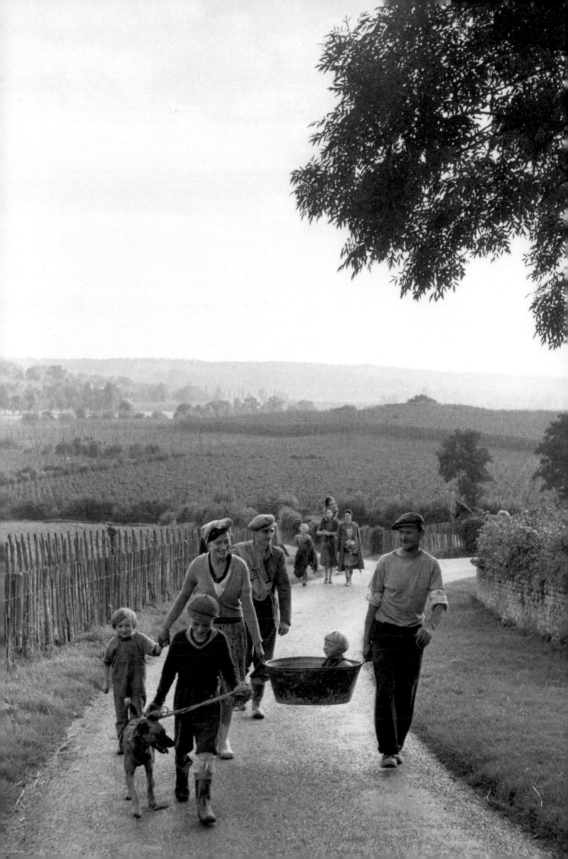

OF MIXED DESCENT II

The Smiths were an average, respectable East End family, with a rub-along sort of marriage. Cyril was a skilled pilot in the docks, and Doris worked in a hairdressers, as her five children were now of school age. They were not hard up, but took their holidays in the hop-picking fields of Kent. Both Cyril and Doris had enjoyed such holidays all through their childhood. Their own children enjoyed the healthy country air, the camaraderie of the other children, the open spaces to run around in, and the chance to earn some pocket money if they filled their baskets with hops. The family met the same people, year after year, who came from other areas of London, and friendships were formed and renewed every year.

Each family had to take their own bedding, primus stove, and cooking equipment. They were allocated a space considered sufficient for the size of each family in sheds or barns, where they dwelt for a fortnight. Food was bought from the farm shop. Some took tents and camped. The adults worked all day in the fields, picking the hops for which they were paid, and most of the children joined in. In the 1950s, poverty was not as extreme as it had been for earlier generations, so the necessity to earn the pittance which was euphemistically called a wage had largely passed. In days gone by, children had had to work from morning to dusk to earn a few pennies which, added to their parents' money, would help the family through the winter. The hop-picking

Opposite: Families enjoy a hop-picking holiday in the Kent countryside (c. 1951).

holidays had also been lifesavers for many East End children, because they were exposed to the sunshine, which prevented rickets.

By the 1950s, the children were mostly free to play, and to join in the picking only if they wanted to. Many farms had a stream or river running through them, which was the centre of childhood fun. The evenings were a great time for the whole temporary community, as they would light fires in the open air, sing songs, flirt and tell stories, and generally make believe that they were country folk and not city-dwellers at all.

Before the war the annual hop-pickers consisted almost exclusively of East Enders, Romany gypsies, and tramps. After the war, with increased mobility of population worldwide, a more varied group of people turned up at the farms each year. (Mechanisation of hop-picking put an end to this annual activity for so many people.)

Doris and Cyril settled with their children in the shed, occupying the seven-foot square space that had been chalked on the floor for them. They were given a straw palliasse to sleep on, and with the primus stove and a hurricane lamp, it was all considered very comfortable. There were a lot of new people at the farm that year, and several families from the West Indies, which was quite a surprise. At first Doris was stand-offish. She had never met or spoken to a black person before, much less slept in the same barn as a group of them, but the children immediately made friends, as children always do. The women were laughing and friendly, and Doris quickly found her inhibitions breaking down.

In fact the holiday proved to be a real eye-opener for Doris and Cyril. They had never before realised that West Indian people could be so much fun. It is said that East Enders are good-humoured. Well, beside the West Indians, Cockneys look positively dour. Doris and Cyril laughed from morning to night, and the hard work of hop-picking was barely felt. Tired but elated in the evenings, Doris would leave the fields to prepare a meal for her family, and then join the groups sitting around the fires. The songs were new this year. She had never heard West Indian singing before, with its blend of beauty and tragedy, and it stirred deep and nameless longings in her heart. She joined in the choruses and the round songs with an ear for music that she never knew she possessed. Cyril didn't think much of the music, and nothing on earth would have induced him to open his mouth and sing, so he joined one of the other groups around another fire where the blokes were more to his liking.

Time passes all too quickly when you are enjoying yourself, and no one wanted to leave at the end of the fortnight. But their time was up, and they all declared it was the best holiday of their life, and that they would meet again next year. The children cried at parting.

The humdrum life of work and school and neighbours and gossip started again, and gradually the memory of the Kentish holiday faded into a dream.

No one was surprised when Doris announced at the Christmas party that she was pregnant again. She was only thirty-eight, and five children was not considered to be a large family. Cyril was told that he "wasn't 'alf a lad", and they were both given everyone's good wishes.

She went into labour early one morning. Cyril rang us on his way to work. Doris was able to get the children up and off to school, and a neighbour came in to be with her for a while. I arrived around 9.30 a.m. to find everything in good order. The house was clean and tidy. The baby things were ready and immaculate. All the requirements we asked for, such as hot water, soap, and so on, were ready. Doris was calm and cheerful. The neighbour left as I arrived, and said that she would pop in later. Labour was uneventful, and fairly quick.

At twelve noon she delivered a baby boy, who was quite obviously black.

I, of course, was the first to see him, and didn't know what to say or do. After I had cut the cord, I wrapped him in a towel, and placed him in the cot whilst I attended to the third stage. This allowed me a little time to think: should I say something? If so, what? Or should I just hand her the baby, and let her see for herself? I decided upon the second course.

The third stage of labour usually takes at least fifteen to twenty minutes, so during that time I simply picked the baby up, and put him in Doris's arms.

She was silent for a long time, and then said, "He's beau'iful. He's so lovely, 'e makes me wanna cry."

Tears silently came to her eyes and coursed down her cheeks. She sobbed inwardly to herself as she clung to the baby.

"Oh he's so beau'iful. I never meant to, but wha' could I do? An' now wha' am I goin' to do? He's the lovelies' baby I ever seed."

She could speak no more for crying.

Overleaf. Any child able to do without a mother, irrespective of race, could be left at any of the London County Council's welfare centres while his or her parent went to work (September 1958).

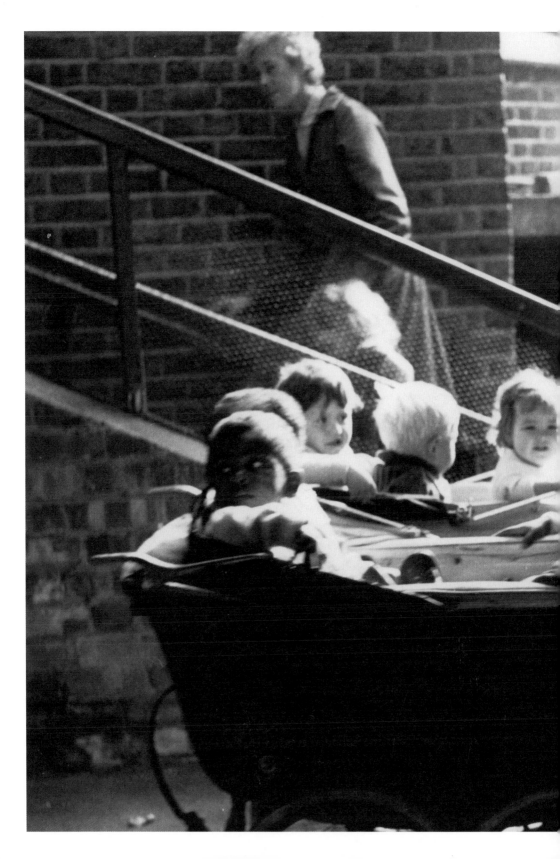

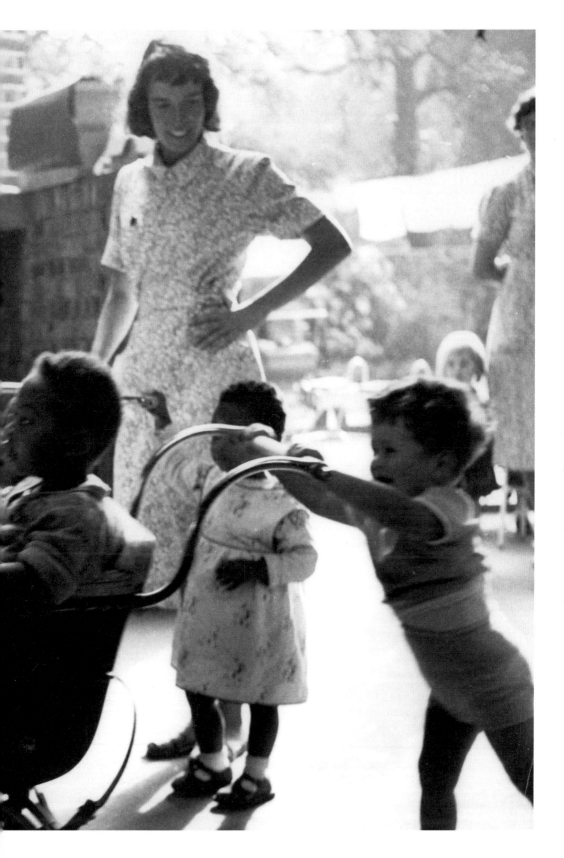

I was shaken by the unexpected turn of events, but had to attend to my job. I said, "Look, I think the placenta will come soon. Let me put the baby back in the cot, only for a few minutes, so that we can complete your delivery safely, and clean you up. We can talk after that."

She allowed me to take the baby, and within ten minutes everything was complete.

I put the baby back in her arms, and silently attended to my clearing up. I felt it better not to initiate any conversation.

She held him quietly for a long time, kissing him, and rubbing her face against his. She held his hand, and flexed his arm, and said, "His fingernails is white, yer know."

Was this a cry of hope? Then she continued, "Wha' am I goin' to do? Wha' can I do, nurse?"

She sobbed in broken-hearted anguish, and clung to the baby with all the fervour and passion of a mother's love. She couldn't speak; she could only groan, and rock him in her arms.

I couldn't reply to her question. What could I say?

I finished what I was doing, and checked the placenta, which was intact. Then I said, "I would like to bath the baby, and weigh him, is that all right?"

She gave the baby to me quietly, and watched every move as I bathed him, as though she was afraid that I might take him away. I think she knew in her heart what was going to happen.

I weighed and measured him. He was a big baby: 9lb 4oz, twenty two inches long, and perfect in every way. He certainly was beautiful; his skin was a dusky tawny colour, fine, dark curly hair already showed on his head. The slightly depressed bridge of his nose, and splayed nostrils accentuated his high, broad forehead. His skin was smooth and unwrinkled.

I gave him back to his mother, and said, "He is the loveliest baby I have ever seen in my life, Doris. You can be proud of him."

She looked at me with bleak despair. "Wha' am I goin' to do?"

"I don't know. I really don't. Your husband will be coming home from work this evening, thinking he is the father of a new baby. He will ask to see him, and you cannot hide him. I don't think you should be alone when he comes home. Can your mother come round to be with you?"

"No. That would make fings worse. He hates my mum. Can you be 'ere wiv me, nurse? You're right. I'm frightened of Cyril seeing 'im."

And she clutched the baby to her, in a desperate gesture of protection.

"I'm not sure that I would be the right person", I replied. "I'm a midwife. Perhaps you need a social worker to be here. I definitely think you need someone for your own protection, and that of the baby."

I promised to look into it, and left.

I imagine she had one happy afternoon with her baby, dozing, cuddling, kissing him, forging with him that unbreakable bond that is a mother's love for her baby, which is every baby's birthright. Perhaps she knew what was coming, and tried to cram a lifetime of love into a few short hours. Perhaps she crooned to him the West Indian spirituals that she had learned around the camp fire.

I reported to Sister Julienne, and expressed my fears. She said, "You are right that someone must be there when her husband sees the baby. However, I think it would be better for a man to be present. All the social workers in this area are women. I will speak to the Rector."

In the event, the Rector sent a young curate to be at the house from five o'clock onwards. He did not go himself, because he thought it would look too portentous if he arrived at the house.

The curate reported that events had transpired very much as I had expected. Cyril took one silent, horrified look at the baby, and made a great swipe at his wife with his fist. The blow was deflected by the curate. Then he made to grab the baby and hurl it against the wall, and was only prevented from doing so by the curate. He said to his wife, "If this bastard stays in the 'ouse one single night, I'll kill 'im, an' you an' all."

The savage gleam in his eye showed that he meant it. "You jest wait, yer bitch."

An hour later the curate left carrying the baby in a small wicker basket, with a bundle of baby clothes in a paper bag. He brought the baby to Nonnatus House, and we cared for him overnight. He was received into a children's home the next morning. His mother never saw him again.

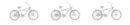

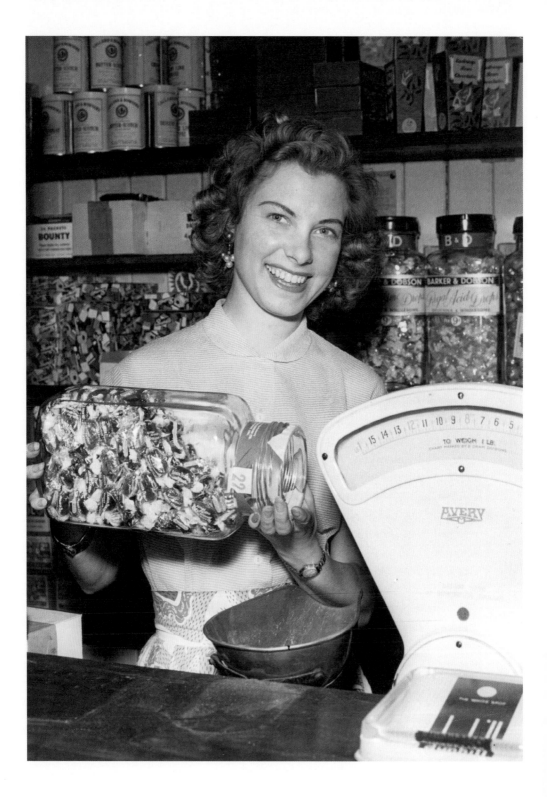

OF MIXED DESCENT III

Ted was fifty-eight when his wife died. She developed cancer and he nursed her tenderly for eighteen months. He gave up his job in order to do so, and they lived on his savings during her illness. They had a happy marriage, and were very close. No children had been born to them, and they had depended entirely on each other for companionship, neither of them being particularly extrovert or sociable. After her death, he was very lonely. He had few real friends, and his mates at work had largely forgotten him since his leaving. He had never cared for pubs and clubs, and was not going to start trying to be the clubby sort at the age of nearly sixty. He tidied the house but couldn't bring himself to clear his wife's room. He cooked scrappy meals for himself, went for long walks, frequented the cinema and the public library, and listened to the radio. He was a Methodist, and attended church each Sunday, and although he tried joining the men's social club, he couldn't get on with it, so he joined the Bible class instead, which was more to his liking.

It seems to be a law of life that a lonely widower will always find a woman to console and comfort him. If he is left with young children he is even more favourably placed. Women are queueing up to look after both him and the children. On the other hand, a lonely widow or divorcee has no such natural advantages. If not exactly shunned by society, she is usually made to feel

Opposite: A woman in a newsagents, tobacconist and confectionery shop (1956). Widowers often had limited opportunities to meet women. Ted met Winnie in a local newsagents, where she worked.

decidedly spare. A lonely widow will usually not find men crowding around anxious to give her love and companionship. If she has children, the men will usually run a mile. She will be left alone to struggle on and support herself and her children, and usually her life will be one of unremitting hard work.

Winnie had been alone for longer than she cared to remember. Her young husband had been killed early in the war, leaving her with three children. A meagre pension from the State barely covered the rent, let alone compensated for the loss of her husband. She took a job in a paper shop. The hours were long and hard – from 5 a.m. to 5.30 p.m. She got up each morning at 4.30 a.m. to get down to the newsagents to receive, sort, pack, and put out the newspapers. Her mother came in each day at 8 a.m. to get the children up and off to school. It meant that they were alone for about four hours, but it was a risk that she had to take. Winnie's mum suggested that they should all come and live with her, but Win valued her independence, and refused unless, as she said, "I jes' can't cope any more". That day never came. Winnie was the coping sort.

They met in the paper shop. She had served him for many years, but never noticed him particularly amongst all her other customers. It was when he started hanging around in the shop for longer than necessary to buy a morning paper that she, and the other staff, began to take note. He would buy his paper, then look at another, then look at the magazine shelves, sometimes buying one. Then he would pick up a bar of chocolate and turn it over in his hand, sigh, and put it back, and buy a packet of Woodbines instead. The staff said to each other, "Somethink's up with that old geezer".

One day, when Ted was holding a bar of chocolate, Winnie went up to him and asked kindly if she could help.

He said, "No, dearie. There's nothing you can do for me. My wife used to like this chocolate. I used to get it for 'er. She died last year. Thank you for asking, dear".

And their eyes met with sympathy and understanding.

After that Winnie always made a point of serving him. One day Ted said, "I was finkin' o' goin' to the flicks tonight. How about comin' wiv me – if yer 'usband don't object".

She said, "I ain't got no 'usband, an' I don't mind if I do".

One thing led to another, and within a year he asked her to marry him.

Winnie thought about it for a week. There were over twenty years between them; she was fond of him, but not really in love with him. He was kind and good, though not wildly exciting. She consulted her mother, and the outcome of the female deliberations was that she accepted his offer of marriage.

Ted was overjoyed, and they had a Methodist Church wedding. He did not want to take his new bride to the house which he had shared for so long with his first wife, so he gave up the rental and took another terraced property. Winnie was able to give up the tiny cheap flat where she had brought up her children, so the terraced cottage was just for her and Ted. It seemed like a palace to her. As the weeks and months passed after the marriage her happiness grew, and she told her mother that she had not done the wrong thing.

When he was young Ted had prudently taken out an insurance policy that matured when he was sixty. He now did not have to go out to work ever again. Winnie, on the other hand, did not want to give up the paper shop. She was so used to hard work that idleness would have bored her to tears but, as Ted wanted her at home more, she agreed to cut down her hours. Their life was very happy.

Winnie was forty-four when her periods stopped. She thought it was the menopause. She felt a bit odd, but her mother told her that all women feel a bit funny during the change, and not to worry. She continued in the paper shop, and brushed aside any feelings of queasiness. It wasn't until six months later that she noticed she was putting on weight. Another month passed, and Ted noticed a hard lump in her tummy. Having experienced his first wife dying of cancer, hard lumps were a source of deep anxiety for him. He insisted that she should see the doctor, and went with her to the surgery.

Examination showed her to be in an advanced stage of pregnancy. The couple were shattered.

Why this obvious explanation had not occurred to either of them before is impossible to conjecture, but it hadn't, and they were both knocked sideways by the news.

There wasn't much time to prepare for a new baby. Winnie left the paper shop that day, and booked with the Sisters for her confinement. Hastily, the bedroom was prepared, and baby equipment bought. Perhaps it was buying the pram and little white sheets that affected Ted so profoundly. Overnight he changed from a bemused and bewildered elderly man to an intensely excited and fiercely proud father-to-be. Suddenly he looked ten years younger.

317

A fortnight later Winnie went into labour. We had arranged for a doctor to be present at the delivery, because there had been so little time for antenatal preparation, and because Winnie, now forty-five, was decidedly old for having a baby.

Ted had taken note of our requirements and advice about preparation. He couldn't have planned it more carefully or thoroughly. He had told Win's mother not to come but that Ted would inform her when the baby was born. He had obtained books on childbirth and babycare, which he read all the time. When she went into labour he called us, full of joy and anticipation, tinged only with a little anxiety.

The doctor and I arrived at almost the same time. It was early first stage, and it had been agreed that I should stay with her throughout labour, from the time of arrival to the third stage completion. The doctor examined her and said he would leave and call back just before evening surgery to assess progress.

I sat down to watch and wait. I advised that she should not lie down, but walk about a bit. Ted took Win's arm and gently and carefully led her up and down the garden path. She could quite easily have walked it by herself, but he wanted and needed to be protective, quite forgetful of the fact that only two weeks earlier she had been dashing off to the paper shop. I suggested she should have a bath. The house boasted a bathroom, and so he heated up the water, and gently helped her in. He washed her, carefully helped her out and then dried her. I advised a light meal, so he poached an egg. He couldn't have done more.

I looked at his library books: Grantley Dick Read's *Natural Childbirth*; *Margaret Myles's Midwifery*; *The New Baby*; *Positive Parents*; *The Growing Child*; *From Birth to Teens*. He had been doing his homework.

The doctor returned just before 6 p.m., and there was no real change in the early labour pattern. We agreed that, in view of her age, if the first stage continued for longer than twelve hours, Winnie should be transferred to the hospital. Both Ted and Winnie agreed to this, but hoped it would not be necessary.

Between 9 and 10 p.m. I observed a change in the labour pattern. Contractions were more frequent and stronger. I started her on the gas and air machine, and asked Ted to go out and phone for the doctor.

When he arrived the doctor gave her a mild analgesic, and we both sat down and waited. Ted courteously offered us a meal, or tea, or drinks, whatever we wanted. We did not have long to wait. Just after midnight the second stage of labour commenced, and within twenty minutes the baby was born.

It was a little boy, with unmistakably ethnic features.

The doctor and I looked at each other, and the mother, in stunned silence. No one said a word. I have never known such an unnerving silence at a delivery. What each of us was thinking the others never knew, but our thoughts must all have been about the same question: "What on earth is Ted going to say when he sees the baby?"

The third stage had to be dealt with, and this was conducted in dead silence. While the doctor was busy with the mother, I bathed, checked, and weighed the baby. He certainly was a beautiful little thing, of average weight, clear dusky skin, soft curly brown hair. A picture perfect baby – if you are expecting to see a baby of mixed racial origins. But Ted wasn't. He was expecting to see his own child. I shut my eyes in a futile attempt to obliterate the scene to come.

Everything was finished and tidied up. The mother looked fresh in a white nightgown; the baby looked beautiful in a white shawl.

The doctor said, "I think we had better ask your husband to come up now."

They were the first words to be spoken since the delivery.

Winnie said, "I reckons as 'ow we'd best get it over wiv".

I went downstairs and told Ted that a baby boy had been safely born, and would he like to come up.

He shouted, "A boy!" and leaped to his feet like a youngster of twenty-two, not a man of over sixty. He bounded up the stairs two at a time, entered the bedroom and took both his wife and the baby in his arms. He kissed them both and said, "This is the proudest and happiest day of my life."

The doctor and I exchanged glances. He hadn't noticed yet. He said to his wife, "You don't know what vis means to me, Win. Can I 'old ve baby?"

She silently handed him over.

Ted sat on the edge of the bed, and cradled the baby awkwardly in his arms (all new fathers look awkward with a baby!) He looked long at his little face, and stroked his hair and ears. He undid the shawl, and looked at the tiny body. He touched his legs, and moved his arms, and took his hand. The

Overleaf: Rubber aprons are a necessity! A group of children play together outside a nursery (1958).

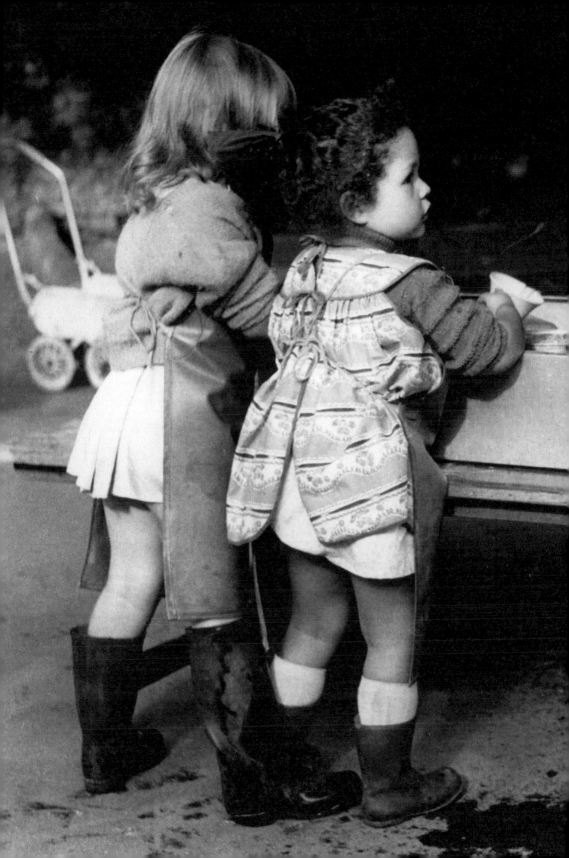

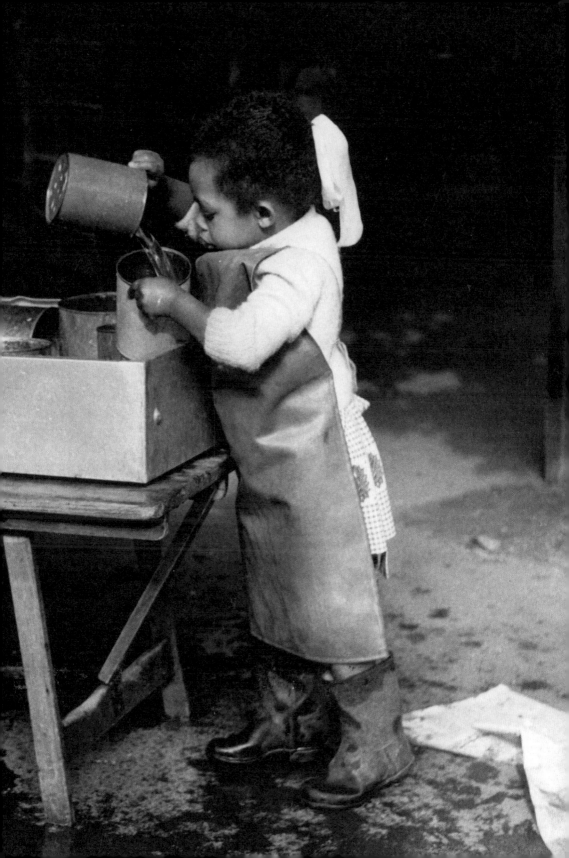

baby's face puckered up and he gave a little mewing cry. Ted gazed at him silently for a long time. Then he looked up with a beatific smile:

"Well, I don't reckon to know much about babies, but I can see as how this is the most beautiful in the world. What's we going to call him, luv?"

The doctor and I looked at each other in silent amazement. Was it really possible he hadn't noticed? Winnie, who had seemed unable to breathe, took a large shuddering breath, and said, "You choose, Ted, luv. He's yourn."

"We'll call 'im Edward, then. It's a good ol' family name. Me dad's an' gran'dad's. He's my son Ted."

The doctor and I left the three of them sitting happily together. Outside, the doctor said, "It is possible that he just hasn't noticed yet. Black skin is pale at birth, and this child is obviously only half-black, or even less than that, because his father may have been of mixed racial descent. However, pigmentation usually becomes more marked as the child ages, and at some stage Ted is certainly going to notice and start asking questions."

Time went by, and Ted didn't notice or, in any event, didn't appear to notice. Win must have had a word with her mother and other female relatives to say nothing to Ted about the baby's appearance, and indeed nothing was said.

Win went back to work part-time at the paper shop after about six weeks. Ted had longer each day with the baby and assumed most of the parenting. He bathed and fed him, and proudly took him out in the pram, greeting passersby and inviting them all to look at "my son Ted". As the baby grew older, he played with him all the time, inventing learning games and toys. In consequence, by the age of eighteen months, little Ted was very bright and advanced for his age. The relationship between father and son was lovely to see.

By the time the child reached school age, his features were noticeably black. Yet still Ted did not appear to notice. He had made a wider circle of friends than he had ever had in his life before, largely due to the fact that he took the child everywhere, and people responded to this bright, handsome little boy, whom Ted introduced proudly as "my son Ted". The child was just as proud, in his own way, of his father and as he clung to his big protective hand, gazed up adoringly with his huge black eyes. At school he always spoke of "my dad" as though he were the king himself.

Ted, approaching seventy, had no inhibitions about waiting outside the school gates along with young mothers nearly half a century his junior.

Only two or three little black or mixed race children would come running out of school, to black mothers, but one of them would fling himself into Ted's arms with the cry, "Daddy."

"Lets go down the docks today, son," he would say, kissing him. "There's a big German vessel jes' come in vis mornin' wiv three funnels. Yer don' see 'em very often. An' yer mum will 'ave tea ready when we gits back."

Yet still he didn't seem to notice.

Of course there were whisperings and gossip amongst neighbours and acquaintances, but none of them actually said anything to Ted. The more unkind would snigger and say, "There's no fool like an old fool." And the rest would laugh and agree, "Yer can say tha' again".

I have a different theory.

In the Russian Orthodox Church there is the concept of the Holy Fool. It means someone who is a fool to the ways of the world, but wise to the ways of God.

I think that Ted, from the moment he saw the baby, knew that he could not possibly be the father. It must have been a shock, but he had controlled himself, and sat thinking for a long time as he held the baby. Perhaps he saw ahead.

Perhaps he understood in that moment that if he so much as questioned the baby's fatherhood, it would mean humiliation for the child, and might jeopardise his entire future. Perhaps, as he held the baby, he realised that any such suggestion could shatter his whole happiness. Perhaps he understood that he could not reasonably expect an independent and energetic spirit like Winnie to find him sexually exciting and fulfilling. Perhaps an angel's voice told him that any questions were best left unasked and unanswered.

And so he decided upon the most unexpected, and yet the simplest course of all. He chose to be such a Fool that he couldn't see the obvious.

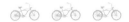

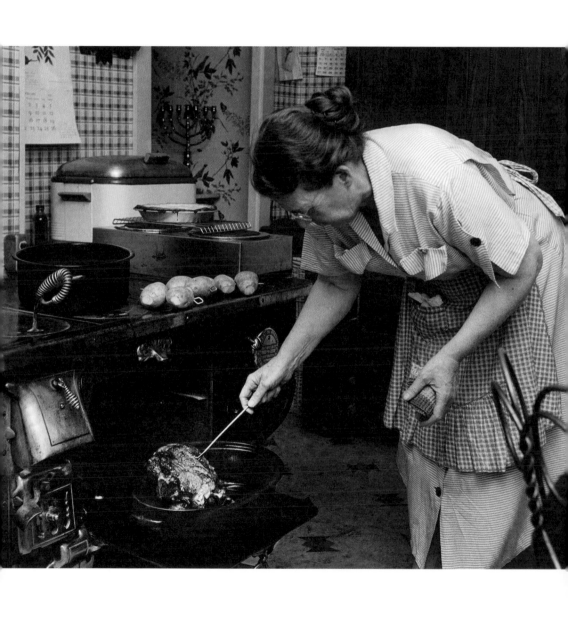

THE LUNCHEON PARTY

"No Jimmy, not this time. You and Mike are *not* camping out in the boiler room at Nonnatus House. I may have deceived the Home Sister at the Hospital, but I am not going to deceive Sister Julienne. Besides, I don't trust you. I don't believe for a moment that there is *another* emergency. I think you just want to be able to boast to the boys that you have slept in a convent!"

Jimmy and Mike looked a trifle crestfallen. They had been plying me with beer and soft talk, in the confident expectation that I would swallow a load of rubbish about them being down on their luck and out of their digs, and would I smuggle them in the back door of Nonnatus House? The male of the species is sweetly naive.

The evening had been fun – a change and relaxation from the rigours of daily work. The beer had been pleasant, and the conversation exuberant, but it was time to go. It was a long way back to the East End, buses were not plentiful after 11 p.m., and I would have to be up at 6.30 a.m. the next morning for a full day's work. I stood up. An idea had come to mind. It seemed a pity to disappoint them altogether.

"But how would you like to come to lunch one Sunday?"

Their enthusiastic agreement was immediate.

"OK. I will ask Sister Julienne, and will ring you to fix a date. I must be off now."

Opposite: What Sunday lunch would be complete without a roast? A woman tests it to make sure it's cooked, just as Mrs B. would have done for Jennifer and her guests.

I spoke to Sister Julienne next day. She had heard about Jimmy before, on the occasion when I had taken a 3 a.m. swim in the sea at Brighton and arrived for work at ten in the morning. She agreed at once to a luncheon party for the boys.

"It would be delightful. We usually entertain retired missionaries, or visiting preachers. A couple of lively young men would be a pleasure for us all."

She fixed a date for three weeks ahead, when there were no other guests for Sunday lunch, and I telephoned Jimmy to firm up the arrangements.

"Do you think the nuns could run to three of us for lunch? Alan wants to come. He thinks he might get a story."

Alan was a reporter, scraping a modest living on his first job in Fleet Street. I thought it highly likely that Sister Julienne could find one more chair at the refectory table, but was not at all sure that Alan would get much of a story out of the lunch. However, hope always runs high in a young reporter's heart – until the iron enters his soul, that is.

The girls were in a flutter of excitement about three young men coming to Sunday lunch. We were all single nurses with a seemingly endless working week and were often hard put to meet eligible young men. Expectations ran high.

I wondered, with a good deal of amusement, how the meal would go. What would the boys make of us? How would they react to the nuns, particularly to Sister Monica Joan? And it would be interesting to see Alan's "story".

The day arrived, warm and bright, and none of our patients was expected to go into labour, which would have disrupted the luncheon party. Everyone was in a flurry of excitement. Had the boys known the flutter they were causing in so many female hearts, they would have been deeply flattered. Or perhaps not. Perhaps they would have regarded it as no more than their devastating charms were due.

They arrived at about 12.30 p.m., just after the Sisters had entered chapel for Tierce, the midday Office.

I opened the door. They certainly looked very spruce, in grey suits, newly washed shirts, and highly polished shoes. I had never before seen them look like that on a Sunday morning. Obviously lunch in a convent was a novel experience for such dedicated young men-about-town. They looked a little unsure of themselves, though.

We kissed, but slightly more formally than usual – no hugs, no laughter, no badinage about nothing much – just a formal kiss, a polite "How are you?", and "Did you have a good journey?"

I felt a trifle uncomfortable, having never found conversation easy. We all know people in a certain context, and outside the familiar, often find them to be completely different. I had known Jimmy since childhood, but normally met up with the others in London pubs. I didn't know what to say, and just stood around looking awkward, thinking the whole thing was not such a good idea after all. The boys could find nothing to say either.

Cynthia saved the day. She always did, without knowing how or what she had done. She stepped forward, her soft smile dispelling the tension and filling the rather strained atmosphere with warmth. When she spoke, the slow sexy voice just knocked them over. All she said was: "You must be Jimmy and Mike and Alan. How lovely – we've been looking forward to this. Now which of you is which?"

Was it the way she said it, or the wide smiling eyes, or the unaffected warmth of her welcome? The boys must have met scores of girls who were more beautiful, with more self-conscious allure, but they could seldom, if ever, have met a girl with a voice quite like that. They were absolutely bowled over and all three stepped forward at the same time, crashing into each other. She laughed. The ice was broken.

"The Sisters will be here soon, but come into the kitchen and have a coffee, and we can have a chat."

Coffee, nectar, ambrosia? They followed eagerly; anything with this glorious girl would be heaven. I, thankfully, was forgotten and I breathed a sigh of relief. The luncheon would be a success.

Mrs B. had neither sex appeal nor an alluring voice, "Now don' you make a mess in 'ere. I've got lunch to serve."

Jimmy smiled confidently at her. "Don't you worry, madam; we won't mess up this beautiful kitchen, will we boys? What a magnificent kitchen, and what glorious smells! All your own home cooking, I take it, madam?"

Mrs B. sniffed, and eyed him suspiciously. She had grown-up sons of her own, and was not susceptible to their particular charms. "You jes' watch it, tha's all I'm sayin'."

"Oh, watch it we certainly will," said Mike, whose eyes had not left Cynthia as she filled the kettle. The water pipes all around the kitchen rattled and shook as she opened the tap.

She laughed and said, "That's just our plumbing system. You'll get used to it."

"Oh, I'd like to get used to it", said Mike with enthusiasm.

Cynthia laughed and blushed a little, brushing back the hair that had fallen over her face.

"Allow me," said Mike gallantly, taking the kettle from her and carrying it over to the gas stove.

Chummy appeared in the doorway, her head buried in *The Times*.

"I say, gels, did you know that Binkie Bingham-Binghouse is getting spliced at last? Jolly good show, what? Actually, her Mater will be frightfully chuffed, don't you know. They thought she was on the shelf. Good old Binkie, haw haw!"

She looked up and saw the boys. At once she went red, and jerked the arm holding the newspaper. It crashed into the dresser, setting the cups rattling and shaking. The paper caught behind a couple of plates and sent them crashing to the floor, smashing them into a dozen pieces.

Mrs B. rushed forward, snarling:

"You clumsy great ... you – you – jest get out o' my kitchen, you clumsy ... you!"

Poor Chummy! It always happened that way. Social situations were a nightmare for her, particularly when men were around. She just didn't know what to say to a man, nor how to behave.

Cynthia again saved the day. She grabbed a dustpan and brush, saying, "Never mind, Mrs B. Luckily it was the plate with the crack in it. It needed throwing out, anyway."

Deftly she swept up the bits, Mike appreciatively studying her neat little bottom as she bent down.

Chummy stood in the doorway, abashed and tongue-tied. I tried to get her to come over and join us for a cup of coffee, but she flushed scarlet and muttered something about going upstairs to wash her hands before lunch. The boys looked at each other in wonder. Lunch in a convent was an unknown, but a female giant hurling plates around was the last thing they had expected. Alan took out his notebook and started scribbling furiously.

We heard the bell sound from the chapel and a little later the Sisters' footsteps. Sister Julienne walked briskly into the kitchen, small, plump, and motherly. She looked at the boys with true affection, and held out both hands.

"I've heard so much about you, and this is a real treat for us all to have you here. Mrs B. has prepared roast beef and Yorkshire pudding, followed by apple pie. Will you like that, do you think?"

Three cool, sophisticated young men responded like three small boys taking sweets from a favourite auntie.

We entered the refectory. After grace, during which the boys eyed each other with amusement, and muttered a self-conscious "Amen", we sat at the large square table and Mrs B. brought in the luncheon trolley. Sister Julienne served as usual, and Trixie took around the plates.

Alan was outrageously handsome. He had perfect, regular features, clear skin, dark curly hair, and soft dark eyes fringed with eyelashes that any girl would kill for. I had met him a couple of times, and when the girls flocked around him in droves, trying to win a glance from his bright eyes, I had noticed that he treated them as pleasing but inconsequential toys. He regarded himself as a "leader of opinion". With a degree in philosophy from Cambridge University, he had already formed conclusions about life which he had picked up secondhand, without having lived much of it himself. The troubles and turmoils that befall most of us had yet to disturb his assumption of superiority. He had a huge regard for his own intelligence which, I had concluded, was adequate but not outstanding. He placed his notebook and pencil beside him on the dining table, which was rude, but Alan was not troubled by propriety; he was on a job, not a guest at a luncheon party.

He had been placed next to Sister Monica Joan and was slightly annoyed about this, probably regarding her as being too old to be of interest to his readership. He had wanted to sit next to Sister Bernadette and talk about the impact of the new National Health Service upon the older style of medicine. However, he was not one to be deflected from his purpose and called across the table to Sister Bernadette.

"As nuns are the servants of God, and the State has now taken over your midwifery service, do you now see your role as servants of the State?"

He had planned this carefully, as he wanted to portray the futility of religion in his story. This would appeal to his editor.

Sister Bernadette was contemplating her Yorkshire pudding with pleasure, and was unprepared such a question. In the ten seconds that it took for her to think of a suitable reply, Sister Monica Joan addressed him.

"In the puny compass of our wit the Silver Cord is loosed. The State is the servant of the Orb. The servant is wiser than the organic process of growth differentiated by truth at the fountain head. Do you see your role as one of the forty-two Assessors of the Dead?"

"What?"

Alan stopped eating, mouth open, fork raised.

"Eh, that is … I mean … pardon?"

"Kindly don't wave your fork at me like that, young man. Put it down," said Sister Monica Joan sharply. She eyed him imperiously. "We were discussing the role of the free spirit, released by the confluence of the several centres, until you so rudely poked your fork in my ear. But what is that to me? Let us go with God, and accept the unacceptable. It is a lonely walk into the mind's retreat. Is there another roast potato? A soft one, and a little more onion gravy, if you please."

She passed her plate, and looked sideways at Alan, with a certain amount of distaste. But she was prepared to continue the conversation.

"Do you regard your role as a new form of sanctity without precedent, or an equivalent revelation of the universe, also without precedent?" she enquired politely.

The whole table was looking at Alan as he struggled for words. I was quietly killing myself. This was better than expected.

"I really don't know. I hadn't thought about it."

"Oh, come now. A young man of your genius must surely consider the impact of your thought as the exertion of energy released by the activities of your several centres. Your thought is the vibration of the horizontal, the centralisation of the polarities of positive and negative. I cannot believe that you have not thought about your thought. It is the duty of every great man to reflect upon the excellence of the intellect or, to put it more simply, the auditory impact of the divine consciousness, within the limits of fragmentation. Wouldn't you agree?"

Mike spluttered, and Cynthia quietly nudged him. Trixie nearly choked, and sent a shower of peas across the table. Jimmy and I looked at each other with secret delight. Poor Alan, aware that all eyes were upon him, had the grace to blush.

Sister Monica Joan murmured, as though to herself, but loud enough to be heard by all, "How sweet. Old enough to know it all, and young enough to blush. Perfectly charming."

Having neatly disposed of Alan, she turned her attention to the roast potato.

Sister Julienne looked brightly round the table. "Who would like some more roast beef? And I'm sure Mrs B. has another Yorkshire pudding in the oven. Mike, you look like a good carver. How about you carving for those who want seconds?"

Mike took up the carving knife, sharpened it with a flourish, and sliced generous helpings. Mrs B. came in with another Yorkshire pudding, piping hot. The boys had brought wine with them, and glasses were found. We were not accustomed to wine with lunch at Nonnatus House, but Sister Julienne said that on such a special occasion, all rules would be waived. The nuns giggled like schoolgirls drinking their wine, murmuring "Ooh, what a treat – delicious – you must come again".

Jimmy and Mike were in sparkling form. It had to be owned that they had great charm and *savoir faire* and the luncheon was a huge success. Even

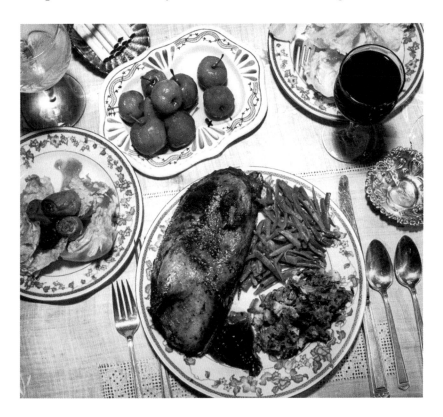

Above: At Nonnatus House, wine was not usually served with lunch but when Jimmy and his friends came to eat there, Sister Julienne declared that on such a special occasion "all rules would be waived".

Sister Evangelina was relaxed and laughing with Jimmy; but then it's not hard to laugh with dear Jimmy, I reflected. Only Chummy was quiet. She didn't look unhappy, just cautious, aware that at any moment she might knock over a glass of wine, or send a tureen flying. She did not dare to join in the fun. But she smiled all the while, and seemed to enjoy herself in her own way.

The only person who did not look happy was Alan. In fact he looked downright furious. Sister Julienne tried several times to draw him into the conversation, but he would have none of it. He had been made to look a fool by a nun of ninety, and he wasn't going to forgive her, or any of them for that matter. He never did produce his story, I was told.

To my great alarm Mike told the story of when they had lived in the drying room of the nurses' home for three months, and how they had climbed that treacherous fire escape twice a day, in the dark of winter. I had long since left the hospital involved, so could not be sacked, but I felt alarmed about what the Sisters would think of my sins. One glance at Sister Julienne's face, a little flushed with wine, reassured me. She looked towards me and laughed.

"You were taking a chance. I remember when a young man was caught in a nurse's bedroom at St Thomas's. The girl was immediately dismissed. She was a good nurse, too. It was a pity. However, a few months later, four young men were found in the broom cupboard – or was it the laundry room, I forget – and no one ever discovered who was responsible. It's just as well, because goodness knows how many nurses would have been lost to the profession if they had been found out. That was just before the war, when we needed all the trained nurses we could get."

Puddings arrived, and Sister Julienne rose to serve them. A strange noise from across the table caught my attention, and I looked in that direction. To my astonishment, it was Sister Evangelina, laughing! In fact she was laughing so much, she was spluttering into her napkin. Her neighbour Jimmy, kind and gentlemanly, patted her on the back and handed her a glass of water. She gulped it down, and sat, dabbing her eyes and nose, muttering through chokes and giggles.

"Oh dear. This is too much for me … it takes me back to the time when … oh, I shall never forget …"

Jimmy set to work seriously slapping her back, which seemed to help, but it caused her veil to slip sideways.

We were all determined to get to the bottom of this. Never before had Sister Evangelina been seen laughing convulsively in the Convent, and it obviously had something to do with young men in nurses' bedrooms.

"What happened? Tell us."

"Come on, now. Be a sport."

Sister Julienne paused, serving spoon in hand.

"Oh come on, Sister. You can't leave us in suspense like this. What's the story? Jimmy, give her another glass of wine."

But Sister Evangelina couldn't, or wouldn't, tell. She blew her nose, and wiped her eyes. She spluttered and gurgled and coughed. But she wouldn't say any more. She just grinned mischievously at everyone. A grin from Sister Evangelina was unheard of, never mind a mischievous one!

Sister Monica Joan had been watching this little exhibition with half-closed eyes, and a tiny smile playing round her lips. I wondered what she was thinking. Sister Evangelina certainly looked a mess, with her veil askew, her face bright red, moisture seeping from every orifice. I feared an icy comment and so, I think, did Sister Evangelina, for she looked at her tormentor with apprehension. But we were both wrong.

Sister Monica Joan waited until the laughter had subsided, and with the timing of an instinctive actress recited slowly and dramatically, "'Oh – I shall remember the hours that we spent, In age I'll remember, and not to repent.'"

She paused for effect, then leaned across the table towards Sister Evangelina, and winked. In a stage whisper that could be heard by all, she said confidentially, "Don't say another word, my dear, not another word. The nosy lot. They clamour and clatter. They chatter and natter. Don't feed their idle expectations, my dear, 'twill only debase your memories!"

She looked Sister Evangelina straight in the eyes, and winked again, with warmth and understanding. Was it possible? Did I imagine it? Was it a trick of the light? Did Sister Evangelina, or did she not, wink back?

Sister Evangelina never told. I daresay she went to her grave with the story locked in her heart.

The puddings were a masterpiece of Mrs B.'s creative skills. Sister Monica Joan had two helpings of ice cream with chocolate fudge sauce and a little apple pie. She was in brilliant form.

"I remember a young man shut in a wardrobe at Queen Charlotte's Hospital," she recalled. "He was locked in for three hours. It would have been perfectly all right, and no one would have found out, but the foolish fellow had borrowed his father's horse, and tied it to the hospital railings. Now you can hide a young man in a wardrobe or under a bed. But how, I ask, can you hide a horse?"

With a gasp I realised that these memories dated back to the 1890s! What happened? But she wouldn't remember.

"I only remember the horse tied to the railings."

What a pity! Life is so fleeting, and the past so rich. I wanted to hear more. Her mind was perfectly clear at that moment, and knowing how it could cloud over, I asked if she had not found the discipline and petty restrictions of nursing to be intolerable.

"Not a bit of it. After the confinement and restraints of family life, nursing was freedom and adventure. We did not have the licence you young people enjoy today. It was the same for all of us. I recall my cousin Barney. His mother, my aunt, had a French maid. One day – in the middle of the day, my dears – she, my aunt, stepped out on to the terrace to find the French maid seated on a chair, and Barney on his knees placing the shoe on to the foot of the gel. The shoe."

She paused and looked around her.

"Not the petticoat, or anything like that. Just the shoe. My aunt screamed and fainted, I was told. The maid was immediately dismissed, and the family was so scandalised that Barney was given a ten pound note, and a one-way ticket to Canada. He was never seen or heard of again."

Mike speculated that being sent off to Canada was probably the best thing that could have happened to him.

Sister Monica Joan looked very thoughtful before replying, "I would like to think that. But it is just as likely that poor Barney died of hunger or disease in the Canadian winter."

It was a sobering thought. I asked for more stories. She smiled at me indulgently.

"I am not here for your entertainment, my dear. I am here by the grace of God. Four score years and ten, it has been. A score too long … too long."

She fell silent for a minute, and no one dared speak. She had seen so much, done so much in life – fighting for independence in her youth; entering a religious order in middle age, wartime nursing and midwifery in the London Docks when she was nearly eighty years old. Who could match such experience?

With a slightly amused, slightly quizzical expression in her fine eyes, she looked around at us, so young, so frivolous, so superficial. Her elbow was resting on the table, her slender fingers supporting her chin. We were spellbound by her presence.

"You are all so young," she mused reflectively. "Youth is the first fair flower of spring."

Lifting her head, she spread out her eloquent hands towards us. Her face was radiant, her eyes shining, her voice joyful and triumphant.

"Therefore … 'Sing, my darlings, sing, Before your petals fade, To feed the flowers of another spring.'"

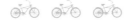

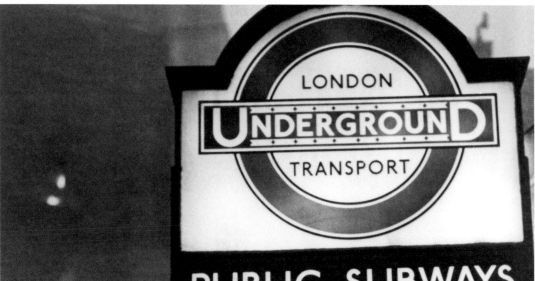
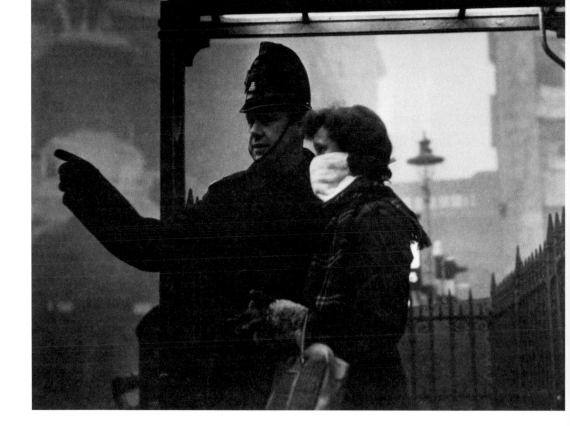

SMOG

Conchita Warren was expecting her twenty-fifth baby. I had seen quite a lot of the family during the past year because Liz Warren was the dressmaker of my dreams. She was the oldest daughter, twenty-two years old, and had been making clothes since she first had a doll. It was all she had ever wanted to do, she told me. On leaving school at fourteen, she went straight into an apprenticeship with a firm of high-class dressmakers, with whom she still worked. She did not usually take private clients at home because she said the mess was such that she couldn't ask ladies to come to the house for fittings. However, as I was accustomed to the house, it did not bother either of us. She was an expert in her trade, and enjoyed making garments for me over many years.

I had always loved clothes, and took a good deal of time and trouble over them. My clothes were specially made for me, and I turned my nose up at ready-to-wear stuff. Today this would be unusual and terribly expensive, but it was not the case in the 1950s. In fact it was cheaper. Really good quality clothes could be made for a fraction of what they cost in the best shops. Beautiful materials could be found in the street markets, going for a song. I usually designed my own things, or adapted styles. When I lived in Paris, I would attend the catwalk shows of the great French couturiers – Dior, Chanel, Schiaparelli. The opening of the season was, of course, reserved

Opposite: People often covered their faces, just like the woman in this 1953 photograph, to protect themselves from the dense and heavily polluted smog that descended on London.

for the press and the very rich, but after about two or three weeks, when the excitement had settled down, the fashion shows continued, perhaps twice weekly, and anyone could attend. I loved them, and made careful notes and sketches of what I knew would suit me, in order to have them made for me later. The only trouble was finding a dressmaker skilled enough to make her own paper patterns. Liz was perfection. She not only made up her own patterns, but she had a real stylish flair, and often suggested or adapted things to suit the cloth or the cut. We were about the same age, and it was a happy collaboration.

During one of these visits Liz told me, with a wry smile, that her mother was expecting again. Together we speculated on how many more Conchita was likely to have. Her precise age was not known, but she was probably about forty-two, so she could have another six to eight babies. Going on past form, we put our money on a total of thirty babies.

Conchita booked again with the Sisters for another home confinement, and requested antenatal visits at home. For continuity's sake, I was asked to take the case. She was in perfect condition again. She looked radiant, and did not really look pregnant until about twenty-four weeks, although once again her dates were uncertain. The youngest little girl was one year old. Len was all excitement and anticipation, as though this were only his second or third baby.

It was winter, and very cold and icy. Heavy snow clouds hung over the city, trapping the smoke fumes from all the coal fires, steam trains, and steam engines, the profuse smoke from the ocean-going vessels, and above all the factories, which were largely fuelled by coal. A thick London smog developed. One can have no conception these days of what they were like. The air would be heavy, foul-smelling, and a thick yellowish-grey colour. It was impossible to see more than a yard ahead, even at midday. Traffic was virtually at a standstill. The only way a vehicle could move would be for a man to walk ahead of it, carrying two bright lights – one to shine ahead of him, so that he could find his way, and the other shining behind him for the vehicle to follow. These smogs were a feature of many winters in London at the time, and lasted until the atmospheric pressure lifted, allowing the trapped fumes to escape.

Opposite: Throughout her life, the author maintained a keen interest in fashion, as this photograph illustrates (Jennifer as a bridesmaid in 1962).

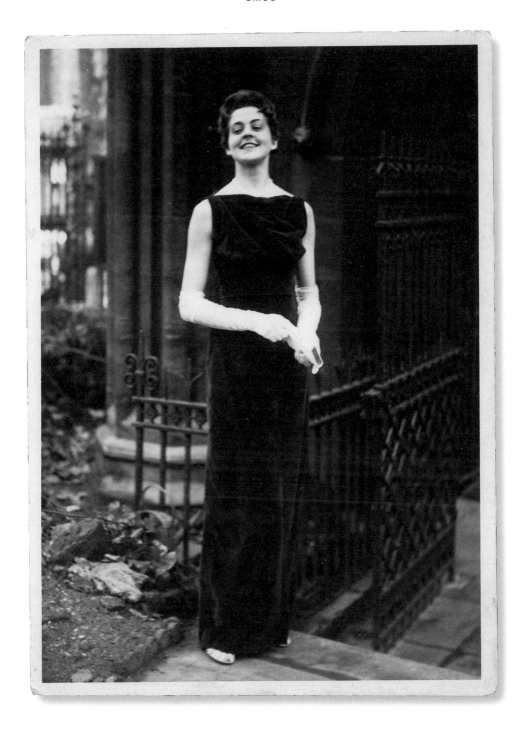

Conchita must have gone into the backyard for something. She either slipped on the ice, or tripped over something she could not see. She must have fallen heavily and lay partly concussed on the freezing concrete for some time. The only children in the house were the little ones under five. She was found by the other children when they came home from school. Apparently she was sufficiently conscious to crawl and with the help of her children, all under eleven, she got back into the house. There was evidence that she had tried to do so before but, being unable to see through the smog, had actually crawled away from the house. It is a miracle that she did not die of exposure. She was in a bad way. A small child went to get a neighbour, who wrapped her in blankets and gave her hot brandy and water. Older children began returning home after 4 p.m. and learned of their mother's accident. Len and the oldest boys were last to return, because they had been on a job in Knightsbridge and the journey home had taken two and a half hours.

That night Conchita went into labour.

The phone rang at about 11.30 p.m. I was called to the phone, as it was my case. I was aghast – firstly because of the premature labour, and secondly because of the weather conditions. How on earth was I to find my way to Limehouse? I was speaking to one of the elder sons, who briefly explained the circumstances. My first question was, "Have you called the doctor?" Yes, he had, but the doctor was out. "Well, you must keep on trying," I said, "because your mother may be ill. If she was concussed, and her temperature dropped a lot, she may need medical treatment, quite apart from the pregnancy. Ring the doctor again now. He may have difficulty getting to you, but so will I."

I replaced the telephone, and looked out of the window. I couldn't see a thing. Thick grey swirls of fog seemed to be circling the window panes, trying to get in. I shivered, as much with apprehension for Conchita's awful plight as reluctance to go out at all. The sirens from the river boats, and those in the docks, moaned a hollow call.

We had hardly been out of the house for three days, hoping and praying that no one would go into labour before the smog lifted. It was a situation I could not, should not, handle alone.

I went up to the Sisters' floor to call Sister Julienne. Nuns go to bed at about nine o'clock because they get up before 4 a.m. for the first Office of the day, so eleven-thirty would be the middle of the night for them. Nonetheless, with the first light tap on the door, Sister was awake.

"Who is it?," she called out.

I said my name, and that Conchita Warren was in premature labour.

"Wait a minute."

I waited thirty seconds, and Sister joined me in the corridor, shutting the door of her cell behind her. She was wearing a coarse brown wool dressing gown, and, amazingly, her veil. The question, does she go to bed in the thing? flashed through my mind. It must be damned uncomfortable.

But there was no time to reflect upon the habit of a nun. I told her briefly the story that had been given to me over the telephone.

She thought for a moment and said, "Limehouse is over three miles away. You might not get there. There is no point in me, or any of the midwives, coming with you, because two people can get lost just as easily as one. You must have a police escort. Go now and ring the police, and God be with you, my dear. I will pray for Conchita Warren and her unborn baby."

The knowledge that Sister Julienne would be praying for us had an extraordinary effect. All the tension and anxiety left me, and I felt calm and confident. I had learned to respect the power of prayer. What change had come over the headstrong young girl who, only a year earlier, had found the whole idea of prayer to be a joke?

I spoke to the police and told them it was an emergency. I was told that the safest way to get there would be to walk, but the quickest would be by bicycle. The policeman said: "There is no point in sending a car, because you can't see further than the bonnet, and we would have to have a man walking ahead. We will send a bicycle escort."

I said I would be ready within ten minutes. My delivery bag was already packed and ready. All my thoughts were with Conchita – I did not think that the baby was likely to survive at around twenty-eight weeks gestation. Finding the bicycle shed in the smog and loading up my bike was a tricky business, but I was at the front of Nonnatus House in less than ten minutes.

Two policemen arrived shortly after on bicycles with very powerful lights, front and rear, which illuminated about two yards ahead. One rode ahead of me, and I was instructed to follow him. The other rode beside me, I being on the kerb side. Thus we progressed with surprising speed, because there was no other traffic around.

Looking back over nearly half a century it seems absurd to be racing to an emergency labour on bicycles at about ten miles per hour. But even today

I can think of no better way. What would be the advantage of the most powerful police car with nil visibility?

We arrived at the Warren household in less than fifteen minutes. I could not have done it alone. The men said they would wait, in case I needed them further, and a couple of the Warren girls took them down to the kitchen for a cup of tea.

I went upstairs to Conchita. She looked ghastly, deathly white, with bright pink splodges under her eyes. She moaned. I took her temperature, which was 103°F. At first I could not feel her pulse, but, on careful counting, I found it to be 120, and intermittent. Her blood pressure was barely perceptible. Her breathing was shallow and rapid, at around forty breaths per minute. I watched her in silence for a couple of minutes, as a contraction came on. It was powerful, and her features distorted in pain, a high-pitched groan emanating from her throat. Her eyes were open, but I don't think she could see anyone.

Len was cradling her in his arms. The suffering on his face was enough to break your heart. He was stroking her hair, and murmuring to her, neither of which she seemed to feel or hear. Liz was in the room.

I enquired if the doctor had been called. He had, but was still out on a call. The call had been put through to another doctor, who was also out with a patient. All doctors worked terribly hard at these times. The London smogs were notorious killers.

I said that we should arrange for a hospital admission as soon as possible. "Is she tha' bad?" Len asked.

It is astonishing how people do not see what they don't want to see. To me it was obvious that Conchita could easily die, especially if complications arose from labour and delivery. But Len couldn't see this.

I went and spoke to the policemen. One said he would telephone the hospital. The other one undertook to try to find one of the local GPs and escort him to the house, if possible. How an ambulance would get there and back was an open question. I returned to Conchita, and started to lay out my delivery things. It was possible that I would be alone with a premature delivery, and a sick and possibly dying woman.

Suddenly I remembered that Sister Julienne was praying for us. Again, the relief was overwhelming. All my fears vanished, and the calm certainty that all would be well flooded my mind and body. I remembered the words of Mother Julian of Norwich:

"All shall be well, and all will be well
and all manner of things shall be well."

I must have given a great sigh of relief, which Len picked up. He said, "You reckons as how she'll be all right then, do you?"

Should I tell him that Sister Julienne was praying for us? It seemed so silly, almost irrelevant. But I did; I felt I knew him well enough. He didn't dismiss it.

"Well, I reckons as 'ow its goin' to be all righ', then, too."

His face was brighter than it had been since I entered the room.

It would have been advisable to examine Conchita vaginally to see how far she was in labour, but I couldn't get her into the right position. She wouldn't allow Len or me to move her. Liz explained to her in Spanish what was required, but she didn't understand or respond in any way. I could only assess the progress of labour from the strength and frequency of contractions, which were approximately every five minutes. I listened for the foetal heart, but couldn't hear a thing.

"Is the baby alive, then?" asked Len.

I didn't like to say a straight "No," so I hedged my bets.

"It's unlikely. Remember your wife got very, very cold today, and has been unconscious. Now she has a fever. All this will affect the baby. I cannot hear a heartbeat."

One of the real problems of premature delivery at the stage of pregnancy Conchita had reached is that the foetus is often lying transversely across the uterus. A human baby ideally should be born head first. A breech delivery is possible, but difficult. A transverse or shoulder delivery is impossible. The head does not normally descend into the pelvis until after thirty-six weeks. A foetus of around twenty-eight weeks is quite large enough to block the cervix completely if contractions push it downwards in the transverse position. In that event, without surgical intervention, the death of the baby is inevitable. I palpated the uterus trying to find out the baby's position, but it was no use, I could not tell. A vaginal examination might have enlightened me, but there was no way that we could persuade Conchita to cooperate.

All I could do was wait. The minutes between contractions ticked by slowly. They were coming every three minutes now. Her pulse was more rapid, 150 per minute; and her breathing seemed to be more shallow. Her blood pressure was quite imperceptible. I prayed for a knock on the door to announce the arrival of a doctor or the ambulance, but none came. The house was silent, save for the low moaning of Conchita as each contraction came and went.

Inevitably the contractions became stronger, and it was then that Conchita began to scream. I have never in my life, before or since, heard such terrifying sounds. They came from the depths of her suffering body with a force and power that I would have thought impossible, given her fevered, debilitated state. She screamed on and on, wild terror in her unseeing eyes, the sound reverberating wave after wave against the walls and ceiling of the room. She clung to her husband, tore at him, until his face and chest and arms were bleeding. He tried to hold her, to comfort her, but she was quite beyond comfort.

I felt helpless. I did not dare to give her an analgesic to lessen the pain and quieten her, because her pulse and blood pressure were so abnormal, and I knew that any drugs would probably kill her. I thought that if it was a normal delivery she had a chance of living; if it was a transverse presentation she would die, unless an ambulance were to arrive quickly. I could not get near her to feel the uterus, or even to hold a leg, as she was throwing herself around the bed with the strength of a wild animal in a trap.

Poor Liz looked terrified. Len, with unconditional love, was still trying to hold her in his arms and console her. She sank her teeth into his hand with the strength of a bulldog, and hung on. He didn't cry out, but winced with pain, sweat and tears falling from his forehead and eyes. He didn't even try to force her jaw open or to pull away. With alarm, I thought that she would sever a tendon. Eventually she loosed the hand, and flung herself to the other side of the bed.

Then, as suddenly as it had started, it was all over. She gave a terrible cry, and a massive push, and water, blood, foetus, placenta – everything – was delivered on to the bed sheets at once. She fell back exhausted.

I could feel no pulse at all. Her breathing seemed to have stopped. But I could feel a flutter of a heartbeat, so I listened with my stethoscope. It was faint and irregular, but it was there. The foetus was blue, and looked quite dead. I snatched a large kidney dish from the dresser, scooped everything into it, and dumped it on the dresser.

"Now we must quickly get her warm," I said, "cleaned up and comfortable, if she is to stand a chance. You help me, Liz – clean warm sheets, a couple of hot water bottles. I will check the placenta in a minute to see if it is complete.

If we can get her to drink something hot it will help. Hot water and honey would do; a teaspoon of brandy in it would be even better. The main thing is to treat the shock. And let us all hope and pray that the bleeding won't get worse."

Len went out to issue some instructions, and to pacify the terrified family gathered around the door. Liz and I started to clean the dirty sheets and linen from under Conchita. Len soon returned with clean sheets and hot water bottles, and Liz and I started to make the inert body comfortable.

Len must have gone over to the dresser. Liz and I had our backs to it, busy with Conchita. We heard a gasp.

"It's alive!"

"What!" I cried.

"It's alive, I sez. Ve baby's alive. It's movin'."

I rushed over to the dresser, and looked at the gory mess in the kidney dish. It moved. The blood actually moved. My heart stood still. Then I saw the tiny creature in the pool of blood, and its leg moved.

Oh, dear God, I could have drowned it! I thought.

I lifted the tiny body out with one hand and tilted it upside down. It seemed to weigh nothing. I have held a new born puppy of about the same size. My head raced.

"We must clamp and cut the cord quickly. Then we must get him warm."

It was a little boy.

I felt desperately guilty. The cord should have been clamped five minutes earlier. If he dies now, it will be all my fault, I thought. I had discarded this tiny living soul to drown in a dish of blood and water. I should have looked more closely. I should have thought.

But wallowing in self-reproach gets us nowhere. I clamped and cut the cord. I felt the fragile ribcage. He was breathing. He was a survivor. Len had warmed a small towel on a hot water bottle, and we wrapped him in the cloth. He moved his head and arms a little. All three of us were stunned by the life in the baby. None of us had seen a human child quite so tiny. A baby that is two months premature usually weighs about four pounds, and seems tiny enough. This baby was about one and a half pounds and looked like a tiny doll. His arms and legs were much smaller than my little finger, yet a miniscule nail completed each digit. His head was smaller than a ping-pong ball, and looked disproportionately large. His rib cage looked like fish-bones. He had tiny ears, and his nostrils were the size of a

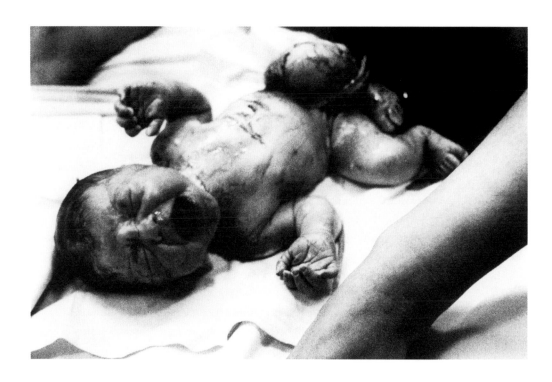

Above: A newborn baby lies on a sheet, waiting for the midwife to cut her umbilical cord.

pin-head. I had never imagined that a baby of around twenty-eight weeks could be so lovely. I felt I ought to suck the mucus from his throat, but was terrified of hurting him. Anyway, when I got the catheter, it was far too large, and would never have gone into his mouth. To force a hosepipe into a normal baby's mouth would have been just as inappropriate. So I just held him nearly upside down with one hand, and gently rubbed his back with one finger.

I had no experience of caring for a premature baby, and did not know what to do. All my instincts told me that he must be kept warm and quiet, preferably in the dark, and with frequent feeding. No cot was ready. Where could we put him? Just then Conchita, who was lying quietly, spoke.

"*Niño. Mi niño. Dónde está mi niño?*" (Baby. My baby. Where is my baby?)

We looked at each other. We had all thought she was semi-conscious or asleep, but obviously she knew exactly what had happened, and wanted to see her baby.

"We've gotta give 'im to 'er. Liz, you tell her he's very little and we've gotta be very careful with him."

Liz spoke to her mother, who smiled slightly and sighed with weariness. Len took the baby from me and sat down beside his wife. He held the baby in one hand so that the child lay within her gaze. Her eyes had been vacant and unfocused for several moments and I don't think she saw or understood at first; she had expected to take a full term baby into her arms. Liz spoke to her again, and I heard the words.

"*El niño es muy pequeño.*" (The baby is very small.)

Conchita struggled to adjust her vision to the minute scrap held in Len's hand. You could almost see the struggle and the effort it cost her. Gradually she became aware, and with a sharp intake of breath put out a shaking hand to touch the child. She smiled, and murmured "*Mi niño. Mi querido niño,*" (my baby, my darling baby) and drifted off to sleep, her hand resting on Len's hand and the baby.

Just then, the Flying Squad arrived.

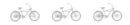

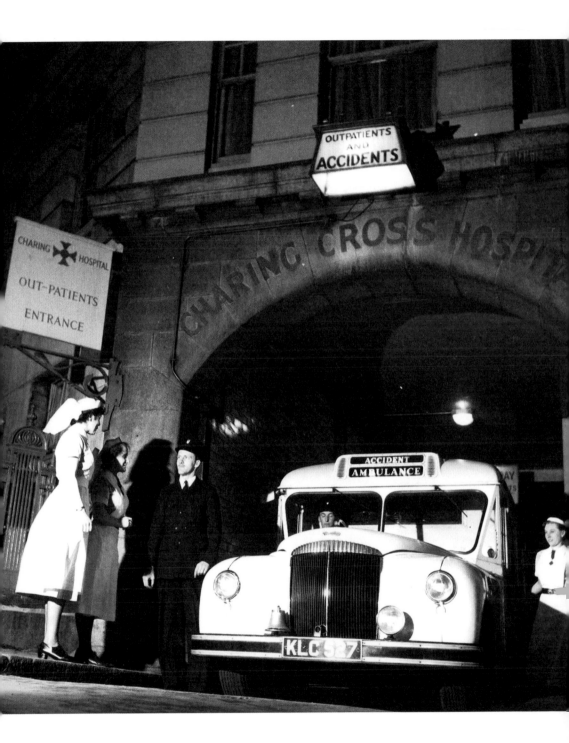

THE FLYING SQUAD

$\mathbf{A}$n Obstetric Flying Squad was provided by most big London hospitals, and I believe by all regional hospitals, as an emergency backup for domiciliary midwifery. The service must have saved thousands of lives, because before the 1940s, when no service existed, a midwife could find herself entirely alone with any obstetric emergency – such as a mal-presentation, haemorrhage, cord prolapse, or placenta previa – and all she could do would be to call in the local GP who might or might not be skilled in midwifery.

It was the proud boast of the Flying Squad of the London Hospital that it could reach any obstetric emergency in twenty minutes. But that was reckoning without a London smog. When the policeman contacted the hospital about Conchita no ambulance had been available to bring the Flying Squad. The smog caused acute and deadly respiratory failure in thousands of old people each year, and every doctor and ambulance was out on these cases. When one finally did return to the depot, the driver, who had been working non-stop for sixteen hours, was sent off duty, and another had to be found. Even then, a policeman had to cycle in front of the ambulance to guide it – hence the delay of nearly three hours. However, a registrar, a houseman, and a nurse from the obstetrics department had been sent by the hospital.

Everything happens at once, so they say, and within minutes a GP also arrived on foot. God bless him, I thought. He looked exhausted. He had

Opposite: The driver of an ambulance chats with nursing staff at Charing Cross Hospital (1954).

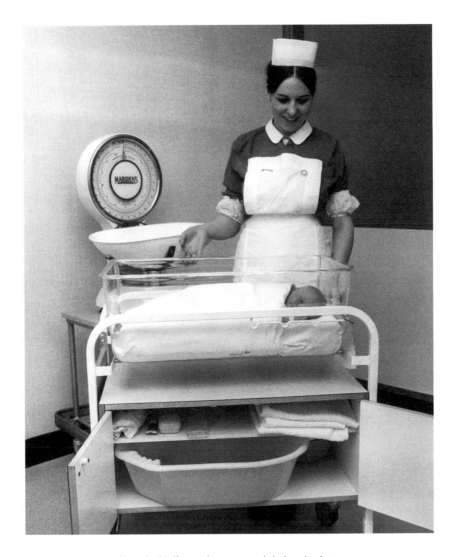

Above: A midwife attends a premature baby in an incubator.

been working all day and all night, and very likely most of the night before, yet he had the professionalism and the courtesy to apologise for being late.

With so much medical know-how in the house, it was necessary to have a case conference to decide the best course of action for mother and baby. We went down to the kitchen for this, and I asked Len to accompany me. Liz was left with her mother and the baby. The two ambulance men and the

350

policemen joined us too – they couldn't be asked to sit outside in the cold, and there was nowhere else for them to sit in the house. Sue, one of the older girls, made tea all round.

I gave my case history, and handed over the recorded notes. All doctors were agreed that mother and baby must be transferred to hospital at once. Len was alarmed.

"Does she 'ave to go? She won't like it. She's never been away from home before, she hasn't. She'd be lost an' frightened. I knows as 'ow she would. We can look after 'er. I'll stop at home, an' the girls can muck in an all, till she's better."

The doctors looked at one another and sighed. Fear of hospital was commonplace. Among the older generation, it arose mainly from the fact that most of the hospital buildings were converted workhouses, which had been feared more than death itself. The doctors agreed that as Conchita was now safely delivered, if no post-natal complications arose, she probably could be treated at home. A course of antibiotics would clear the infection that was causing fever. The head injury, causing concussion and delirium, would heal with rest and quiet. They tried to point out that she would get more rest in hospital than at home, surrounded by children, but Len would have none of it, so they capitulated.

However, the baby was another matter. He hadn't been weighed, but my guess of between one and a half and two pounds was accepted. They all said twenty-eight weeks was barely viable, and that a living baby of that gestation must have hospital treatment, with the latest technological equipment, and twenty-four hour expert nursing and medical care. They suggested that he should be transferred at once to Great Ormond Street Hospital for Sick Children. Len looked dubious, but when they told him that without such care the baby would die, he readily agreed.

We all went upstairs to the bedroom. I don't know what these hospital doctors thought of having to squeeze past all the prams in the hallway and parting the washing flapping around their heads as they climbed the wooden stairs. Nor did I ask. But I smiled to myself.

Conchita was sleeping, the tiny baby lying on her chest. One hand was protectively over it, the other lay limp by her side. She was smiling, and her breathing, although shallow, was regular and less rapid. I approached the bed and felt her pulse. It was slightly stronger, and regular, but still rapid. I counted 120 per minute, which, though abnormal, was an improvement. Liz was cleaning up quietly and efficiently, and the whole scene was peaceful.

The baby looked even smaller now that the entire hand of the mother covered it. Only its head was visible. It did not really look as if it were alive, although its colour did not suggest death.

The registrar wanted to examine Conchita. I told him that I had not yet examined the placenta, as I had not had time between delivery and the arrival of the ambulance. We examined it together; it was very ragged. "Not hopeful," he muttered, "and it all came out at once, you tell me? I must have a look at her."

He pulled back the bedclothes to examine her abdomen and see the vaginal discharge. Conchita seemed quite unconscious and didn't move as he palpated the uterus. Some blood rushed out.

"Another pad," he said, and, to the houseman, "Draw me up 0.5 cc of ergometrine for injection."

He sank the needle deep into her gluteus muscle, but she didn't move. He covered her and said to Len: "I think part of the placenta has been left behind. She may have to go to hospital for a D and C. It would only be for a few days but we cannot risk a haemorrhage occurring at home. In her condition it would be very serious."

I saw Len turn white and he had to grab the back of a chair to prevent himself from falling.

"However," continued the registrar kindly, "it may not be necessary. The next five minutes will tell if the injection is going to be effective."

He then took Conchita's blood pressure.

"I can hear nothing," he said, and the three doctors exchanged significant glances. Len groaned and had to sit down.

His daughter put her hand on his shoulder, and he squeezed it.

We all waited. The registrar said, "There is no point in examining the baby. It is obviously alive, but we are none of us paediatricians. Examination must wait for the experts."

He asked for the telephone, to ring Great Ormond Street Hospital, but there was no telephone in the house. He cursed silently under his breath and asked where he could find the nearest phone box. It was two hundred yards down the road, on the other side. The long-suffering houseman was

Opposite: Great Ormond Street Hospital in London in the 1950s.

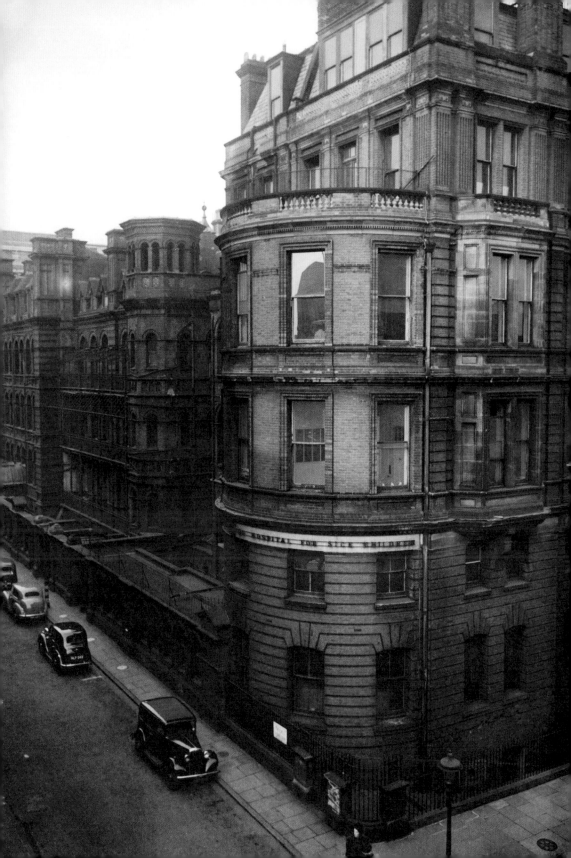

dispatched out into the freezing fog and icy roads with a pocket full of pennies gleaned from us all, to ring the hospital and make the necessary arrangements.

We continued waiting. There was no sign of an abdominal contraction. Five minutes slipped by. The houseman returned to say that Great Ormond Street would send a paediatrician and a nurse with an incubator and special equipment to collect the baby at once, although the time of their arrival depended on visibility.

Another five minutes passed. There was steady vaginal bleeding, but no contractions.

"Draw up another 0.5cc," the registrar said. "We must give it intravenously. There is something in there that has to come out. If we can't get it this way," he said to Len, "we will have to take her back with us for a scrape. And if you value her life, you must agree to this."

Len groaned, and nodded dumbly.

I clamped the upper arm and endeavoured to pump up a vein for injection, but nothing showed. Her blood pressure was so low that the venous return could not be found. The registrar tried, with a couple of stabs, to locate the vein and on the third attempt blood showed in the syringe. He emptied the 0.5cc into her vein, and I released the arm.

Within a minute Conchita winced in pain and moved her legs. A large quantity of fresh blood spurted from her vagina, and then, mercifully, several large, darker lumps. There was a pause, then a second contraction. The registrar grasped the fundus and pressed the uterus hard, downwards and backwards. More blood and placenta were evacuated.

All this time Conchita was inert, but I thought I saw her hand tighten over her baby.

"That might be it," said the registrar, "but we must wait a bit longer to see."

He was more relaxed now and started chatting with anyone who would listen about the excellent golf down at Greenwich and the house he was buying at Dulwich, and his holiday in Scotland.

Over the next ten minutes there was no further blood loss, and no more contractions. Thanks to modern obstetrics, the danger of post-partum haemorrhage had been overcome for Conchita. But she still looked very ill indeed. Her breathing and pulse were rapid, her blood pressure abnormally low, and her temperature high. She did not appear to be conscious, although as her eyes were now closed, she might have been asleep. Nonetheless, her hand was still firmly placed over the baby, and any attempt to remove it was resisted.

With difficulty Liz and I cleaned up the bed again, and the houseman was given the messy job of checking the bits of placenta against the larger piece that had first been delivered, and measuring the blood that we had managed to contain.

"Placenta seems to be all here, sir, and I measure one and a half pints of blood. Add to that about eight ounces lost in the bed, and you could say around two pints of blood loss."

The registrar muttered to himself, then said aloud, "She really needs a transfusion. Her blood pressure is already low. Can we do it here?" he added, turning to the GP.

"Yes, I'll take a sample now for cross-matching."

I had wondered why the GP had remained all the while, when he could have left. Now it became clear to me. He anticipated having ongoing responsibility for Conchita if she was to be cared for at home, and he wanted full cognisance of the facts.

At that moment the ambulance arrived from Great Ormond Street to collect the baby.

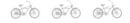

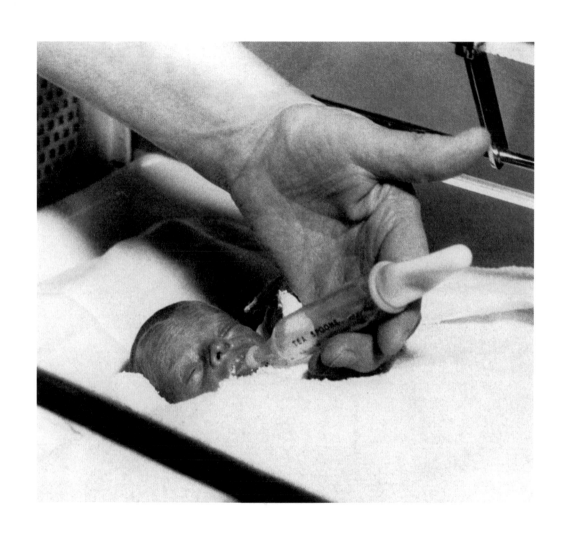

A PREMATURE BABY

It was a thousand pities, I thought, from the point of view of the good gossips of Limehouse, that all this had been carried out in a London smog. Had it been a clear night, every move would have been witnessed and reported – a midwife, police, teams of doctors, ambulances, each with a police escort. Such a sensation would have kept the gossips in business for a year at least. As it was, not even the next-door neighbour would have been able to see the two ambulances parked outside the Warren house, and police coming and going throughout the night. Their only consolation might have been that the whole street was wakened by the blood-curdling screams that lasted for about twenty minutes.

The paraphernalia and personnel that emerged from the second ambulance was overwhelming. A doctor came hurrying past, carrying an incubator. Another followed with a ventilating machine. A nurse followed with a huge box. Two ambulance men and the policeman came last, each carrying oxygen cylinders. All this equipment had to be manoeuvred past the three coach prams and two ladders lining the hallway. The washing hanging overhead didn't help, because it got caught up on the equipment and several small, dainty items, personal to the young ladies of the house were transported upstairs. The children, who had been in and out of bed

Opposite: A three-week old baby is fed. Although the midwives and doctors would have done everything possible to save Conchita Warren's premature baby, hospitals such as Great Ormond Street had special units dedicated to dealing with such cases.

all night, hung over the banisters, and hid in doorways, to get the full impact of the procession.

On reaching the bedroom, the medical staff entered whilst the policeman and the ambulance men were directed down to the kitchen to join their colleagues for tea. Nevertheless, the bedroom, of average size, now contained five doctors, two nurses, a midwife, and Len and Liz. There was equipment everywhere. My delivery instruments still covered the dresser. The obstetrician's was on the chest of drawers. The paediatrician's had to be left on the floor, whilst we hastily cleared space.

"I think we'll push off, now," said the registrar to his colleague. "I'm very glad to see you. The mother is to be nursed at home. Good luck with the baby."

They left, but the GP remained.

The paediatrician looked at the baby and gasped.

"Think he'll make it, sir?" asked the young doctor.

"We'll have a damn good try," said the paediatric registrar. "Fix up the oxygen, and the suction, and heat up the incubator."

The team got busy.

The paediatrician leaned over Conchita to take the baby. You could not tell whether she was asleep or semi-conscious, but the muscles of her arm tightened, and she held the baby fast.

He said to Len, "Would you tell her to let me have the baby, please? I've got to examine him, before we can transport him."

Len leaned over his wife and murmured to her, trying to loosen her hand. It tightened, and her other hand came up to cover the first.

"Liz, luv, you tell yer mum we've got to 'ave the baby, to take to hospital."

He shook her gently, trying to waken her. Her eyes flickered, and opened a little.

Liz bent over her and spoke to her in Spanish. None of us could tell what she said. Conchita opened her eyes more, and tried to focus on the little creature lying on her chest.

"No," she said.

Liz spoke to her again, more persuasively and urgently this time.

"No," said her mother.

Liz tried a third time.

"*Morirá! Morirá!*" (He will die.)

The effect on Cochita was dramatic and immediate. She opened her eyes wide, desperately trying to focus on the people around her. She saw the equipment and the white coats. I think her clouded brain took it all in and she struggled to sit up. Liz and Len helped her. She looked wildly round at everyone, thrust the baby down between her breasts, and folded her arms over him.

"No", she said. Then repeated louder, "No."

"Mama, you must," said Liz softly. "*Si no lo haces, morirá.*" (If you don't, he will die.)

Conchita's face was blank with anguish, but something was going on in her mind. One could almost see her struggling to get her thoughts under her command. Struggling to think, to remember, she held her breasts and the tiny baby fast, and glanced down at his head. The sight of it must have been the catalyst that brought it all together for her. Her mind seemed to clear, and a fierce, determined look came into her huge black eyes.

She looked round at each of the people in the room, her eyes finally clear and focused, and said with perfect confidence: "*No. Se queda conmigo.*" (He stays with me). "*No morirá.*" Then, with more emphasis: "*No morirá.*" (He will not die.)

The doctors didn't know what to do. Short of tearing her arms apart with brute force, which Len would not have allowed, and grabbing the baby, there was nothing they could do.

The paediatrician said to Liz, "Tell her that she can't look after it. She hasn't got the equipment or the know-how. Tell her the baby will be taken to the finest children's hospital in the world, and will have expert treatment. Tell her he cannot live without an incubator."

Liz started to speak, but Len stepped in, and showed his true strength and manliness. He turned to the doctors and nurse.

"This is all my fault, an' I must apologise. I said the baby could go to hospital without consultin' my wife. I shouldn't 'ave done that. When it comes to the kiddies she must always 'ave the last word, she must. An' she don't agree to it. You can see she don't. An' so the baby's not goin' nowhere. He'll stop 'ere with us, and he'll be christened, an' if he dies, he'll have a Christian burial. But he's not goin' nowhere without 'is mother's consent."

He looked at his wife, and she smiled and stroked the baby's head. She seemed to understand that he was on her side, and the battle was over. She looked at him with confident love, and said quietly, "*No morirá.*"

"There you are," said Len buoyantly, "he won' die. If my Connie says that, then he won't die. You can take it from me."

And that was that. The doctors knew they were defeated, and started to pack up their equipment.

Len graciously apologised a second time, thanked them for the trouble they had taken, and said again that it was all his fault. He offered to pay for the expense of the ambulance, and the time of the medical and nursing staff. He offered them a cup of tea in the kitchen. They declined. He gave them one of his winning smiles and said:

"Go on, 'ave a cup. Yer got a long journey and it'll warm yer."

He had such an engaging way about him, that everyone agreed to accept the hospitality, even though they were cross about the wasted journey.

He and Liz helped the team downstairs with all their equipment, and the GP and I were left alone. He had hardly spoken during the past three hours or so, and I liked him for this. We knew that we had a huge responsibility, and that both mother and baby could still die. Conchita's condition had been serious, but now, with the loss of two pints of blood, it was critical.

"She must have blood," said the GP. "I have taken a sample for cross-matching, and as soon as the blood bank can supply it, I will set up an I.V. We will need a district nurse to stay with her while it is going in. Can you Sisters provide one?"

I told him I was sure of it. He said, "I'm going to start antibiotics at once, because she is breathing only into the upper lobes. I would like to listen to her chest, but I doubt if she will let me, because of the baby."

He was right – she wouldn't. So he drew up an ampoule of penicillin and injected it into the thigh.

"She must have one ampoule I.M. for seven days b.d.," he said, as he entered it on the notes, and wrote out a prescription.

"Now I'm going to try to see about this blood. That's as much as I can do at present. Frankly, nurse, I don't know what to do about the baby. I think I will have to leave it to you and the Sisters. They are sure to have more experience than I have."

"Or me," I said. "I have never handled a premature baby before."

We looked at each other with shared helplessness, and he left. Bless him, I thought. He hadn't had any sleep for God knows how long; it was about 5 a.m., it was a filthy morning; and now he was leaving, on foot in thick fog, to try to get the blood sorted out. No doubt he had a surgery at 9 a.m. and a full day's work after that.

I was so tired I could scarcely think. The adrenalin had been pumping all night, and now my body was drained. Conchita was sleeping; the baby could have been alive or dead for all I knew. I tried to think if there was anything I could do, but my brain wouldn't work. Should I go back to Nonnatus House? How could I get there? The policemen had gone, and I couldn't face the prospect of cycling alone in the fog.

Just then Liz came in with a cup of tea.

"Sit yerself down, luvvy, and 'ave a rest," she said.

I sat down in the armchair. I remembered drinking half a cup of tea, and then the next moment it was daylight. Len was in the room, sitting on the bed, brushing Conchita's hair and murmuring sweet nothings to her. She was smiling at him and the baby. He saw me waken and said, "Feel better now, nurse? It's ten o'clock, an' it said on ve news tha' the fog'll start to lift today."

I looked at Conchita who was sitting up in bed, the baby still between her breasts. She was stroking his little head and cooing to him. She looked pathetically weak, but her skin colour and her breathing had improved. Above all, her eyes were still focusing and she looked collected. The delirium from concussion had quite gone.

From then on she improved rapidly. No doubt the penicillin helped, but alone it could not have effected the astonishing transformation, within a few hours, from someone close to death who didn't even know her own husband, to a calm competent woman who knew exactly what she was doing and why.

I have a theory that it was the living baby that cured her, and that the crisis had occurred when she thought that they were going to take him away. In that moment, her powerful maternal instincts had kicked in, and told her that she was the protector, the provider. She didn't have time to be ill. She couldn't afford to be woolly minded. His life depended on her.

Had the baby died at birth, or had he been taken away to hospital, I think Conchita would have died also. The animal world is full of such stories. I have heard that a sheep or an elephant will die if the baby dies, and live if the baby lives.

Overleaf: A group of doctors and nurses give a blood transfusion to a baby in an oxygen tent.

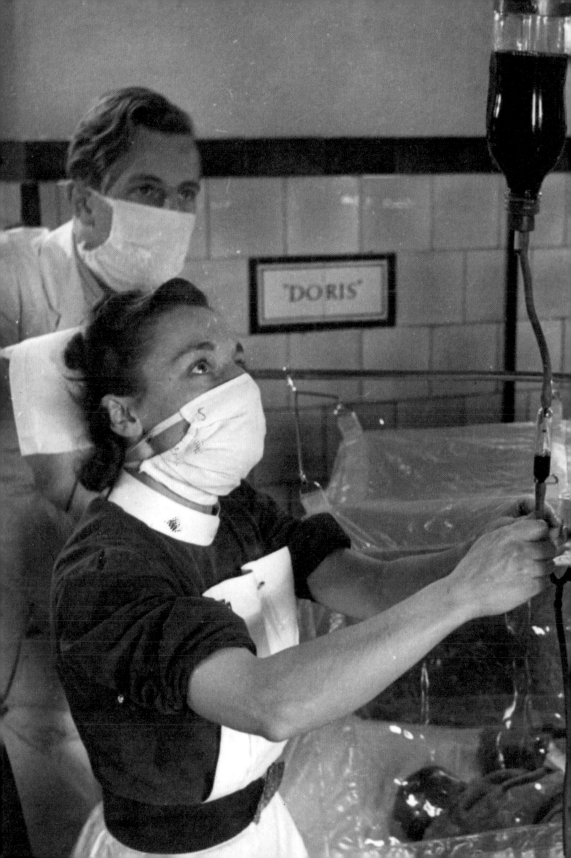

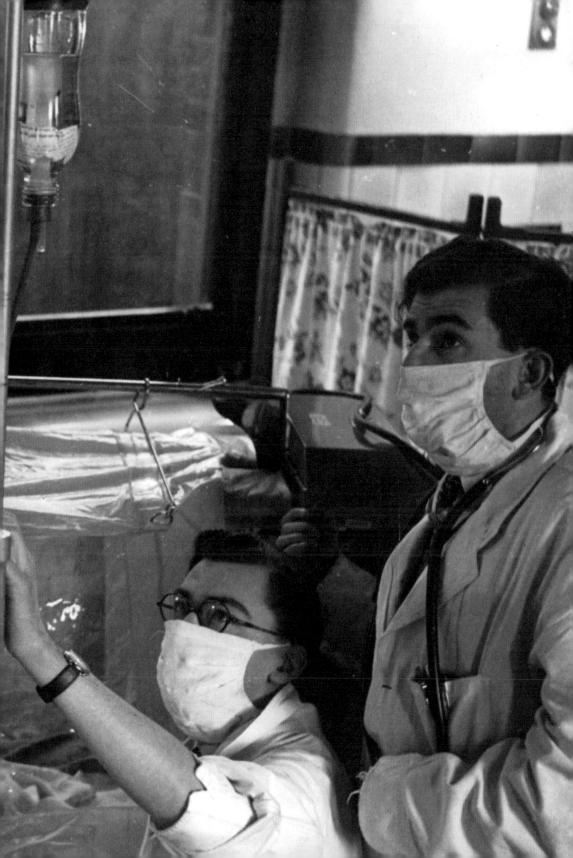

The level of consciousness or unconsciousness is also deeply interesting. Having sat with many dying patients over the years, I am not at all convinced that what we call "unconscious" is anything like the state of unknowingness we think it to be. Unconsciousness can be profoundly knowing, and intuitive. Conchita had seemed quite unconscious, yet her hand tightened over her baby when the paediatrician tried to take him. She could not have seen who was in the room, because her eyes were not focusing, nor known what had been said, because she did not understand the language. Yet somehow she understood that they were planning to take her baby away, and she fought back with every ounce of her strength. This had cured her.

Douglas Bader, the Battle of Britain flying ace, tells a similar story. After an air crash and bi-lateral mid-thigh amputations, he heard a voice say, "Hush, a young airman is dying in that room." The words focused his mind, and he thought, "Die? Me? I'll bloody well show you." The rest is history.

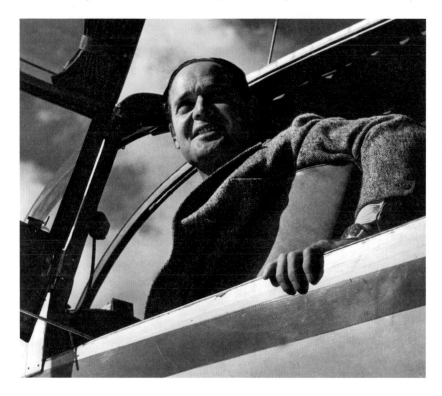

Above: Douglas Bader, who presented the awards at Jennifer's nurse graduation ceremony in 1957.

* * *

Conchita reached for a saucer at the side of her and began to squeeze her nipples, pressing out a few drops of colostrum, which fell into the saucer. Then she took a fine glass rod which was used by one of her daughters for icing cakes. She held the little baby in her left hand and, having suspended a drop of colostrum on the glass rod, touched his lips with it. I watched, fascinated. His lips were no bigger than a couple of daisy petals. A tiny tongue came out and licked the fluid. She repeated this about six or eight times, then tucked him back between her breasts.

Len said: "She's bin doin' this every 'alf 'our since six o'clock. Then they both 'ave a little sleep, an' she does it agen. She said 'e won't die, and 'e won't, yer know. She knows 'ow to look after 'im."

I checked that she was not bleeding unduly, and left. I had to get back to Nonnatus House to report, and to request a district nurse to monitor the blood transfusion when it arrived. The smog was beginning to lift, and one could just about see across the road. It felt as though the world was filling with new life as the foul smog cleared, and I cycled back with a light heart.

Sister Julienne herself prepared a huge breakfast of double bacon and eggs for me "to keep the wolf from the door", as she put it, and then took my report in the dining room whilst I was eating. She said, "I have never cared for such a premature baby myself, but a Sister in one of our other Houses has experience. We will consult her. Conchita will have to be watched very carefully for further blood loss."

She found the whole story astonishing, and said, quietly, "God's will be done." She then went away to make arrangements for covering the blood transfusion.

Conchita didn't lose any more blood. After the transfusion colour returned to her cheeks, and also to Len's. She was weak, but all danger had passed. The baby lay on her breast, day and night, fed in the manner that I have described about every half hour. All the lay staff and Sisters from Nonnatus House came to see the two of them, it was such a beautiful and unusual sight. On the fourth day I weighed the baby in a handkerchief. He was 1 lb. 10 oz.

After three weeks, Conchita began to get up for short periods. I had thought ahead, and had wondered what would happen to the baby. Obviously Conchita had also been thinking ahead, and knew exactly what was to be done. She had asked Liz to acquire from the dressmakers several lengths of the finest unbleached silk. With the help of her skilled eldest daughter, she fixed a kind of sling or firm blouse around her shoulders and breasts, tight underneath, but loose above. The baby was carried in this for five months, between his mother's breasts, never leaving her.

Who had taught her this? I have never before or since, in any literature, heard of such a way of caring for a premature baby. Was it purely maternal instinct? I remembered back to the delivery, and to her monumental struggle when they tried to take the baby. I had the impression then that she was trying to think, trying to remember something; and the sudden clarity and conviction with which she said, " *No morirá.*"

Had she remembered seeing a peasant or gypsy woman carrying a tiny premature baby like this when she was a child in Southern Spain? Had this fleeting memory of times half forgotten been the cause of her conviction that her baby would not die?

Some years later, when I was night sister at the Elizabeth Garrett Anderson Hospital in Euston, I cared for several premature babies of about the same gestation and weight. They were all nursed in incubators, and I do not remember any fatalities. The hospital staff prided themselves on the excellent modern care which preserved the life of the baby. The hospital way, and Conchita's way, are poles apart. Incubator babies are alone, day and night, lying flat on a firm surface, usually in strong light. Only hands and clinical equipment touch the baby. Food usually comes as formula cow's milk. Conchita's baby was never alone. He had the warmth, the touch, the softness, the smell, the moisture of his mother. He heard her heartbeat and her voice. He had her milk. Above all, he had her love.

Possibly today, her decision to refuse hospitalisation for the baby would have been over-ruled by Court Order, the assumption being that only trained staff and advanced technology can adequately care for a premature child. In the 1950s we were less intrusive into family life, and parental responsibility was respected. I am forced to the conclusion that modern medicine does not know it all.

Admittedly Conchita was lucky. The speed of delivery might have caused brain damage to the baby, but this did not occur. Apart from that, the great danger for a premature baby arises from immature vital organs, especially lungs and liver. The baby did indeed become very jaundiced, more than once, in the first few months, but each time it passed. It was a miracle, after I had heedlessly left the baby in a kidney dish, that his lungs were not wholly, or even partly collapsed from birth. I can take no credit for that. However, the fact is, he breathed. I like to think that by holding him upside down, and tapping his fragile back with a finger, I facilitated his first breath. His mother was advised to do the same after each feed, because, if fluid enters the trachea, a premature baby cannot cough as a full-term baby would. She was also given a very fine suction tube, and shown how to use it.

Apart from that, which was very little, the baby received no medical treatment. The constant temperature of his mother's skin kept his body temperature stable. Possibly the constant rise and fall of her breathing helped him over the first critical weeks. I am sure that her feeding policy – a few drops of breast milk placed on the lips at frequent intervals – was the right one. She even did this all through the night, I was told. Conchita took no precautions about sterilising her feeding equipment. I doubt if she had ever heard of such a thing. The saucer and the glass rod were simply wiped clean after each use, ready for the next time. The baby survived. Either he is the ultimate survivor, or we put far too much emphasis on technology and techniques, I thought.

We visited three times a day every day for six weeks, then twice a day for a further six weeks. Domiciliary care was good in those days. At four months he weighed six and a half pounds and was responding with smiles, and turning his head. He reached out a tiny hand to grasp a finger. He gurgled and chuckled to himself. I was told he hardly ever cried.

Several times in those post-natal months I thought of that dreadful night when he was born, and remembered Sister Julienne's words to me as I left. "God be with you, my dear. I will pray for Conchita Warren and her unborn baby." She had not just said that she would pray for Conchita. Nor had she assumed that the foetus would be born dead. She had said, with equal emphasis, that she would pray for them both. In fact, she prayed for us all.

One happy day in midsummer I made a routine call to check the weight of the baby. Laughter was coming from the downstairs kitchen as I descended the stairs. The baby was lying in a cot with his brothers and sisters around him. They were all laughing. A delicious smell wafted towards me. Conchita, smiling and in full command, was standing over the steaming copper boiler making plum jam. The copper boiled ferociously as she stirred with a huge wooden spoon. Thank God she had had the wisdom and the strength not to let the baby go, I thought. Had she done so, I felt sure that she would have died, and all the happiness of the household would have died with her.

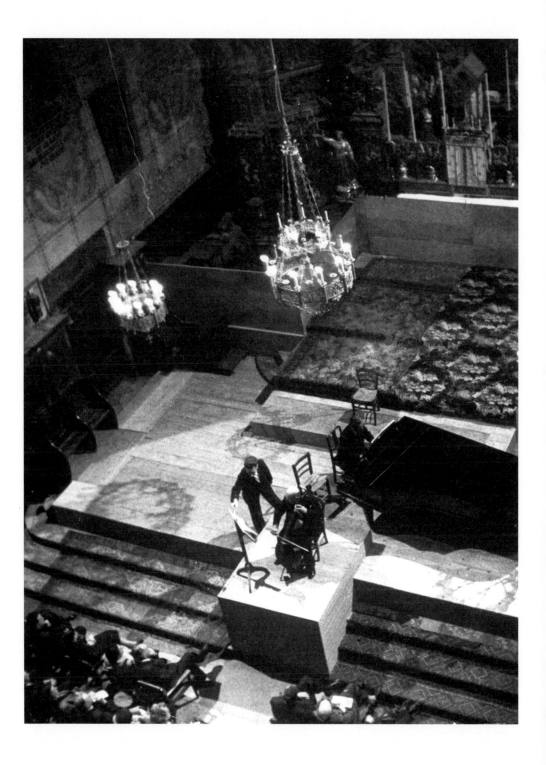

OLD, OLD AGE

Whilst I was fascinated and captivated by Sister Monica Joan, I could not for the life of me decide if she really was verging on senility or not. I could not avoid the suspicion that she might craftily be manipulating us all, in order to get her own way – an old lady's prerogative down the ages! Without doubt she was highly intelligent, well informed, and in some ways deeply learned, though it was often hard to disentangle the muddled strands of her discourse. In view of her history, fifty years professed nun, nurse and midwife in the East End of London, there could be no doubt of her Christian vocation. Yet her behaviour was often far from Christian. She was often selfish and inconsiderate. Flashes of brilliance and flashes of senility crossed and recrossed each other in lightning streaks; goodness and cruelty rubbed shoulders; memory and forgetfulness were intertwined. The old are deeply interesting and I watched her often. Which was the real Sister Monica Joan? I could not tell.

No doubt she had always been eccentric. Even the manner in which she went to church was singular. She would leave Nonnatus House, walk swiftly down Leyland Street, round the corner and straight across the East India Dock Road, without so much as glancing to right or left. Lorry drivers would slam on their brakes, tyres would scream, lorries would come to a shuddering halt, whilst this elderly nun, gown and veil billowing out behind her, crossed the busiest road in London.

Opposite: A cellist performs in the beautiful setting of a church.

One day a mounted policeman on a jet black horse was proceeding sedately down the centre of the road. He wore a magnificent white helmet and long white gauntlets, which gave him a kind of Ruritarian, operatic appearance. He saw Sister Monica Joan and, anticipating what would happen, turned his horse sideways in the road, raised his gloved hands to halt the traffic in both directions and indicated that she could cross. As she passed, Sister turned, looked up at the horse and rider, and said, quite clearly and loudly, "Thank you, young man, that is very kind. But you need not trouble yourself. I am perfectly safe. The angels will take care of me." She tossed her head and walked swiftly on.

That incident occurred years before I knew her, so clearly her idiosyncrasies had always been there although perhaps they had become more accentuated as she grew older. Sometimes I wondered, though, if her celebrated eccentricity was not an affectation, assumed for the childish delight of drawing attention to herself. Like the incident with the cellist. Poor fellow, it must have shattered him, and I tremble to think what it must have done to the pianist.

All Saints, East India Dock Road, was and still is a prestigious church, commanding a favoured position in the diocese. Built in classical Regency style, and beautifully proportioned, the interior is a gem and the acoustics beyond reproach, making it an excellent place for concerts.

The Rector had managed to persuade a world famous cellist to perform. Cynthia and I were given the evening off in order to attend the concert. At the last minute we thought how nice it would be to take Sister Monica Joan. Never again!

To begin with, she insisted on taking her knitting. Neither Cynthia nor I remonstrated as we should have done, but that was only with the wisdom of hindsight. We entered the church, which was full, and Sister Monica Joan wanted to sit in the front row. Like a dowager duchess she sailed down the central aisle, with Cynthia and me trotting after her like a couple of lady's maids. She sat down middle centre, directly opposite the chair placed in readiness for the cellist, and we sat on either side. Everyone knew Sister Monica Joan, and from the outset I felt conspicuous and uncomfortable.

The chairs were too hard. Sister Monica Joan fidgeted and grumbled, trying to adjust her bony bottom to the wooden chair. We offered her a kneeling pad, but that was no good. Cushions had to be found. Curates ran hither and thither poking into sacristy cupboards, but with no luck. Church paraphernalia contains everything but soft cushions. The nearest thing was a length of velvet curtaining. This was folded up, and placed under her bony prominences. She sighed at the young curate, who was new and eager to please.

"If that's the best you can do, I suppose it will have to do." Her sharp tone erased the smile from his face.

The Rector stepped forward to welcome the audience, and said that coffee would be served in the interval.

"And now it is my great pleasure to welcome—"

He was cut short.

"Do you have decaffeinated for those who do not drink coffee?"

The Rector stopped. The cellist, one foot on stage, paused.

"Decaffeinated? I really don't know, Sister."

"Perhaps you would be good enough to find out?"

"Yes, of course Sister."

He signalled to a curate to go and find out. I had not seen the Rector look uncertain before; it was a new experience.

"May I continue, Sister?"

"Yes, of course." Very graciously she inclined her head.

"… my pleasure to welcome to All Saints the renowned cellist and pianist …" They bowed to the audience. The pianist seated herself at the piano. The cellist adjusted his stool. Silence fell on the audience.

"She's wearing brocade, my dear."

Sister Monica Joan's articulation was faultless, and, as I have said, the acoustics at All Saints are superb. Her stage whisper, which at its best could penetrate a railway station at rush hour, reached every corner of the church.

"We used to do that in the 1890s; cut down some old curtains, and make a second best dress out of them. I wonder whose curtains she got hold of?"

The pianist glared, but the cellist, being a man, had noticed no insult, and started tuning up. Sister Monica Joan was fidgeting beside me, trying to get comfortable.

Satisfied, the cellist smiled confidently at his audience and raised his bow.

"It's no good. I can't sit like this. I shall have to have a cushion at my back."

The cellist let his arm fall. The Rector gazed helplessly at his curates. A lady from the back came forward. She had providently brought a cushion for herself, and Sister Monica Joan was welcome to use it.

"How very kind. It is greatly appreciated. So kind."

Her regal graciousness could have out-queened the Queen Mother. She felt the cushion, and decided she would sit on the cushion and have the cloth at her back. Cynthia and the Rector adjusted all this, whilst the cellist and pianist sat quietly looking at their instruments. I was squirming, trying in vain not to be noticed.

The recital started and Sister Monica Joan, comfortable at last, took out her knitting.

Knitting during a recital is not common. In fact I have never seen anyone do it. But Sister Monica Joan was not concerned with what other people did or did not do. She always did exactly as she chose. Nor is knitting generally considered to be a noisy occupation. I had frequently seen Sister Monica Joan knitting in absolute serenity and silence. But not on this occasion. The knitting was of a lacy pattern, requiring three needles, and this produced absolute mayhem.

She dropped the needles repeatedly. They were steel knitting needles, and each time they fell they clattered on to the wooden floor. Cynthia or I had to retrieve them, depending on which side the needle had dropped. The ball of wool fell and rolled under several chairs. Someone about four chairs down kicked it back towards her, but the trailing piece of wool caught around the leg of a chair and pulled tight, thus pulling several stitches off the work in Sister Monica Joan's hands. "Be careful," she hissed at us as the cellist approached a particularly difficult cadenza, his eyes closed in rapture. He opened his eyes sharply, and an unexpected bum note sounded from the strings. Seeing Sister Monica Joan fumbling after the wool, the cellist, with true professionalism, launched into his cadenza. He finished the movement in masterly fashion.

The slow movement started very quietly and peacefully, but the ball of wool was not so easily dealt with. The person four chairs down tried to retrieve it and push it back the way it had come, without success. The ball rolled backwards, and got tangled around the feet of someone sitting behind, who picked it up, causing the trailing end to pull tight again, pulling several more stitches off Sister Monica Joan's needle.

"You are ruining it," she spat out to the man behind.

The pianist was playing a hauntingly tender passage. She turned from the piano and looked daggers at the first row.

As the final cadence approached another needle dropped to the floor with a resounding clatter, destroying the plaintive cry of the cello in the dying fall of the movement.

The Rector, with a desperate look on his face, came forward and whispered to Sister Monica Joan to be quiet. "What did you say, Rector?" she said loudly, as though she were deaf – which she wasn't. He backed off in alarm, fearing that he might make things worse.

The third movement was an *allegro con fuoco*, and the duo played it faster and with more fire than I have ever heard.

Cynthia and I, who were just about dying with mortification, were counting the minutes until the interval when we could take Sister home. I was grinding my teeth in fury, and plotting murder in my heart. Cynthia, who has a sweeter nature than mine, was patient and understanding. But worse was to come.

The musicians brought the third movement to a triumphant close. With a magnificent gesture the cellist swept the bow upwards, and raised his arm aloft, smiling confidently at the audience.

Only a few seconds were to elapse before the applause began, but it was time enough for Sister Monica Joan to make her exit. She stood up abruptly.

"This is too painful. I cannot put up with this a moment longer. I must go."

With knitting needles dropping all around her she passed the musicians and, in full view of the entire audience, swept down the central aisle towards the door.

Tumultuous applause broke out from the Poplar audience. Stamping, cheering, whistling – no musicians could have asked for a greater ovation. But they knew, and we knew, and they knew that we knew, that the applause was not for them or their music. They bowed stiffly, faces set in a grim smile, and left the platform.

Black fury took possession of me. I greatly respect musicians, knowing their years of intensive training, and I could not excuse this last gratuitous insult, which I saw as deliberate.

I could have hit Sister Monica Joan, hard, in front of a couple of hundred people. I must have been shaking with rage, because Cynthia looked at me in alarm.

"I'll take her home. You stay and find a chair at the back somewhere, and enjoy the second half."

"I can't enjoy anything after that," I hissed through clenched teeth; my voice must have sounded strange.

She laughed her soft, warm laugh. "Of course you can. Get yourself a cup of coffee. They are playing the Brahms Cello Sonata next."

She gathered up the knitting needles, extricated the wool from around the chair legs, put it all into the knitting bag, blew a kiss with a whispered "cheerio", and ran off after Sister Monica Joan.

For many days, or perhaps it was weeks, I could not bring myself to speak to Sister Monica Joan. I was convinced that she had deliberately set out to wreck the recital, and to humiliate the musicians. I remembered her petulance when she did not get her own way, her sulks when she was thwarted, and above all her relentless torment of Sister Evangelina. I made up my mind that the apparent senility was no more than an elaborate game she was playing for her own amusement. I decided that I wanted nothing more to do with her. I could be as haughty as Sister Monica Joan if I chose to be, and whenever we met, I turned my head away and said not one word.

But later an incident occurred that left me in no doubt at all about the reality of her mental condition.

It was about 8.30 in the morning. The Sisters and other staff had all left for their morning visits. Chummy and I were the last to leave, and were just stepping out when the telephone rang.

"Is that Nonnatus 'ouse? Sid ve Fish 'ere. I thought you ought'a know Sister Monica Joan has jus' gone past me shop in 'er nightie. I've sent ve lad after 'er, so she won't come to no 'arm."

I gasped in horror, and quickly told Chummy. We dropped our midwifery bags, grabbed a Sister's cloak from the hall-stand, and sprinted down towards Sid's fish shop. Sure enough, weaving a zig-zag line down the East India Dock Road, the fish boy a couple of paces behind, was Sister Monica Joan. She was wearing only a long white nightie with long sleeves. Her bony shoulders and elbows stuck out under the thin cloth. You could have counted every vertebra in her spine. She wore no dressing gown, no slippers, no veil, and the wind blew thin white strands of hair upwards from a head that was nearly bald. It was a cold morning, and her feet and ankles were blue-black with cold and bleeding. From behind I saw these sad old feet, like skeleton's bones, clad only in mottled blue skin, doggedly, determinedly trudging on to a destination known only to her clouded mind.

Without her veil and habit she was almost unrecognisable, and looked vaguely grotesque. Her rheumy, red-rimmed eyes were watering. Her nose was bright red, and a dew-drop hung on the tip. My heart gave a lurch, and I realised how much I loved her.

We caught up and spoke to her. She looked at us as though we were strangers, and tried to push us aside.

"Mind, out of my way. I must get to them. The waters have broken. That brute will kill the baby. He killed the last one, I swear it. I must get there. Out of my way."

She took another few steps on bleeding feet. Chummy threw the warm woollen cloak around her shoulders, and I took off my cap and put it on her head. The sudden warmth seemed to bring her to her senses. Her eyes focused, and she looked at us in recognition. I leaned towards her and said slowly, "Sister Monica Joan, it's breakfast time. Mrs B. has made some nice hot porridge for you, with honey in it. It will be getting cold if you don't come now."

She looked at me eagerly and said, "Porridge! With honey! Ooh, lovely. Come along, then. What are you standing there for? Did you say porridge? With honey?"

She took two steps, and cried out in pain. Obviously she had not been aware of her cut and bleeding feet. Thank God for Chummy, her size and strength. She picked Sister Monica Joan up in her arms as though she were a child, and carried her all the way back to Nonnatus House. A crowd of curious children followed.

We alerted Mrs B., who was full of concern.

"Oh, the poor lamb. Get her up to bed. She mus' be froze, poor dear. She'll catch 'er death o' cold. I'll get a couple of 'ot water bottles, and make her some porridge, an' some 'ot chocolate. I knows as wha' she likes."

We got her to bed and left her in Mrs B.'s capable hands. We both had a morning's work to attend to, and had to go.

I attended my morning visits as though in a dream. Now and then in life, love catches you unawares, illuminating the dark corners of your mind, and filling them with radiance. Once in a while you are faced with a beauty and a joy that takes your soul, all unprepared, by assault. As I cycled around that morning, I knew that I loved not only Sister Monica Joan, but all that she represented: her religion, her vocation, her monastic profession, the bells, the constant prayers within the convent, the quietness, and the selfless work in the service of God. Was it perhaps – and I nearly fell off my bike with shock – could it be the love of God?

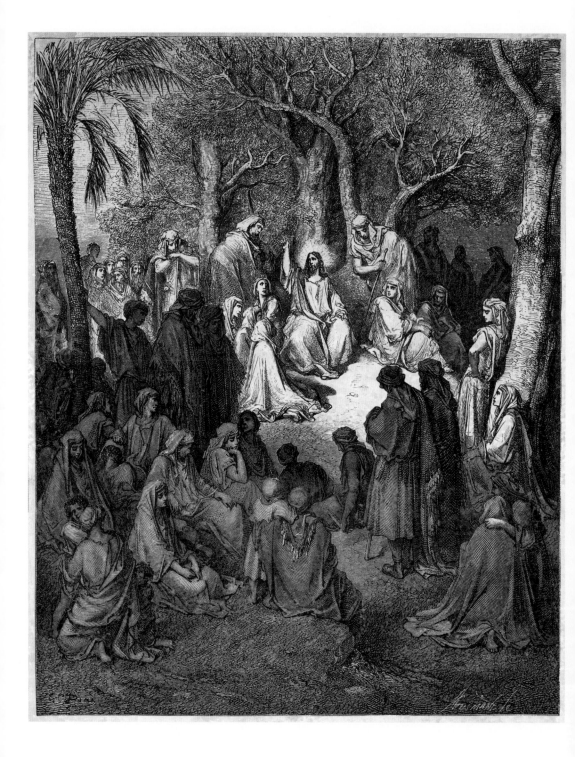

IN THE BEGINNING

Sister Monica Joan developed pneumonia. She fell deeply asleep when Chummy, Mrs B. and I placed her into bed that cold morning, and remained apparently unconscious for the whole day. Her temperature was high, her pulse full and throbbing, and her breathing laboured. Nonnatus House was sad and subdued. The chapel bell, calling the Office of the day, sounded like the portent of a funeral bell. We all thought that she would die. However, we had not taken into account two significant factors: antibiotics, and her own phenomenal stamina.

Today, antibiotics are as common as a cup of coffee. In the 1950s they were relatively new. Today, over-use has reduced their efficacy but in the 1950s they really were a miracle drug. Sister Monica Joan had never had penicillin before, and responded immediately. Within a couple of shots her temperature dropped, her pulse returned to normal, the murmur in her chest vanished, and she opened her eyes. She looked around. "I really don't know why you are all standing there doing nothing. Haven't you got any work to do? I suppose you think I am going to die. Well, you are wrong. I'm not. You can tell Mrs B. that I will have a boiled egg for breakfast."

Her stamina and physical strength became apparent during the next few weeks. Had she led a life of luxury and idleness, as her aristocratic birth would have allowed, I am quite sure that she would have died, in spite of the penicillin. However, a life of intense hard work had rendered her as tough

Opposite: The artist Gustave Doré illustrated many of the Gospels, including The Sermon on the Mount (1865).

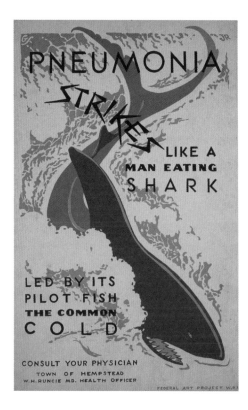

Left: A pneumonia warning poster from c. 1936–7 encourages people to consult their doctors about common colds.

as old boots. A mere touch of pneumonia could not kill her. She recovered quickly, and became very peevish about being kept in bed, which the doctor insisted upon. She thought she had a slight cold, and had no memory of the incident that had brought her to bed in the first place. She did not actually call the doctor a fool, but she looked at him in such a way that left no doubt in his, or anyone else's mind.

"I do not pretend to understand your superior wisdom, doctor, but we will go with God in all things. Am I to understand that I can have visitors?"

Yes indeed, Sister Monica Joan could have visitors (as long as they did not tire her), whatever she wanted to read (provided it did not strain her eyes), and whatever she wanted to eat (provided it did not upset her digestion).

Sister Monica Joan settled back on her pillows, contented. Books were provided and Mrs B. was instructed to attend to her every wish.

A nun's bedroom is properly called a cell and is small, bare, and plain, without comfort. However, since her retirement from active midwifery, Sister Monica Joan had managed to wangle things so that her cell was comparatively large, comfortably furnished, and pretty: an elegant bedsitting-room would be the more appropriate description. Lay people are not normally admitted to a nun's cell, but Sister Monica Joan had just extracted the doctor's assurance that she could have visitors, and thus began a very happy period of my life.

Every day I visited her, and as I entered the room, an almost tangible feeling of peace and tranquillity surrounded me. She was always sitting up in bed, with no outward signs of illness or fatigue, her veil perfectly adjusted, her white nightie high in the neck, her soft skin opaque, and her large eyes clear and penetrating. Her bed was always covered in books, and she had a number of notebooks in which she wrote voluminously in a firm stylish hand.

I discovered that she was a poet. I suppose it should not have surprised me, but it did. All her life she had written poetry, and had in her notebooks a collection of several hundred poems dating from the 1890s.

I am no judge of poetry – I do not have an ear for it. But the consistency of her output impressed me and I asked if I might have a look. She shrugged negligently.

"Take it. I have no secrets, my dear. I am but a spark in the divine fire."

Over many long evenings I studied these poems. I had expected them all to be religious poetry, having been written by a nun, but they were not. Many were love poems, many satirical, and many were humorous, as:

> One of the sweetest things in life to see
> Is a calm, settled fly,
> Cleansing its fastidious face
> On my chosen reading place;
> He twines his legs around his arse
> And takes his time,
> As Beauty with her glass.

or:

Lyric of an Obese Dachshund Bitch

> They are equally pretty,
> My toes or my tittie,
> To ramble or gallop upon;

Whatever will happen
When I must re-cap'em
The days that my nipples wear out
And are gone?

This is my favourite:

It's OK to be tight on
The seafront at Brighton
But I say, by Jove
Watch out if it's Hove.

It may not be great poetry, but I thought it had charm. Or perhaps it was the charm of Sister Monica Joan that coloured my assessment.

I found a revealing poem about her father, which told a lot about her early life:

Fretful, unloving, mannerless Papa,
What a crustaceous old boy you are –
How you do go it!
Blowing your bugle, like a ham stage-star,
How you do blow it!
And where does it get you, Papa?
Or is it wasted breath?
"Leave everything to me"
Vainly the old man saith.

With an arrogant, domineering father her struggle to assert herself and to leave home must have been monumental. A weaker character would have been crushed.

For a lovesick young girl, her love poems spoke to my heart, and brought tears to my eyes. As:

To an Unknown God

I sang to you
In the day of my bliss
And you were near

I thought of you
In my lover's kiss
And felt you there

I turned to you
When our love was too brief
And found your strength.

I needed you
In the years of my grief
And knew you, at length.

"Our love was too brief." Oh, I knew all about that. Does one have to suffer so dreadfully in order to know the unknown God? Who, when, what was the story of Sister Monica Joan's lost love? I longed to know, but dared not ask. Did he die, or did her parents object? Why was he unobtainable? Was he already married, or did he just cease to care, and leave her? I longed to know, but could not ask. Any intrusive questions would deserve, and receive, a caustic comment from that barbed tongue.

Her religious poetry was surprisingly slender, and as I was eager to know more about her religion, I asked her about this aspect of her poetry. She replied with these lines from Keats' *Ode to a Grecian Urn*:

"Beauty is truth, truth beauty" – that is all
Ye know on earth, and all ye need to know.

"Do not ask me to immortalise the great mystery of life. I am just a humble worker. For beauty, look to the Psalms, to Isaiah, to St John of the Cross. How could my poor pen scan such verse? For truth, look to the Gospels – four short accounts of God made Man. There is nothing more to say."

She looked unusually tired that day and, as she lay back on the pillows, the wintry light from the window accentuating her pale, aristocratic features, my heart filled with tenderness. I had come to a convent by mistake, an irreligious girl. I would not have described myself as a committed atheist for whom all spirituality was nonsense, but as an agnostic in whom large areas of doubt and uncertainty resided. I had never met nuns before, and regarded them at first as a bit of a joke; later, with astonishment bordering on incredulity. Finally this was replaced by respect, and then deep love.

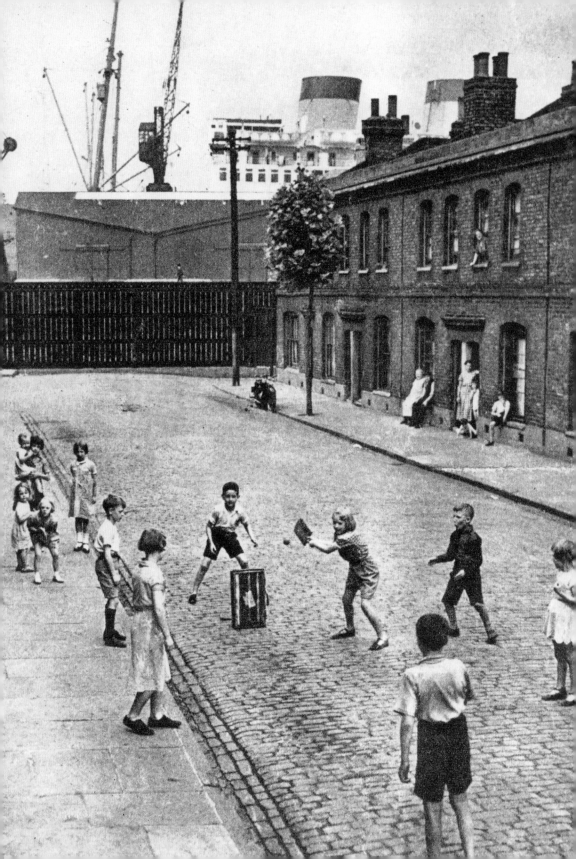

What had impelled Sister Monica Joan to abandon a privileged life for one of hardship, working in the slums of London's Docklands? "Was it love of people?" I asked her.

"Of course not," she snapped sharply. "How can you love ignorant, brutish people whom you don't even know? Can anyone love filth and squalor? Or lice and rats? Who can love aching weariness, and carry on working, in spite of it? One cannot love these things. One can only love God, and through His grace come to love His people."

I asked her how she had heard her calling, and come to be professed. She quoted lines from *The Hound of Heaven*.

> *I fled Him, down the nights and down the days;*
> *I fled Him down the arches of the years;*
> *I fled Him down the labyrinthine ways*
> *Of my own mind; and in the midst of tears*
> *I hid from Him.*

I asked her what was meant by "I fled Him", and she became cross.

"Questions, questions – you wear me out with your questions, child. Find out for yourself – we all have to in the end. No one can give you faith. It is a gift from God alone. Seek and ye shall find. Read the Gospels. There is no other way. Do not pester me with your everlasting questions. Go with God, child; just go with God."

She was obviously tired. I kissed her and slipped away.

Her constant phrase, "Go with God", had puzzled me a good deal. Suddenly it became clear. It was a revelation – acceptance. It filled me with joy. Accept life, the world, Spirit, God, call it what you will, and all else will follow. I had been groping for years to understand, or at least to come to terms with the meaning of life. These three small words, "Go with God", were for me the beginning of faith.

That evening, I started to read the Gospels.

Opposite: Mothers watch children play in the streets in the Docklands.

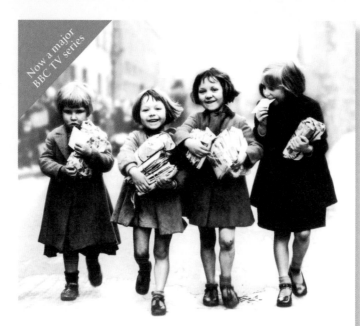

Now a major
BBC TV series

a true story of the east end
in the 1950s

Call the Midwife

JENNIFER WORTH

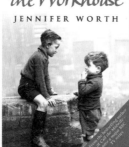

Shadows of
the Workhouse

JENNIFER WORTH

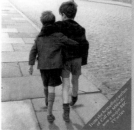

Farewell to the
East End

JENNIFER WORTH

Jennifer Worth

Why I wrote *Call the Midwife*

In January 1998 the *Midwives Journal* published an article by Terri Coates entitled "Impressions of the Midwife in Literature". After careful research, Terri was forced to conclude that midwives are virtually non-existent in literature. Why, in heaven's name? Fictional doctors strut across the pages of books in droves, scattering pearls of wisdom as they pass. Nurses, good and bad, are by no means absent. But midwives? Whoever heard of a midwife as a literary heroine?

Yet midwifery is in itself the very stuff of drama and melodrama. Every child is conceived either in love or lust, is born in pain and suffering followed by joy or tragedy and anguish. A midwife attends every birth; she is in the thick of it, she sees it all. Why, then, does she remain a shadowy figure, hidden behind the delivery room door?

Terri Coates ended her article with the words: "Maybe there is a midwife somewhere who can do for midwifery what James Herriot did for veterinary practice." I read those words and took up the challenge.

This text originally appeared as the preface in the 2002 edition of *Call the Midwife*.

The original midwife,
Jennifer Worth

Based on the experiences of Jennifer Worth, née Lee, who worked as a midwife and district nurse in late 1950s' East End London, *Call the Midwife* has been lauded as doing as much for midwifery as Alf Wight's popular James Herriot books have done for the veterinary profession. The trilogy, which begins with *Call the Midwife* (originally published in 2002; reissued 2007) and continues on with *Shadows of the Workhouse* (2005; reissued 2008) and *Farewell to the East End* (2009), has sold almost 2 million copies worldwide. It is also now the subject of an acclaimed BBC television series.

Jennifer Lee was born in Clacton-on-Sea, Essex, on 25 September 1935. She grew up in Buckinghamshire and attended Belle Vue School in Little Chalfont. She excelled in music, which remained a great passion throughout her life, but her interests lay beyond academia and she left school at the age of 14. A shorthand and typing course followed, after which she was employed at Dr Challoner's Grammar School, in Amersham, Buckinghamshire, for a year as secretary to the headmaster.

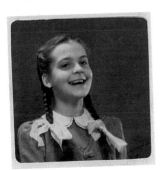

Before she began to train as a nurse at the Royal Berkshire Hospital in Reading, Jennifer hitchhiked around Britain, taking odd jobs, including waitressing in Blackpool. At the age

Left. Jennifer aged 8 or 9 years old.

of 19, however, she turned to nursing and, in doing so, seemingly discovered her natural calling. Jennifer's caring nature and innate compassion towards other people made her an excellent nurse.

She qualified on 30 December 1957 and moved to London shortly afterwards to begin her midwife Part 1 training in March 1958. Due to a shoulder injury, it took Jennifer a year and a half to get her midwifery qualification and she worked briefly as an au pair in Paris during this period. In September 1959, however, she was awarded the certificate, while working as a district nurse and midwife in the East End.

Jennifer was in her early 20s when she moved to Poplar to work with the nuns of the Anglican Community of St John the Divine (renamed the Midwives of St Raymond Nonnatus in the books). The St John the Divine community had been created in 1848 as a nursing sisterhood and had sent nuns to work with Florence Nightingale, nursing soldiers wounded in the Crimean War (1853–6). After the creation of the NHS (National Health Service) in 1948, the sisters worked alongside district nurses and doctors in the East End. They continued in that capacity until 1978.

The world that Jennifer entered, when she first went to live and work in the East End, was one still reeling from the horror of the Second World War (1939–45). Many people lived in slum conditions, inhabiting overcrowded tenements or bombed-out buildings. Others just existed on the streets as best they could. Employment rates were high and skilled workers were relatively well paid; yet the majority of unskilled labourers, often employed in the docks, endured long hard days for comparatively little pay.

People tended to marry young and the large families that often resulted – such as the 24 children of Len and Conchita Warren in *Call the Midwife* – had to be supported somehow. Gang warfare and organized crime were prevalent in the East End and prostitutes – often young girls like Mary in this book, lured into selling their bodies by the promise of a better life – could be found on most street corners or in the backrooms of the special cafés located in and around Cable Street.

Initially, Jennifer was shocked by what she found – the extreme conditions under which people lived, the neglect and degradation that the young and old, in particular, suffered. However, as she worked side-by-side with the sisters and treated her patients, she began to recognise and respect the strong sense of community and loyalty among the local population. Dealing on a day-to-day basis with women, who fought so courageously to bring new life into such a challenging world, struggling to bring up their families as best they could in truly adverse circumstances, Jennifer came to see them as true "heroines". She said that being a midwife was "a privilege beyond any other privilege".

Call the Midwife features real people and locations, although in most cases the names have been changed to protect true identities. One notable exception, however, is Cynthia, Jennifer Lee's close friend and fellow midwife in the books. Cynthia remained a lifelong friend of Jennifer and her family and her photograph appears in this book courtesy of Cynthia's stepson, Adrian Pickering. Similarly, the character Sister Julienne in the book is based on Jennifer's great friend, Sister Jocelyn.

In *Call the Midwife*, Jennifer allows us precious insight into a lost world, recounting stories that are, by turn, funny, moving and heartbreaking, and it is perhaps for those reasons that the book is so popular with modern audiences. As Jennifer herself said, "So many of those great characters have stayed with me. Most people in London at that time didn't know the East

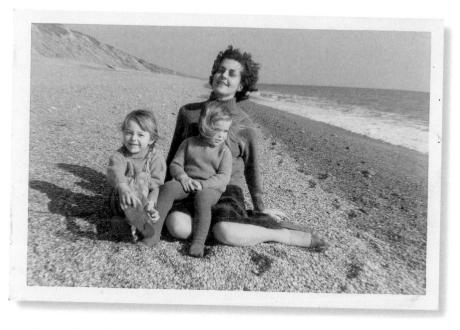

Above: Jennifer loved the sea and spent many family holidays with her husband and daughters, Suzannah *(left)* and Juliette *(right)* on the coast (1968). She particularly loved Dorset.

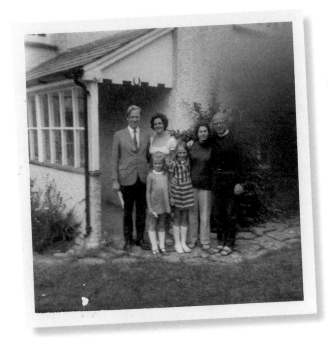

Left: Cynthia and her husband (*pictured far right*) were close familly friends of the Worths (1972).

End – they pushed it aside. There was no law, no lighting, bedbugs and fleas. It was a hidden place, not written about at all."

In the early 1960s, Jennifer left the nuns to become a staff nurse at the Royal London Hospital in Whitechapel. Later, she became a ward nurse at the Elizabeth Garrett Anderson Hospital in Euston and the Marie Curie Hospital in Hampstead.

In 1963, she married schoolmaster and artist Philip Worth, with whom she had two daughters, Suzannah and Juliette. She left nursing in 1973 to study music and became a licentiate of the London College of Music in 1974. She was awarded a fellowship in 1984 and for many years performed solo and with choirs in the UK and around Europe.

In the last decade or so of her life, Jennifer dedicated her time to writing, and the unprecedented success of the *Call the Midwife* trilogy brought Jennifer to the notice of international audiences. Her last book, *In the Midst of Life*, was published in 2010.

Jennifer died on 31 May 2011. She is survived by her husband, daughters and three grandchildren, Dan, Lydia and Eleanor.

ACKNOWLEDGEMENTS

All nurses and midwives, many long since dead, with whom I worked half a century ago; Terri Coates, who fired my memories; Canon Tony Williamson, President of The Wellclose Trust; Elizabeth Fairbairn for her encouragement; Pat Schooling, who had courage to go for original publication; Naomi Stevens, for all her help with the Cockney dialect; Suzannah Hart, Jenny Whitefield, Dolores Cook, Peggy Sayer, Betty Howney, Rita Perry; All who typed, read and advised; Tower Hamlets Local History Library and Archives; The Curator, Island History Trust, E14; The Archivist, The Museum in Dockland, E14; The Librarian, Simmons Aerofilms.

PICTURE CREDITS

The publisher would like to thank Jennifer Worth's family, especially Philip Worth and Suzannah Hart, for allowing it access to the private family archives, and Adrian Pickering for allowing publication of the images of his stepmother, Cynthia.

IMAGES FROM THE WORTH FAMILY:
Pages iv; vi–vii; 21; 27; 149; 292; 386; 388.

IMAGES FROM ADRIAN PICKERING:
Pages 48; 389.

IMAGES FROM PICTURE LIBRARIES/ARCHIVES:
Alamy: Pages122–123 (Trinity Mirror/Mirrorpix).

With permission of The Bank of England: Page187.

Getty Images: Pages 18, 36–37 (SSPL), 44, 54–55, 67 (David Lees), 94 (Merlyn Severn), 106 (SSPL), 114, 124 (Lambert), 138, 144, 152 (*Time & Life Pictures*), 156–157 (Thurston Hopkins), 160, 172, 184 (Harry Kerr), 200, 218 (Thurston Hopkins), 246–247 (SSPL), 250 (Popperfoto), 282, 294 (SSPL), 304 (Hulton Collection), 306, 314, 331 (*Time & Life Pictures*), 336 (Popperfoto), 348 (Popperfoto), 353, 356 (*Daily Herald Archive*/SSPL), 362–363, 364 (Popperfoto), 368 (*Time & Life Pictures*).

Photograph courtesy of The Island History Trust: Page 383.

Library of Congress: Page 87.

Mary Evans Picture Library: Pages 28 (Classic Stock/H. Armstrong Roberts), 50 (Onslow Auctions Limited), 84 (Illustrated London News Ltd), 89 (Mark Furness), 100–101, 110–111, 202 (Roger Mayne), 209 (Photo Union Collection), 224, 226, 234–235, 238 (Onslow Auctions Limited), 254–255 (Peter Higginbotham Collection), 262 (Roger Mayne), 264 (John Gay/English Heritage.NMR), 272, 274 (National Archives, London), 284 (Onslow Auctions Limited), 324 (Classic Stock/H. Armstrong Roberts), 346 (Roger Mayne), 376 (INTERFOTO/Bildarchiv Hansmann), 378 (Library of Congress).

Photographs courtesy of the Museum of the Docklands, PLA Collections: Pages 14–15.

Courtesy of Raleigh: Page 64.

Rex Features: Page 42 (Herbert Mason/*Daily Mail*).

© Royal College of Midwifes; reproduced with permission: Pages 70, 102, 134–135, 350.

© Science Museum/Science & Society Picture Library: Page 8.

Topfoto: Pages 146-147, 164, 310–311, 320–321.

Courtesy of Tower Hamlets Local History Library and Archives: Pages 52, 73, 116, 180, 270, 278–279.

Courtesy of The Wellclose Trust (Photos by Frank Rust): Pages 31, 80–81, 190, 196–197, 205, 214.

The Wellcome Library, London: Pages ii, viii, 175.

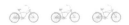

First published in Great Britain in 2002 by Merton Books

This illustrated edition published in 2012
by Weidenfeld & Nicolson
10 9 8 7 6 5 4 3 2 1

This is work of non-fiction, and the events it recounts are true. However, certain names
and identifying characteristics of some of the people who appear in its pages have
been changed. The views expressed in this book are the author's.

A CIP catalogue record for this book is available from the British Library.

ISBN: 978 0 297 868 781

Weidenfeld & Nicolson
The Orion Publishing Group
Orion House
5 Upper St Martin's Lane
London WC2H 9EA

An Hachette UK Company

Editorial: Aruna Vasudevan and Jane Sturrock
Text design and layout: Carrdesignstudio.com
Picture Researcher: Susannah Jayes
Proofreader: Nick Ascroft

"The original midwife, Jennifer Worth" Copyright © A.Vasudevan 2012

Printed and bound in Germany by Mohn Media

The Orion Publishing Group's policy is to use papers that are natural, renewable and
recyclable products and made from wood grown in sustainable forests. The logging and
manufacturing processes are expected to conform to the environmental regulations of
the country of origin.

www.orionbooks.co.uk